Saunders

MEDICAL ASSISTING EXAM REVIEW

Saunders

MEDICAL ASSISTING EXAM REVIEW

Deborah E. Barbier Holmes
RN, BSN, RMA, CMA (AAMA)

Medical Assistant Program Director
Vatterott College – Sunset Hills
Saint Louis, Missouri

THIRD EDITION

ELSEVIER
SAUNDERS

ELSEVIER
SAUNDERS

3251 Riverport Lane
Maryland Heights, MO 63043

SAUNDERS MEDICAL ASSISTING EXAM REVIEW,   ISBN: 978-1-4377-2236-9
THIRD EDITION

Notices

Knowledge and best practice in this field are constantly changing. As new research and experience broaden our understanding, changes in research methods, professional practices, or medical treatment may become necessary.

Practitioners and researchers must always rely on their own experience and knowledge in evaluating and using any information, methods, compounds, or experiments described herein. In using such information or methods they should be mindful of their own safety and the safety of others, including parties for whom they have a professional responsibility.

With respect to any drug or pharmaceutical products identified, readers are advised to check the most current information provided (i) on procedures featured or (ii) by the manufacturer of each product to be administered, to verify the recommended dose or formula, the method and duration of administration, and contraindications. It is the responsibility of practitioners, relying on their own experience and knowledge of their patients, to make diagnoses, to determine dosages and the best treatment for each individual patient, and to take all appropriate safety precautions.

To the fullest extent of the law, neither the Publisher nor the authors, contributors, or editors, assume any liability for any injury and/or damage to persons or property as a matter of products liability, negligence or otherwise, or from any use or operation of any methods, products, instructions, or ideas contained in the material herein.

ISBN: 978-1-4377-2236-9

Executive Editor: Susan Cole
Developmental Editor: Jennifer Bertucci
Publishing Services Manager: Julie Eddy
Senior Project Manager: Andrea Campbell
Project Manager: Kiruthiga Kasthuriswamy
Designer: Jessica Williams

Printed in the United States of America

9 8 7 6 5 4 3 2 1

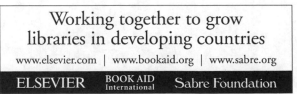

To Granny and Jon,
my biggest fans and guardian angels,

and to my students,
who teach me something new every day.

Reviewers

I am extremely grateful to the people who shared their suggestions, comments, and thoughts on this edition (as well as on previous editions). Reviewing a book takes an amazing amount of time and energy, and I am so pleased that we could find willing and capable colleagues to help make this book better and better with every edition. The reviewers give us valuable feedback and opinions, and it is with their help and guidance that this book is what it is today. I would like to especially thank the following editorial reviewing team, who reviewed and contributed to the second and third editions of this book:

Joyce Combs, BS, AAS, CMA (AAMA)
Coordinator/Professor
LSAA AH – Medical Assisting
Central Kentucky Technical College
Lexington, Kentucky

Tammy Gant, CMA (AAMA), CPC, RHIT, AHI
Medical Office Administration and Medical
    Assisting Instructor
Surry Community College
Dobson, NC

Jeanette Goodwin, BS, BSN, CMA (AAMA)
Program Chair/Instructor
Health Division
Southeast Community College
Lincoln, Nebraska

Edith Hamelin, BSN, RN, CMA (AAMA)
Director
Medical Department
Latter Day Saints Business College
Salt Lake City, Utah

Rose Hecht, BS, CMAC
Program Director/Medical Assistant Instructor
Health Science and Medical Technology
Southern California Regional Occupational Center
Torrance, California

Christine Hollander, CMA (AAMA), BS
Medical Department Director
Health Careers Division
Westwood College of Technology
Denver, Colorado

Tracy Thomas, RMA, BS
Medical Assisting Instructor
Saint Louis College of Health Careers
Saint Louis, MO

Skilled. Compassionate. Healer. Competent.
These are words that come to mind when describing the medical assistant. As the profession of medical assisting continues to change, the medical assistant must meet these new challenges. Earning a medical assistant credential is the first step.

There are many reasons to achieve this credential. It shows that the student is recognized by the credentialing organization as having met predetermined qualifications. It shows proof of competency, and it shows others a commitment to the profession. This credential will be even more important in the coming years as medical assistants become more and more recognized for the versatile allied health professionals that they are.

Saunders Medical Assisting Exam Review was written to aid the student in studying for a medical assisting credentialing exam and was developed with today's busy student in mind. This textbook presents simplified study materials that focus on all the General, Administrative and Clinical topics from the medical assisting curriculum in preparation for either the Certified Medical Assistant or the Registered Medical Assistant examination.

The book features the following:
- A single, comprehensive guide. This allows for information to be found easily in one text, and

eliminates the need for many big, bulky textbooks and stacks of notes.
- An easy-to-follow outline format. Information is organized and presented in this format to allow the student to identify key concepts and facts. All subject areas typically included in a Medical Assistant Program are covered.
- Three practice pre-tests and a post-test, complete with answers and rationales. These may help assess weak and strong areas. A CD-ROM with different practice exams (as well as the pre-tests from the text) and review questions offers more practice.
- Simple pictures and diagrams to illustrate the text. These may help to clarify concepts.
- Study and test-taking tips to help the student be successful. Included are suggestions on how to prepare to study, how to study, and how to take a multiple-choice exam.

As the practicing medical assistant moves on in his/her career, this text may be used as a source of reference. It is also useful as a reference for educators in creating lecture material, curriculum, or review courses.

I wish the best of luck to all who use this text to achieve their credential. Hopefully it helps make the process a little easier.

Deborah E. Barbier Holmes, RN, BSN, RMA, CMA (AAMA)

Acknowledgments

I am deeply grateful to the following people who have given me ideas, encouragement, praise, and support.

My students, past, present, and future—they are THE reason for this project. They have been an endless source of ideas, criticism, support, and inspiration.

Michael Ledbetter, Susan Cole, and Jennifer Bertucci at Elsevier—for supporting, understanding, listening to ideas, and helping tremendously. This project started as a discussion at a national convention, wound up as this book, and each edition has gotten better and better.

David, Robert, and Jennifer—the loves of my life.

Madelyn, Chris, Amy—additions to the Holmes family.

Tyler Mathis—the newest addition to the Holmes family.

Deborah E. Barbier Holmes, RN, BSN, RMA, CMA (AAMA)

Contents

Study Tips: Taking the Medical Assistant Examination

GENERAL EXAMINATION DESCRIPTIONS

CMA EXAM

The CMA exam is administered on the last Friday in January, the last Saturday in June, and the fourth Friday in October of each year. The exam is also available to take online. Individuals who meet the requirements set by the American Association of Medical Assistants (AAMA) are eligible to sit for this exam. The exam consists of 200 questions in multiple-choice format. Three subject areas are covered on the exam, with the content of each area broken down as follows:

General Medical Knowledge
- Medical terminology
- Anatomy and physiology
- Law
- Ethics
- Patient relations
- Communications

Administrative Knowledge
- Keyboarding concepts
- Correspondence
- Mail
- Appointments
- Phone management
- Filing and records management
- Banking
- Bookkeeping
- Payroll
- Medical coding
- Insurance
- Office automation
- General office management concepts

Clinical Knowledge
- Patient interviewing
- Charting and documentation
- Physical measurements and examinations
- Nutrition
- Physical therapy
- Radiography
- Electrocardiography
- Surgical treatment
- First aid
- Cardiopulmonary resuscitation
- Laboratory orientation
- Urinalysis
- Hematology
- Chemistry
- Serology/Immunology
- Microbiology

You are given four hours to complete the exam. All questions are assigned equal weight. Guessing at answers is not counted against you; the exam is scored according to the number of correct answers versus the total number of questions given. An overall minimum standard score of 445 must be attained to pass the exam. On successfully passing the exam, the medical assistant may wear the CMA credential. For more information on taking the CMA exam, visit the American Association of Medical Assistants Web site at www.aama-ntl.org.

RMA EXAM

The RMA exam is administered throughout the year either by paper and pencil or by computerized test. The paper test is administered at the school with a proctor, and the school sets the time and dates. The computerized test is administered at Pearson Vue locations nationwide any day of the year except Sundays and holidays. Individuals who meet the criteria set forth by the American Medical Technologists (AMT) are eligible to sit for this exam. The exam consists of 200–210 questions in multiple-choice format, covering the same three general areas as the CMA exam. The approximate percentage of material covered from each section and its content is broken down as follows:

General Medical Knowledge
- Anatomy and physiology
- Medical terminology
- Medical law
- Medical ethics
- Human relations
- Patient education

1

Administrative Knowledge
- Insurance
- Financial bookkeeping
- Medical secretarial-receptionist

Clinical Knowledge
- Asepsis
- Sterilization
- Instruments
- Vital signs
- Physical examinations
- Clinical pharmacology
- Minor surgery
- Therapeutic modalities
- Laboratory procedures
- Electrocardiography
- First aid

A minimum scaled score of 70 must be attained to pass the exam. On successfully passing the exam, the medical assistant may wear the RMA credential. For more information on taking the RMA exam, visit the American Medical Technologists Web site at www.amt1.com.

STUDY TIPS FOR THE EXAM

Taking the medical assistant certification (CMA) or registration (RMA) examination is an important event in the medical assistant's career. This section will guide you in preparing for the examination by offering study techniques and tips and by describing the exam itself and what to expect when exam day arrives.

A great deal of commitment is required on your part to study for the exam. Your performance on the exam will reflect your study habits. If you give an effort of 100%, you should do well; if you halfheartedly study for the exam, you will not do well. The earlier you begin studying for the exam, the better.

It is up to you to determine what study methods work best for you. Once you have done this, discipline yourself and stick to your plan!

1. **Assess your learning capabilities.** This will help you to determine the amount of time you will need to study.
2. **Request a content outline from your certifying agency.** Review the outline and determine the amount of time you will need for your own learning capabilities.
3. **Plot a study schedule.** Divide the outline into subjects. Place the subjects into a study schedule. Allow extra time for subjects that are more difficult for you.
4. **Set up a time schedule.** Retention levels are higher when you study in short sessions.
5. **Prepare to study.**
   - Create the environment
     Select a place with a desk or table, straight-backed chair, and good lighting. Being too comfortable may encourage sleep.

Keep the room temperature comfortable—not too warm or too cool.
Avoid interruptions from family, friends, and telephone.
Avoid unnecessary noise.
   - Gather study tools
     Gather all books, notebooks, and flashcards. Have extra pens, pencils, and flashcards handy.
6. **Commit to study.** You are preparing to take a national exam for your medical assistant credential!
7. **Study!**
   - Study material you do not know. Do not waste time on the material you do know.
   - Take a break halfway through each session.
   - Study the subject you dislike or are weakest in first and the subject you like or are strongest in last.
   - Do not study after a heavy meal.
   - Take your review book, notes, and/or flashcards with you and answer questions at lunch time, coffee breaks, and in your spare time.
   - Attend an exam review class or join a study group.

The Day Before the Exam
1. Be familiar with the directions and the route to the test site.
2. Review your notes briefly. Do not cram!
3. Go to bed early and get a good night's sleep.
4. Plan to arrive early at the test site. Doors will be locked to latecomers after a certain amount of time.
5. Have pencils and supplies ready to take with you to the exam.

The Day of the Exam
1. Eat a light breakfast.
2. Avoid caffeinated drinks. Caffeine can decrease the attention span and can over-stimulate the metabolism. This reduces concentration!
3. Dress comfortably in layers.
4. Listen to traffic and weather reports beforehand.
5. Bring your flashcards for a last review while waiting to take the exam.
6. Bring test material, photo identification, admission card, and several No. 2 pencils with erasers.

Taking the Exam
As you sit down to take the CMA or RMA exam, remember these important points.
1. Take a deep breath before starting.
2. Read all directions before starting.
3. If permissible, make notes on the exam booklet.
4. Read each question carefully and analyze what is being asked.
5. Pay attention to words that are emphasized by underline, capitalization, bold, or italics.
6. Concentrate on each question. Do not wander off to other questions.

7. Do not leave any blank answers. Guessing gives you a chance to get it right.
8. Be careful when making answers on the answer sheet so that you do not skip a line or mark an incorrect circle.
9. Check your time periodically. Allow one hour per section.
10. Multiple-choice questions have one correct answer. Do not overanalyze. Give the *best* answer to the question as it is written.
11. If you do not know the answer immediately, start eliminating choices to at least two possibilities. Highlight/mark the question on the test booklet so you can return to it after finishing the rest of the test.
12. After completing the exam, check the answer sheet to make sure it is complete. Check your exam booklet for highlighted questions and return to them.
13. Before handing in the test booklet and answer sheet, make sure your identification information is on the answer sheet and that it is correct.

MULTIPLE-CHOICE QUESTIONS

1. Statements that contain words such as "always," "every," "never," and "all" are usually too broad and often incorrect.
2. If two choices have the same or almost the same meaning, they are both incorrect; eliminate both choices when you select your answer.
3. Be aware of directional words such as "but," "except," and "however." They signal opposite meanings.
4. Try to answer the test question before looking at the options.
5. If you do not know the answer, eliminate the choices you know are wrong.
6. Read the question with the answer you selected to hear how they sound together.
7. To answer a multiple-choice question, you need to:
   a. find the main idea
   b. find and remember details that support the main idea
   c. draw conclusions

Pre-Test 1

GENERAL

Directions: Each of the following questions is followed by five possible responses. Select the *best* response.

1. An abnormal decrease in the size of a muscle is
   A. Myopathy
   B. Atrophy
   C. Dystrophy
   D. Hypertrophy
   E. Myotrophy

2. The cell from which a muscle develops is called a(n)
   A. Myeloblast
   B. Osteoblast
   C. Myoblast
   D. Myoclast
   E. Erythroblast

3. The abbreviation for right ear is
   A. AD
   B. AS
   C. AU
   D. OD
   E. OS

4. An otoscope is used to
   A. Inspect the nasal cavity
   B. Inspect the exterior ear canal
   C. Measure eyeball pressure
   D. Inspect the oral cavity
   E. Measure oxygen levels

5. This procedure is used to puncture the chest and remove fluid.
   A. Spirometry
   B. Bronchoscopy
   C. Intubation
   D. Thoracentesis
   E. Tracheostomy

6. Which of the following laboratory tests would be abnormal for a patient with anemia?
   A. Differential
   B. Hematocrit and hemoglobin
   C. Blood glucose
   D. Total cholesterol
   E. White blood cell count

7. Hyperparathyroidism may be treated by which medical specialist?
   A. Cardiologist
   B. Emergency medical technician
   C. Endocrinologist
   D. Hematologist
   E. Obstetrician

8. An abnormal increase in total number of white blood cells is called
   A. Anemia
   B. Leukopenia
   C. Leukosis
   D. Leukocytosis
   E. Polycythemia

9. The term for extremely rapid breathing is
   A. Hyperpnea
   B. Hypopnea
   C. Dyspnea
   D. Apnea
   E. Hypertension

10. Which of the following suffixes refers to pain?
    A. –phagia
    B. –desis
    C. –pnea
    D. –algia
    E. –lysis

11. A suffix used to denote a surgical repair is
    A. –pexy
    B. –desis

C. –plasty
D. –lysis
E. –centesis

12. A mammogram is a radiograph of the
A. Chest
B. Bladder
C. Breast
D. Lymph nodes
E. Axilla

13. The term *alopecia* is synonymous with
A. Excessive hair growth
B. Itching
C. Myopia
D. Baldness
E. A whitish pigmentation of the skin

14. Another term for chewing is
A. Mastication
B. Obstipation
C. Deglutition
D. Peristalsis
E. Regurgitation

15. A nevus in the antecubital area is a
A. Mass on the shoulder
B. Polyp on the lower back
C. Wart on the ankle
D. Scar on the knee
E. Mole on the inside of the elbow

16. An inflammation of a joint is called
A. Arthrodesis
B. Arthrodynia
C. Arthroclasis
D. Arthritis
E. Arthrocentesis

17. Fat is the main component of
A. The epidermis
B. Adipose tissue
C. Muscle tissue
D. Tendons
E. Lymphatic tissue

18. The study of the cause of disease is referred to as
A. Biology
B. Epidemiology
C. Pathology
D. Etiology
E. Physiology

19. The main function of the olfactory nerve is
A. Touching
B. Tasting

C. Smelling
D. Seeing
E. Hearing

20. An oophorectomy is a surgical procedure performed on the
A. Uterus
B. Ovaries
C. Knee
D. Vagina
E. Ear

21. The medical specialty that is involved with diseases and treatment of the male and female urinary systems is
A. Nephrology
B. Oncology
C. Urology
D. Proctology
E. Gynecology

22. This diagnostic procedure allows for visualization of the urinary bladder.
A. Urethral dilation
B. Intravenous pyelogram (IVP)
C. Cystography
D. Cystoscopy
E. Transurethral resection of the prostate (TURP)

23. The correct medical term for hives is
A. Urticaria
B. Verruca
C. A nevus
D. Shingles
E. Alopecia

24. The membrane that surrounds the heart is the
A. Endocardium
B. Endometrium
C. Pericardium
D. Perineum
E. Myocardium

25. A mucous membrane
A. Lines closed cavities of the body
B. Covers the lungs
C. Lines the abdominal cavity
D. Lines body cavities that open to the outside
E. Surrounds the heart

26. The ventral region of the body is described as
A. Superior
B. Lateral
C. Medial
D. Anterior
E. Posterior

27. The body cavity that contains the intestines is the
    A. Thoracic
    B. Spinal
    C. Abdominal
    D. Pleural
    E. Peritoneal

28. Movement of a body part toward the midline of the body is
    A. Supination
    B. Pronation
    C. Adduction
    D. Abduction
    E. Rotation

29. The plane that divides the body into front and back halves is
    A. Frontal
    B. Horizontal
    C. Median
    D. Oblique
    E. Transverse

30. Reye's syndrome
    A. Can follow a viral illness in children
    B. Is caused by high fever
    C. Is a symptom of acquired immunodeficiency syndrome (AIDS)
    D. Causes muscular dystrophy
    E. Is the common cold

31. The vertebrae located in the lower back are the
    A. Cervical
    B. Thoracic
    C. Lumbar
    D. Sacral
    E. Coccyx

32. This acute infectious skin disease is caused by staphylococci.
    A. Impetigo
    B. Psoriasis
    C. Athlete's foot
    D. Melanoma
    E. Eczema

33. The bone located in the posterior of the skull is the
    A. Frontal
    B. Ethmoid
    C. Temporal
    D. Occipital
    E. Mandible

34. The type of bone fracture in which the bone is bent and partially broken is a
    A. Simple fracture
    B. Compound fracture
    C. Greenstick fracture
    D. Comminuted fracture
    E. Complete fracture

35. The peripheral nervous system is composed of how many pairs of spinal nerves?
    A. 2
    B. 5
    C. 12
    D. 20
    E. 31

36. The pons and medulla make up the
    A. Brainstem
    B. Cerebellum
    C. Cerebrum
    D. Thalamus
    E. Right hemisphere

37. The failure of bone marrow to produce red blood cells results in which type of anemia?
    A. Aplastic
    B. Hemolytic
    C. Pernicious
    D. Microcytic
    E. Leukemia

38. Protrusion of a part of the stomach through the esophageal opening in the diaphragm is a(n)
    A. Esophageal aneurysm
    B. Esophageal varices
    C. Hiatal hernia
    D. Pyloric stenosis
    E. Gastroesophageal reflux disease (GERD)

39. Another name for the tympanic membrane is the
    A. Ossicle
    B. Cochlea
    C. Auricle
    D. Eardrum
    E. Organ of Corti

40. The largest artery in the body is the
    A. Brachial artery
    B. Temporal artery
    C. Radial artery
    D. Aorta
    E. Femoral artery

41. The sinoatrial node
    A. Stimulates the diaphragm
    B. Is the same as the atrioventricular node
    C. Is the pacemaker of the heart
    D. Divides the heart into right and left sides
    E. Regulates blood flow to the brain

42. An x-ray taken to confirm a fracture of the distal forearm would include the
    A. Tibia and fibula
    B. Radius and ulna
    C. Femur and trochanter
    D. Calcaneus and malleolus
    E. Humerus and scapula

43. Which of the following demonstrates an involuntary muscle action?
    A. Heartbeat
    B. Breathing
    C. Peristalsis
    D. Pupil dilation
    E. All of the above

44. Which of the following organs is located in the right upper quadrant?
    A. Liver
    B. Right ovary
    C. Appendix
    D. Uterus
    E. Stomach

45. Which of the following nerves stimulates the diaphragm?
    A. Trochlear
    B. Accessory
    C. Sciatic
    D. Phrenic
    E. Vagus

46. An abnormal lateral curvature of the spine is known as
    A. Spondylosis
    B. Kyphosis
    C. Scoliosis
    D. Ankylosis
    E. Lordosis

47. The alpha cells in the pancreas are responsible for the production of
    A. Insulin
    B. Glucagon
    C. Hydrochloric acid (HCl)
    D. Pepsin
    E. Gastrin

48. The surgical removal of the gallbladder is a
    A. Cholectomy
    B. Colostomy
    C. Cholecystectomy
    D. Laparoscopy
    E. Gastrectomy

49. Which of the following cranial nerves is involved in blindness?
    A. Abducens
    B. Oculomotor
    C. Trigeminal
    D. Olfactory
    E. Optic

50. The number of permanent teeth is
    A. 20
    B. 24
    C. 28
    D. 32
    E. 36

51. Legally, a physician
    A. May not refuse treatment in an emergency situation
    B. May refuse to provide follow-up care after initial treatment
    C. Must provide a diagnosis to a patient's employer if requested
    D. Must provide a medical history to the patient's insurance company if the insurance company requests it
    E. May refuse to accept a patient if he or she chooses

52. An itinerary
    A. Is a yearly schedule
    B. Is a travel guide
    C. Contains tickets
    D. Is a detailed outline of a trip
    E. Makes travel arrangements

53. Professionalism may best be displayed by
    A. Keeping emotions to one's self
    B. Staying calm when dealing with angry patients
    C. Showing no consideration for other members of the team
    D. Referring all problems to the physician
    E. Arriving late or leaving early

54. The ability to imagine taking the place of the patient and accepting the patient's behavior is
    A. Objectivity
    B. Empathy
    C. Sympathy
    D. Industry
    E. Subjectivity

55. The patient's medical record belongs to
    A. The patient's spouse
    B. The physician
    C. The patient
    D. The patient's attorney
    E. The state medical board

56. A breast mass is found in a woman whose mother and sister have died of breast cancer. She cancels her next three follow-up appointments. Which defense mechanism is she using?
    A. Denial
    B. Anxiety
    C. Acceptance
    D. Isolation
    E. Suppression

57. Personality differences are due to
    A. Age
    B. Experience
    C. Heredity
    D. Environment
    E. All of the above

58. Which of the following is *not* a characteristic desirable in a medical assistant?
    A. Appreciation
    B. Impatience
    C. Flexibility
    D. Friendliness
    E. Concern

59. Which of the following is not an example of stereotyping?
    A. Similar people have similar needs
    B. Elderly patients have hearing deficits
    C. Medicaid patients are lazy
    D. Educated patients have no fear of illness
    E. Young children react differently to stressful situations

60. To release medical information
    A. The physician must sign a waiver
    B. The insurance company must make the request in writing
    C. The patient must sign a release form
    D. A certified record technician must be employed by the office
    E. The patient must deliver the records in person to the requester

61. Which of the following should be reported to the health department?
    A. Otitis media
    B. Strep throat
    C. Influenza
    D. Vaginal yeast infection
    E. Human immunodeficiency virus

62. Which of the following is an example of objective data?
    A. Family history
    B. Vital signs
    C. Past surgical history
    D. Last menstrual period (LMP)
    E. Insurance information

63. Which of the following telephone calls should be given immediately to the physician?
    A. Another physician
    B. An angry patient
    C. A patient's family member
    D. A salesperson
    E. An insurance company

64. In Maslow's hierarchy of needs, the need to be loved and free from loneliness is a
    A. Physiologic need
    B. Safety need
    C. Social need
    D. Self-esteem need
    E. Self-actualization need

65. If a patient refuses to consent to treatment, the medical assistant should
    A. Schedule the patient for another appointment
    B. Force treatment on the patient
    C. Force the patient to consent
    D. Delay treatment and inform or consult with the physician
    E. Terminate the patient

66. An enforceable contract contains
    A. An offer
    B. An acceptance
    C. A consideration
    D. A capacity
    E. All of the above

67. The opposite of anterior is
    A. Distal
    B. Medial
    C. Proximal
    D. Posterior
    E. Lateral

68. Informed consent includes which of the following elements?
    A. Benefits and risks of the treatment
    B. Purpose of treatment
    C. Nature of the patient's condition
    D. Assessment of the patient's understanding of the treatment
    E. All of the above

69. All of the following are reasons for revoking a physician's license *except*
    A. Mental incapacity
    B. Physical incapacity
    C. Conviction of a crime

D. Unprofessional conduct
E. Providing atypical care

70. The control center of a cell is
    A. DNA
    B. Organelles
    C. Nucleus
    D. Ribosomes
    E. Cell membrane

71. Subcutaneous tissue
    A. Is found under the skin
    B. Contains fat
    C. Is an injection site
    D. Connects the dermis to the muscle surface
    E. All of the above

72. Which of the following is *not* a bone of the lower extremity?
    A. Femur
    B. Humerus
    C. Tibia
    D. Fibula
    E. Metatarsals

73. The muscle in the upper extremity that is used as an injection site is the
    A. Deltoid
    B. Biceps brachii
    C. Triceps brachii
    D. Trapezius
    E. Gluteus medius

74. The pacemaker of the heart is the
    A. Septum
    B. Sinoatrial node
    C. Atrioventricular node
    D. Left atrium
    E. Mitral valve

75. Gas exchange in the lungs takes place in the
    A. Pharynx
    B. Bronchi
    C. Trachea
    D. Bronchiole
    E. Alveoli

76. The liver
    A. Makes bile
    B. Detoxifies harmful substances
    C. Produces heparin
    D. Stores glycogen
    E. All of the above

77. The fertilized ovum implants into the
    A. Cervix
    B. Endometrium

C. Myometrium
D. Epimetrium
E. Oviducts

78. In the male, testosterone is produced in the
    A. Ovaries
    B. Testes
    C. Epididymis
    D. Seminal vesicles
    E. Prostate gland

79. The largest portion of the brain is the
    A. Cerebrum
    B. Cerebellum
    C. Medulla oblongata
    D. Brainstem
    E. Hypothalamus

80. There are _____ pairs of spinal nerves.
    A. 100
    B. 10
    C. 12
    D. 25
    E. 31

81. Gustatory receptors are located in the
    A. Mouth
    B. Nose
    C. Eye
    D. Ear
    E. Skin

82. Insulin
    A. Is produced by the liver
    B. Controls metabolism
    C. Increases blood sugar levels
    D. Decreases blood sugar levels
    E. Controls blood calcium levels

83. A decrease in the total number of white blood cells is called
    A. Leukocyte
    B. Leukoderma
    C. Leukocytosis
    D. Anemia
    E. Leukopenia

84. The abbreviation meaning *immediately* is
    A. prn
    B. stat
    C. qod
    D. ad lib
    E. dc

85. The physician is legally obligated to report
    A. Deaths
    B. Births

C. Communicable diseases
D. Abuse
E. All of the above

86. The prefix *brady-* denotes
    A. Slow
    B. Fast
    C. Hard
    D. Soft
    E. Difficult

87. The opposite of superficial is
    A. Ventral
    B. Proximal
    C. Deep
    D. Distal
    E. Dorsal

88. An authorization in advance to withdraw artificial life support is
    A. Assault
    B. Battery
    C. An advance directive
    D. Uniform Anatomical Gift Act
    E. Good Samaritan Act

89. Unconsciously avoiding the reality of an unpleasant event is
    A. Regression
    B. Denial
    C. Repression
    D. Suppression
    E. Rationalization

90. "Tell me more about it" is an example of
    A. An open-ended statement
    B. A closed statement
    C. Clarification
    D. Feedback
    E. Reflection

91. The study of the cause of disease is
    A. Epidemiology
    B. Pathology
    C. Etiology
    D. Symptomology
    E. Risk management

92. Nonverbal communication may be conveyed by
    A. Touch
    B. Eye contact
    C. Body position
    D. Silence
    E. All of the above

93. Bulimia is
    A. A mass of food
    B. An eating disorder

C. Loss of appetite
D. A blood condition
E. An arrhythmia

94. A cerebral vascular accident can also be called a(n)
    A. Arrhythmia
    B. Heart attack
    C. Aneurysm
    D. Stroke
    E. Thrombus

95. Rubeola is
    A. Herpes simplex virus I
    B. Scarlet fever
    C. Whooping cough
    D. Measles
    E. Chicken pox

96. A sexually transmitted disease caused by a protozoal infestation is
    A. Herpes
    B. Gonorrhea
    C. Trichomoniasis
    D. Crabs
    E. Syphilis

97. An electrolyte that has an important influence on the activity of the heart muscle is
    A. Chloride
    B. Magnesium
    C. Peptase
    D. Phosphorus
    E. Potassium

98. Which of the following respiratory disorders is characterized by a loss of lung capacity?
    A. Asthma
    B. Emphysema
    C. Bronchitis
    D. Tuberculosis
    E. Psoriasis

99. The type of membrane that lines cavities of the body that open to the outside is
    A. Cutaneous
    B. Synovial
    C. Mucous
    D. Pleural
    E. Peritoneum

100. Another name for an open fracture is a
    A. Comminuted fracture
    B. Closed fracture
    C. Simple fracture
    D. Greenstick fracture
    E. Compound fracture

ADMINISTRATIVE

Directions: Each of the following questions is followed by five possible responses. Select the *best* response.

1. Which of the following types of scheduling allows for the most efficient use of staff, materials, and facilities?
   A. Open appointments
   B. Double-booking
   C. Wave
   D. Modified wave
   E. Grouping

2. What piece of mail should be placed on top when sorting the physician's mail?
   A. First-class mail
   B. Journals
   C. Envelope marked *Personal*
   D. Bills and statements
   E. Equipment catalogs

3. Open punctuation is characterized by
   A. Enclosure notation
   B. Absence of punctuation after the salutation and a comma after the complimentary close
   C. Modified block style
   D. Use of a colon after the salutation
   E. Block style

4. The federal insurance program that provides for the medically indigent is
   A. CHAMPUS
   B. Medicare
   C. Blue Shield
   D. Medicaid
   E. HMO

5. The process of transferring an amount from the day sheet to the ledger is
   A. Journalizing
   B. Charting
   C. Posting
   D. Crediting
   E. Debiting

6. A numeric filing system requires the use of
   A. Lateral files
   B. An alphabetical cross-reference
   C. Color-coding
   D. A tickler file
   E. Subject headings

7. The file folder label for Jennie Holmes-Mathis should be
   A. Jennie, Holmes-Mathis
   B. Mathis, Jennie Holmes
   C. Holmes, Jennie-Mathis
   D. Holmes-Mathis, Jennie
   E. Mathis, Jennie (nee Holmes)

8. Third-party participation in an office indicates the relationships among the
   A. Physician, patient, and medical assistant
   B. Physician, medical assistant, and insurance company
   C. Physician, patient, and insurance company
   D. Physician, hospital, and insurance company
   E. Physician, patient, and hospital

9. A claim may be rejected by an insurance company because of the omission of
   A. Complete diagnosis
   B. Policy number
   C. Patient birth date
   D. Itemization of charges
   E. All of the above

10. How much postage is required for a first-class letter that weighs 3 oz if the first ounce costs $0.34 and each additional ounce is $0.25?
    A. $1.00
    B. $0.50
    C. $0.34
    D. $0.84
    E. $0.75

11. When the word *Confidential* is to be typed on the envelope, it should be placed
    A. In the lower right corner
    B. Below the zip code
    C. In the lower left corner
    D. Below the return address
    E. Both C and D

12. The most formal of complimentary closings is
    A. Very truly yours
    B. Warm wishes
    C. Sincerely
    D. Sincerely yours
    E. As always

13. When making an appointment, which of the following is *not* needed?
    A. Patient's name
    B. Telephone number
    C. Reason for visit
    D. Insurance information
    E. Availability

14. This type of call allows more than one person in more than one place to talk simultaneously.
    A. Person-to-person
    B. Conference call
    C. Three-party billing
    D. Appointment call
    E. Collect call

15. This procedure protects against the loss of data.
    A. Buffering
    B. Debugging
    C. Backing up
    D. Initializing
    E. Formatting

16. A tickler file is
    A. A guide for processing insurance claims
    B. A list of procedures for equipment maintenance
    C. A type of color-coding
    D. A physician referral service
    E. Future events arranged in chronological order

17. All of the following would require a Current Procedural Terminology (CPT) code *except*
    A. Diarrhea
    B. Mastectomy
    C. Otoplasty
    D. Hysterectomy
    E. Sigmoidoscopy

18. Which of the following characteristics of a receptionist might make an impression on a patient?
    A. Appearance
    B. Professionalism
    C. Manners
    D. Attitude
    E. All of the above

19. A direction to consider additional codes is
    A. NEC
    B. NOS
    C. See also
    D. See condition
    E. See category

20. A V-code
    A. Refers to specific health conditions
    B. Refers to specific body systems
    C. Refers to factors that influence health status
    D. Refers to neoplasms
    E. Refers to injuries

21. Mail that is opened accidentally should be
    A. Hand delivered immediately
    B. Put at the bottom of the stack
    C. Left as is
    D. Resealed with tape and noted as *opened in error*
    E. Placed in another envelope

22. Which of the following are Evaluation and Management (E&M) descriptors?
    A. Physical examination
    B. School physical
    C. Well-baby check-up
    D. Preoperative physical
    E. All of the above

23. Which is an example of a third-party payor?
    A. Health Maintenance Organization (HMO)
    B. Medicare
    C. Preferred Provider Organization (PPO)
    D. Patient's spouse
    E. Patient's parent

24. In the problem-oriented medical record (POMR) system, the initial database includes
    A. A list of past medical problems
    B. A complete physical examination
    C. A numbered list of present problems
    D. The patient's progress
    E. A list of social problems

25. A trial balance is a comparison of
    A. Cash on hand and cash received
    B. Daily charges and payments
    C. Balance sheet and income sheet
    D. Ledger card totals and account-receivable balance
    E. Owners' equity and liabilities

26. When adding information to the medical record, new notes are added
   A. In alphabetical order
   B. In subject order
   C. Newest to the front
   D. Newest to the back
   E. To a newly created file

27. Which of the following calls require immediate transfer to the physician?
   A. A young child with a high fever
   B. A patient with a possible medical allergy
   C. Another physician
   D. An adult with a low-grade fever
   E. A patient with questions about a mammogram

28. Appointments should be scheduled
   A. For 15 minutes each with 15-minute open slots in between
   B. Every 15 minutes
   C. Either all in the morning or all in the afternoon
   D. In consecutive order without large gaps
   E. So that patients with similar problems are seen on the same day

29. Which is *not* part of basic information obtained at the patient's first visit?
   A. Insurance information
   B. Name, address, and telephone number
   C. Name of person who referred the patient
   D. Business address and business telephone number
   E. Diagnosis

30. Standard-size paper and envelope for business correspondence is
   A. 8½ × 11; no. 10 envelope
   B. 7¼ × 10½; no. 7¾ envelope
   C. 5½ × 8½; 3½ × 6 envelope
   D. 6¼ × 9¼; no. 6¾ envelope
   E. 11 × 14; no. 10 envelope

31. Patient's ledger cards should be kept
   A. With the patient's chart
   B. In a general ledger
   C. In a separate ledger file
   D. In a job ledger
   E. With insurance forms

32. The bank statement is reconciled with
   A. The checkbook
   B. The day sheet
   C. Accounts receivable
   D. The payment record
   E. Both A and D

33. The record of the proceedings of a meeting are the
   A. Agenda
   B. *Roberts Rules of Order*
   C. Itinerary
   D. Minutes
   E. Format

34. Which of the following protects data from loss?
   A. Booting up the system
   B. Initializing disks
   C. Backing up
   D. Virus check
   E. Debugging

35. The scheduling system based on scheduling similar appointments or procedures together is called
   A. Wave
   B. Modified wave
   C. Grouping
   D. Double-booking
   E. Open scheduling

36. Appropriate information to include in a patient information brochure would be
   A. Information about the scope of the practice
   B. Physician's fees
   C. Billing information
   D. Employee's names and telephone numbers
   E. Coding information

37. A new employee must complete which of the following?
   A. 501 Form
   B. W-4 Form
   C. W-3 Form
   D. W-2 Form
   E. FICA Form

38. Which of the following abbreviations is not correct?
   A. pH
   B. mEq
   C. PKU
   D. HGB
   E. kg S

39. Patient information that is released without patient's authorization might result in legal charge of
   A. Fraud
   B. Battery
   C. Invasion of privacy
   D. Abandonment
   E. Libel

40. A correctly addressed envelope includes
    A. Omission of all punctuation
    B. Periods after abbreviation
    C. Periods after initials
    D. Comma between city and state
    E. Comma between street name and numbers

41. Which of the following circumstances would waive the need for a written release of medical records?
    A. Requested from other practices
    B. A subpoena
    C. Attorney request
    D. Hospital request
    E. Insurance company request

42. In double-entry bookkeeping, the original entry is put onto the
    A. Patient ledger card
    B. Daily log
    C. General ledger
    D. Account ledger
    E. Appointment book

43. The correct way to indicate an enclosure notation is
    A. encl:
    B. Enclosure
    C. enclosure
    D. enc
    E. encl

44. A superbill provides which of the following?
    A. Insurance claim
    B. Fee schedule
    C. Deposit slip
    D. Dictation
    E. Abnormal test results

45. Which of the following is the purpose of records management?
    A. Storage
    B. Arranging
    C. Accessibility
    D. Classifying
    E. All of the above

46. Which coding system is not associated with medical procedures?
    A. CPT
    B. *International Classification of Diseases*, ninth edition, Clinical Modification (ICD-9-CM)
    C. Health Care Financing Administration Common Procedure Coding System (HCPCS)
    D. Relative value scale (RVS)
    E. Resource-based RVS (RBRVS)

47. Which is *not* an indexing rule?
    A. Unit 1 is the surname

    B. A hyphen is disregarded
    C. Initials come before complete names
    D. Apostrophes are disregarded
    E. Names are divided into units

48. ICD-9-CM codes that refer to factors that may influence the patient's health status are
    A. Human immunodeficiency virus (HIV) codes
    B. Volume I codes
    C. Volume II codes
    D. E-codes
    E. V-codes

49. The smallest piece of information that the computer can process is a(n)
    A. Output
    B. Bit
    C. Byte
    D. Font
    E. Icon

50. The index of files on a disk is the
    A. Window
    B. Menu
    C. Byte
    D. Directory
    E. Icon

51. The appointment system of the office should take into account the needs of the
    A. Staff
    B. Physician
    C. Patients
    D. A and B only
    E. B and C only

52. *Dear Mrs. May:* is an example of
    A. Open punctuation
    B. Mixed punctuation
    C. Block punctuation
    D. Semiblock punctuation
    E. Modified block

53. A master list of equipment inventory includes all of the following *except* the
    A. Date of purchase
    B. Cost
    C. Operating manuals
    D. Estimated life of the piece
    E. Description

54. Which of the following hospital records may be released by the authorization of the attending surgeon only?
    A. Nurses' notes
    B. Operative notes
    C. Laboratory reports

    D. Radiology reports

    E. Billing information

55. An illness that existed before an insurance policy is written is known as a(n)

    A. Special risk

    B. Exclusion

    C. Preexisting condition

    D. Waiting period

    E. Prior authorization required

56. A patient has not been seen in the office for 2 years. The patient's record would be found in the

    A. Basement

    B. Active files

    C. Open files

    D. Inactive files

    E. Closed files

57. An important consideration when deciding how to position the computer monitor at the reception desk is

    A. Patient confidentiality

    B. Staff access

    C. Lighting

    D. Position of the printer

    E. Availability of patient records

58. Which group of patients should be escorted to the examination room and given instructions on what they are to do?

    A. Children

    B. New patients

    C. Established patients

    D. Older adults

    E. All of the above

59. Which information is *not* essential for the surgery scheduler when requesting a surgery date?

    A. Type of procedure

    B. Name of the assisting physician

    C. Name of patient

    D. Age of patient

    E. Telephone number of the patient

60. The notation c: *Julia Jones, MD* means

    A. A copy is made for Dr. Jones

    B. A copy of the letter is sent to Dr. Jones

    C. The receiver had been advised that a copy has been sent to Dr. Jones

    D. Dr. Jones will answer the letter

    E. The copy was sent to Dr. Jones by certified mail

61. A *history and physical usually* contains all of the following except

    A. Results of laboratory tests

    B. Reason for the visit

    C. Vital signs

    D. Review of body systems

    E. General appearance of patient

62. Under a managed care plan, the physician agrees to

    A. Set fees within certain ranges provided by the plan

    B. Accept predetermined fees

    C. Charge fees based on community average

    D. Base fees on the national average

    E. Limit the number of patients seen

63. Which type of insurance organization uses the fee-for-services concept?

    A. Health Maintenance Organization (HMO)

    B. Managed care

    C. Independent practice association

    D. Preferred Provider Organization (PPO)

    E. Medicaid

64. Which factor is *not* included when determining the level of service for E&M codes?

    A. Cost of services

    B. Level of decision making required of the physician

    C. Health history of patient

    D. Type of examination

    E. Type of laboratory tests

65. When money is placed in an account, which of the following documents is prepared?

    A. Check

    B. Statement

    C. Debit slip

    D. Credit slip

    E. Deposit slip

66. The most common color-coding system color codes the

    A. Patient's Social Security number

    B. Patient's date of birth

    C. Patient's given name

    D. Patient's surname

    E. Patient's account number

67. Who is the legal owner of the information in a patient's medical record?

    A. The physician

    B. The patient

    C. The insurance company

    D. The patient and physician

    E. The physician and the insurance company

68. When preparing the appointment matrix, the first action is to indicate

    A. Hospital calls

    B. Times available

    C. Times not available

D. Facilities available
E. Staff available

69. Scheduling patients with the same medical complaints on the same day is
    A. Wave scheduling
    B. Modified wave scheduling
    C. Open hours
    D. Group scheduling
    E. Double-booking

70. A major advantage of using a computer for word processing is
    A. Extensive editing capability
    B. Speed of processing
    C. Spell-check
    D. Column layout
    E. Storage capacity

71. Which is *not* true of certified mail?
    A. Insurance coverage is available
    B. Receipt of delivery can be obtained for a fee
    C. Only first-class mail can be certified
    D. Record of delivery is kept by the post office
    E. Restricted delivery can be obtained for a fee

72. Which of the following must be sent by first-class mail?
    A. Magazines
    B. Books
    C. Printed materials
    D. Personal letters and postcards
    E. Equipment catalogues

73. A Medicare claim for a deceased beneficiary may be paid directly to the physician if
    A. The physician accepts assignment
    B. The spouse assigns benefits to the physician
    C. Social Security verifies Medicare coverage
    D. Charges are paid by the intermediary
    E. The estate is billed

74. All checks received as payment for charges should be endorsed
    A. Immediately
    B. At the end of the day
    C. When they are deposited
    D. After they are posted
    E. Monthly

75. In an alphabetical file, which is filed first?
    A. A. R. Stephenson
    B. John Stephenson
    C. George Stephens
    D. Ann Stephenson-Bailey
    E. Andrew Stephen

76. Which is correct for an inside address?
    A. Dr. David Roberts
    B. Dr. David Roberts, M.D.
    C. Mr. David Roberts, M.D.
    D. Roberts, David, M.D.
    E. David Roberts, M.D.

77. Which is *not* true about a postage meter?
    A. It prints its own postage
    B. Some can seal the envelope
    C. It locks when the postage is used up
    D. The mailer leases the machine and purchases the postage
    E. A license must be obtained from the post office

78. The two-letter abbreviation for Nebraska is
    A. NB
    B. NE
    C. NA
    D. NR
    E. NK

79. Which letter style requires the complimentary closing and typed signature be placed in line with the left margin of the body of the letter?
    A. Block style
    B. Semiblock style
    C. Full block style
    D. Indented style
    E. Semi-indented style

80. Which of the following is *not* included in a memorandum?
    A. Date
    B. Subject
    C. Complimentary close
    D. Writer's name
    E. Reference initials

81. The second page of a two-page letter contains which of the following in the heading?
    A. Name and date
    B. Name and page number
    C. Name, page number, and date
    D. Name, page number, date, and subject
    E. Name, writer's name, subject, and date

82. The complimentary close of a letter is typed how many lines below the last line of the body?
    A. Two
    B. Three
    C. Four
    D. Five
    E. Ten

83. A fee profile is derived from
    A. Insurance payments
    B. Patient's payments
    C. Government payments
    D. Physician charges
    E. Insurance charges

84. Which of the following is demographic information included in a medical record?
    A. Present illness
    B. Date of birth
    C. Laboratory reports
    D. X-ray findings
    E. Complete physical examination

85. Which of the following requires an ICD-9-CM code?
    A. Proctoscopy
    B. Pap smear
    C. Appendectomy
    D. Irritable bowel syndrome
    E. Mastectomy

86. When it is 4:00 pm in New York City, what time is it in Seattle, WA?
    A. 12:00 pm
    B. 1:00 pm
    C. 2:00 pm
    D. 3:00 pm
    E. 4:00 pm

87. Ideally, a telephone should be answered before the
    A. First ring
    B. Third ring
    C. Fourth ring
    D. Fifth ring
    E. Other line picks up the call

88. An E code in the ICD-9-CM coding system
    A. Refers to external causes
    B. Refers to hypertension
    C. Refers to neoplasms
    D. Refers to suicide attempt
    E. Refers to disease

89. The universal claim form developed by Health Care Financing Administration (HCFA) is
    A. Form 1904
    B. ICD-9
    C. Form 1040
    D. CMS-1500
    E. HCFA-1999

90. Patients who are always late or who habitually cancel appointments should be scheduled
    A. First in the morning
    B. Right before lunch

C. Midafternoon
D. At the end of the day
E. On Fridays

91. An error was made in charting the patient's record. The method used to correct the error is to
    A. Erase the error and write in the correction
    B. Reenter the notation on the next line
    C. Draw a single line through the error, write the word *error*, make the correction, and date and initial the entry
    D. Cross out the error, and make the correction in the margin
    E. Cross out the entry, and correct it

92. SOAP is an acronym for
    A. Child protection services
    B. A medical assistant society
    C. Source-oriented medical records
    D. Problem-oriented progress notes
    E. Traditional medical records

93. A patient refuses to follow medical advice and the physician decides to terminate the relationship. The letter to the patient should state all of the following *except*
    A. A referral to another physician
    B. An offer to make records available
    C. That the physician withdraws from the case
    D. A future date after which the physician is not available
    E. That the patient still needs medical care

94. When the medical office works on a fixed appointment schedule and a patient arrives without an appointment requesting to see the physician, the patient
    A. Should be sent away
    B. Should be referred to another physician
    C. Should be called as soon as a cancellation has been made
    D. Should be told to come back tomorrow
    E. Should be squeezed in for a brief visit so the physician can decide what the next treatment step should be

95. If a patient calls to cancel his or her appointment
    A. Express regret
    B. Immediately offer a new appointment time
    C. Have the patient speak to the office manager
    D. Discourage cancellations sternly
    E. All of the above

96. A good telephone technique is a
    A. High-pitched voice
    B. Low-pitched and expressive voice

C. Monotone voice
D. Breathless and excited voice
E. Soft-spoken voice

97. If a patient's account has been turned over to a collection agency and the patient calls about the bill, the patient should be told
A. To remit payment to the physician's office
B. To deal with the collection agency
C. To talk with the office manager
D. To disregard further statements
E. To find another physician

98. The entry, editing, manipulation, and storage of text using the computer is
A. Telecommunications
B. Documentation
C. Interfacing

D. Word processing
E. Formatting

99. When a shipment of supplies is received, the supplies should be checked against the
A. Advertised prices
B. Enclosed packing slip
C. Invoice
D. Requisition slip
E. Inventory

100. A credit balance on an account occurs when
A. The patient's check was returned for insufficient funds
B. The insurance company disallows the claim
C. The patient pays in advance
D. A discount is given
E. The patient's account is sent for collection

CLINICAL

Directions: Each of the following questions is followed by five possible responses. Select the *best* response.

1. *Standard precautions* are designed to be used for
   A. Patients known to be infected
   B. Patients suspected of being infected
   C. All patients
   D. Patients recovering from an infectious disease
   E. Infected health care workers

2. Disposable single use gloves should be worn
   A. When taking a blood pressure
   B. When handling specimens
   C. When performing venipuncture
   D. All of the above
   E. B and C

3. Normal oral temperature, in degrees, is
   A. 96.8°F
   B. 97.6°F
   C. 98.6°F
   D. 36°C
   E. 38°C

4. Normal respiratory rate for an adult is
   A. 10 to 16 breaths per minute
   B. 14 to 20 breaths per minute
   C. 20 to 26 breaths per minute
   D. 30 to 38 breaths per minute
   E. 30 to 60 breaths per minute

5. Vital signs include
   A. Temperature
   B. Blood pressure
   C. TPR
   D. A and B
   E. B and C

6. The pulse rate is
   A. Usually higher in adults than in children
   B. Usually higher in children than in adults
   C. The same for both
   D. Lower at birth than at 1 year
   E. Higher in adults over 60 than in a child under 7 years of age

7. Pulse rate is decreased by
   A. Sleep
   B. Brain injury, causing increased pressure
   C. Hypothyroidism
   D. A and B
   E. All of the above

8. A high temperature is when the body temperature, in degrees, is
   A. 98° to 99°F
   B. 99° to 101°F
   C. 101° to 103°F
   D. 103° to 105°F
   E. 38.3° to 39.5°C

9. The pulse pressure is
   A. The difference between the systolic and the diastolic blood pressure
   B. An occasional missed beat
   C. Absence of a carotid pulse
   D. Alternating weak and strong beats
   E. The difference between apical and radial pulses

10. A patient who weighs 45 kg also weighs how many pounds?
   A. 45
   B. 99
   C. 105
   D. 145
   E. 150

11. A patient who is 72 inches tall is
   A. 6 feet
   B. 6 feet, 2 inches
   C. 6 feet, 4 inches
   D. 5 feet, 2 inches
   E. 5 feet, 6 inches

12. During a physical examination, percussion is most commonly used to examine the
    A. Chest and back
    B. Mouth and throat
    C. Eyes and ears
    D. Breasts
    E. Nose and neck

13. A patient's reaction to stress, use of defense mechanisms, and resources for support would be recorded under
    A. Chief complaint
    B. Past history
    C. History of present illness
    D. Social history
    E. Family history

14. Subjective findings include
    A. How the patient feels
    B. Information about the patient's family
    C. Previous pregnancies
    D. All of the above
    E. A and B

15. Visual acuity is
    A. Pressure in the eyeball
    B. Nearsightedness
    C. Farsightedness
    D. Color vision
    E. Clearness of vision

16. The purpose of a proctoscopy is to examine the
    A. Prostate gland
    B. Uterus
    C. Rectum
    D. Sigmoid colon
    E. Esophagus

17. A patient in the Sims' position is lying on the
    A. Right side, with left leg flexed
    B. Left side and chest, with right leg flexed
    C. Back, with both legs bent
    D. Right side, with right leg flexed
    E. Left side, with left leg flexed

18. A patient lying flat on the abdomen is in the
    A. Dorsal position
    B. Lithotomy position
    C. Supine position
    D. Prone position
    E. Fowler's position

19. The physician uses which of the following to examine the patient's eyes?
    A. Ophthalmoscope
    B. Percussion hammer
    C. Tonometer
    D. Otoscope
    E. Speculum

20. The patient should be placed in which of the following positions for examination of the head and neck?
    A. Standing
    B. Sitting
    C. Prone
    D. Supine
    E. Sims'

21. For an obstetrics examination, urine is routinely checked for the presence of
    A. Glucose and protein
    B. Glucose and ketones
    C. Human chorionic gonadotropin (HCG)
    D. Protein and ketones
    E. Blood and glucose

22. A patient should be taught that the best time to perform breast self-examination is approximately
    A. 1 week after her period
    B. The sixth day of every month
    C. 1 week before her period
    D. 2 weeks after her period
    E. 2 weeks before her period

23. An infection that has a rapid onset, severe symptoms, and subsides in a short period is called
    A. Acute
    B. Chronic
    C. Local
    D. Systemic
    E. Contagious

24. Sterile-wrapped items can be safely stored, and considered sterile, for up to
    A. 7 to 14 days
    B. 14 to 21 days
    C. 21 to 28 days
    D. 28 to 30 days
    E. Indefinitely

25. When removing a pack from the autoclave, you notice that the sterilization indicator has not changed color. You should
    A. Do nothing
    B. Place the pack back in the autoclave and resterilize
    C. Place a new indicator on the pack and resterilize
    D. Place the pack back in the autoclave but in a different location
    E. Unwrap the pack, rewrap the pack, replace the indicator, and resterilize

26. Scrubbing an item with soap and water before sterilization is
    A. Cleaning
    B. Sanitization
    C. Disinfection
    D. Sterilization
    E. Antisepsis

27. The type of immunity that develops from having the disease is
    A. Natural active
    B. Natural passive
    C. Acquired active
    D. Acquired passive
    E. Congenital

28. When opening a sterile pack, the top flap should be opened
    A. Toward the body
    B. Away from the body
    C. Toward the right side
    D. Toward the left side
    E. In any direction

29. The finest suture material of the following list is
    A. 0
    B. 00
    C. 000
    D. 4-0
    E. 8-0

30. A type of instrument that is used to grasp or hold tissues or objects is a
    A. Probe
    B. Scalpel
    C. Scissors
    D. Forceps
    E. Retractor

31. Betadine (povidone-iodine) should not be used on the skin of a patient who is allergic to
    A. Alcohol
    B. Metal
    C. Iodine
    D. Soap
    E. Latex

32. Wound drainage that contains pus is charted as
    A. Serous
    B. Normal
    C. Serosanguinous
    D. Sanguinous
    E. Purulent

33. The angle for the insertion of the needle for an intradermal injection is
    A. 10 to 15 degrees

B. 20 to 30 degrees
C. 45 degrees
D. 90 degrees
E. Not important

34. A medication that is placed under the tongue is being administered by which technique?
    A. By mouth
    B. Buccal
    C. Sublingual
    D. Instillation
    E. Topical

35. To administer an intramuscular injection, which needle would you use?
    A. 1 inch, 25 gauge
    B. 1½ inch, 21 gauge
    C. 1 inch, 18 gauge
    D. ½ inch, 22 gauge
    E. 2 inch, 20 gauge

36. A type of drug that increases urinary output is a(n)
    A. Emetic
    B. Diuretic
    C. Miotic
    D. Cathartic
    E. Antibiotic

37. The physician orders 250 mg amoxicillin intramuscularly. The vial reads *500 mg per 1 mL*. How much would be given to the patient?
    A. 0.5 mL
    B. 1 mL
    C. 2 mL
    D. 3 mL
    E. 5 mL

38. When a specimen is placed in a centrifuge, a tube of similar size containing a liquid of similar weight should be placed
    A. On the counter
    B. Directly opposite from the specimen
    C. Directly beside the specimen
    D. In all empty spaces in the centrifuge
    E. To the right side of the specimen

39. Microscopic examination of a urine sample should be performed
    A. Within ½ hour of collection
    B. Within 1 hour of collection
    C. Within 1½ hours of collection
    D. Within 2 hours of collection
    E. Within 3 hours of collection

40. The absence of urine formation is termed
    A. Anuria
    B. Polyuria

C. Dysuria
D. Oliguria
E. Ketonuria

41. Normal specific gravity is generally between
   A. 1.000 and 1.005
   B. 1.010 and 1.050
   C. 1.025 and 1.500
   D. 1.005 and 1.050
   E. 1.010 and 1.025

42. A complete blood count (CBC) includes
   A. Platelet count
   B. Hemoglobin and hematocrit
   C. White blood cell count
   D. All of the above
   E. A and C

43. Capillary blood is usually obtained
   A. From a skin puncture
   B. From a venipuncture
   C. From an arterial puncture
   D. All of the above
   E. B and C

44. A cholecystogram is used to view the
   A. Urinary bladder
   B. Liver
   C. Gallbladder
   D. Kidneys
   E. Ureters

45. Application of heat
   A. Dilates blood vessels
   B. Constricts blood vessels
   C. Elevates blood pressure
   D. Decreases respiration
   E. Produces weight loss

46. The wave on an electrocardiogram that represents contraction of the atria is
   A. P
   B. QRS
   C. T
   D. V
   E. R

47. The pacemaker of the heart is the
   A. Myocardium
   B. Sinoatrial node
   C. Atrioventricular node
   D. Purkinje fibers
   E. Bundle of His

48. A standard electrocardiogram has how many leads?
   A. 4
   B. 8
   C. 10
   D. 12
   E. 14

49. The standard speed for recording an electrocardiogram is
   A. 5 mm/sec
   B. 10 mm/sec
   C. 20 mm/sec
   D. 25 mm/sec
   E. 50 mm/sec

50. To cauterize a small lesion on the oral mucosa, the physician may use an applicator with
   A. Silver nitrate
   B. Alcohol
   C. Formalin
   D. Betadine
   E. Zephiran chloride

51. A common laboratory test that may be ordered for a patient on Coumadin therapy is
   A. Prothrombin time
   B. Erythrocyte sedimentation rate (ESR)
   C. White blood cell (WBC) count
   D. Hematocrit
   E. Complete blood count (CBC)

52. Which one of the following types of suture material is absorbable?
   A. Steel
   B. Cotton
   C. Catgut
   D. Nylon
   E. Silk

53. The minimum number of cells to be counted in a differential blood smear is
   A. 50
   B. 100
   C. 150
   D. 200
   E. Unlimited; count them all

54. A hemoglobin of 10 g/dL is approximately equivalent to a hematocrit of
   A. 10%
   B. 20%
   C. 30%
   D. 36%
   E. 40%

55. Which of the following laboratory results should be called to the attention of the physician?
   A. White blood cell count: $7200/mm^3$
   B. Red blood cell count: 4.4 million/mm^3
   C. Hemoglobin: 12g/dL
   D. Erythrocyte sedimentation rate: 30 mm/hr
   E. Total cholesterol: 180 mg

56. The stain used to identify bacteria on a prepared slide is the
    A. Gram stain
    B. Wright's stain
    C. Giemsa stain
    D. India ink
    E. All of the above

57. After sitting for a long time, a urine sample becomes
    A. Clear
    B. Alkaline
    C. Acid
    D. Neutral
    E. Darker

58. A blood sample for serum is collected in which of the following tubes?
    A. Blue-stoppered
    B. Lavender-stoppered
    C. Green-stoppered
    D. Red-stoppered (tiger)
    E. Black-stoppered

59. Which of the following are categories to classify instruments used in surgery?
    A. Probing and dilating
    B. Cutting and dissecting
    C. Grasping and clamping
    D. Retracting
    E. All of the above

60. The first thing that should be done in an emergent situation involving an unconscious person is to
    A. Assess the victim's airway
    B. Control any bleeding
    C. Apply a tourniquet
    D. Dial 911
    E. Give the patient breaths

61. A physical examination of a urine sample includes
    A. Odor
    B. Color
    C. Transparency
    D. Specific gravity
    E. All of the above

62. Most drugs are metabolized in the
    A. Lungs
    B. Blood
    C. Stomach
    D. Liver
    E. Intestines

63. The Ishihara test
    A. Tests for visual acuity
    B. Tests for glaucoma
    C. Tests for color-blindness
    D. Tests for presbyopia
    E. Tests for nerve deafness

64. Which is *not* a common symptom of a myocardial infarction?
    A. Nausea
    B. Angina
    C. Dyspnea
    D. Diaphoresis
    E. Polyuria

65. Hemostats are a type of
    A. Forceps
    B. Probe
    C. Applicator
    D. Scissors
    E. Retractors

66. The normal ratio for respiration to pulse is
    A. 1 to 6
    B. 1 to 2
    C. 1 to 4
    D. 2 to 4
    E. 4 to 1

67. Symptoms of insulin shock include
    A. Restless and confusion
    B. Cold, clammy skin
    C. Profuse sweating
    D. Rapid, weak pulse
    E. All of the above

68. Which is the most important route for eliminating drugs from the body?
    A. Kidneys
    B. Skin
    C. Mammary glands
    D. Lungs
    E. Digestive system

69. Prozac is an example of an
    A. Antihistamine
    B. Antidiuretic
    C. Antidepressant
    D. Antifungal
    E. Antibiotic

70. The two most important factors in performing effective hand washing are
    A. Temperature of water and soap
    B. Friction and running water
    C. Position of hands and hot water
    D. Length of time and soap
    E. Friction and soap

71. At which age is the first mumps, measles, and rubella (MMR) vaccination recommended?
    A. Birth
    B. 2 months
    C. 4 months
    D. 12 months
    E. 5 years

72. If a patient describes an aura before the onset of a severe headache, this is often a sign of
    A. Cerebrovascular accident
    B. Migraine
    C. Hay fever
    D. Brain tumor
    E. Seizure

73. A function of hemoglobin is
    A. To repair cells
    B. To destroy cells
    C. To prevent blood loss
    D. To carry oxygen and carbon dioxide
    E. To fight off infection

74. A quality assurance program in the laboratory
    A. Ensures the accuracy of results
    B. Requires less paperwork
    C. Eliminates outside laboratory tests
    D. Increases convenience
    E. Provides quick results

75. The reaction of the purified protein derivative (PPD) test is read
    A. 12 to 24 hours after it has been placed
    B. 48 to 72 hours after it has been placed
    C. Immediately after it has been placed
    D. 24 to 36 hours after it has been placed
    E. 4 to 8 hours after it has been placed

76. The abbreviation for *both ears* is
    A. AS
    B. AD
    C. AU
    D. BE
    E. AS/AD

77. The blood type known as the *universal donor* is
    A. A
    B. B
    C. AB
    D. O
    E. All of the above

78. A lower gastrointestinal (GI) series is performed to outline the
    A. Esophagus
    B. Stomach
    C. Ileum
    D. Duodenum
    E. Colon

79. A technique that provides soft-tissue images in three dimensions is
    A. Ultrasound
    B. Computed tomography (CT) scan
    C. Myelography
    D. Tomography
    E. Intravenous pyelogram (IVP)

80. Massive and prolonged exposure to radiation can result in
    A. Cancer
    B. Increased number of white blood cells
    C. Increased number of red blood cells
    D. Arthritis
    E. Death

81. Which is the first group of leads to be recorded on an electrocardiogram?
    A. Augmented leads
    B. Leads I, II, and III
    C. aVR, aVL, and aVF
    D. Leads V_1 through V_3
    E. Leads V_1 through V_6

82. Streptococci are arranged in
    A. Clusters
    B. Chains
    C. Circles
    D. Pairs
    E. Fours

83. Pulse rate may be increased in all of the following *except*
    A. Fear
    B. Anger
    C. Anxiety
    D. Increasing age
    E. Exercise

84. The electrode that is used for grounding in an electrocardiogram is placed on the
    A. LA
    B. RA
    C. LL
    D. RL
    E. C

85. Which federal agency oversees the safety of health facilities?
    A. OSHA
    B. CLIA '88
    C. CDC
    D. DEA
    E. COLA

86. A drug reference contains all of the following information *except*
    A. Description
    B. Indications
    C. Contraindications
    D. Dose
    E. Cost

87. Ibuprofen has analgesic and antipyretic properties and is used to treat
    A. Pain
    B. Arthritis
    C. Headache
    D. Dysmenorrhea
    E. All of the above

88. Which of the following patient instructions is critical for a successful Holter monitor recording interpretation?
    A. Avoid stress
    B. Refrain from exercise
    C. Keep a written record of all daily activities
    D. Wear the monitor for 5 days
    E. Do not take any medications

89. The involuntary muscular action that moves food along the gastrointestinal tract is called
    A. Digestion
    B. Indigestion
    C. Mastication
    D. Peristalsis
    E. Deglutition

90. The first dose of diphtheria tetanus acellular pertussis (DTaP) vaccine should be administered at
    A. 2 months
    B. 4 months
    C. 12 months
    D. 5 years
    E. 12 years

91. Tissue samples removed during a biopsy would be sent to which department of the laboratory?
    A. Serology
    B. Cytology
    C. Histology
    D. Chemistry
    E. Microbiology

92. Which of the following would be *least* likely to contaminate the sterile field?
    A. Talking over the field
    B. Hair not pulled back
    C. A nonsterile person entering the room
    D. A sterile instrument touching the edge of the field
    E. Moisture on the sterile field

93. An antihistamine that may be used to treat an allergic reaction is
    A. Bactrim
    B. Motrin
    C. Benadryl
    D. Inderal
    E. Indocin

94. Each of the following abbreviations is correctly defined *except*
    A. bid (twice a day)
    B. tid (three times a day)
    C. OD (right eye)
    D. qod (every day)
    E. ac (before meals)

95. Surgical asepsis should be maintained when performing which of the following?
    A. Dipstick urinalysis
    B. Pelvic examination
    C. Snellen test
    D. Needle biopsy
    E. Blood pressure

96. How often should quality control tests be performed in the laboratory?
    A. Daily
    B. Weekly
    C. Monthly
    D. When necessary
    E. Before each test

97. An infectious inflammatory skin disease caused by staphylococci and characterized by vesicles that later crust is called
    A. Vitiligo
    B. Impetigo
    C. Tinea
    D. Cellulitis
    E. Acne

98. A decrease in bone density may indicate
    A. Osteolysis
    B. Osteoclasis
    C. Osteoporosis
    D. Crepitus
    E. Osteomyelitis

99. A disorder of accommodation usually associated with aging is known as
    A. Myopia
    B. Hyperopia
    C. Astigmatism
    D. Presbyopia
    E. Macular degeneration

100. An infection of the middle ear may be charted as
    A. Otitis media
    B. Tinnitus
    C. Conjunctivitis
    D. Mastoiditis
    E. Tympanitis

1 *Medical Terminology*

- Language of medicine
- Mostly Latin and Greek origins
- Made up of word parts:
  1. Root word
     - Core of the word
     - Tells the fundamental meaning of the word
     - More than one root word may exist in a medical term
  2. Suffix
     - Word part attached to the end of a root word
     - Changes or modifies its meaning
     - Can be:
       - Symptomatic: describes evidence of illness
       - Diagnostic: names a medical condition
       - Operative: describes a surgical treatment
       - General: general applications
  3. Prefix
     - Word part attached to the beginning of a root word
     - Changes or modifies its meaning
  4. Combining vowel or form
     - Used between two root words or between a root word and a suffix to make pronunciation easier
     - Not used between a prefix and the root word
     - Usually an *o*
     - Combining form is a root word with the combining vowel attached

To analyze a medical term:
- Divide the word into word parts
- Divide the word by slashes, and label each word part

Example: leukocytosis
leuk/o/cyt/osis
rw/cv/rw/s

rw = root word
cv = combining vowel
s = suffix
p = prefix

To define a medical term:
- Give each word part a meaning
- Begin by defining the suffix, then the prefix, then the root word

To build a medical term, use the same procedure as previously described

A. General Body Combining Forms

1.	anter/o	before, front
2.	bi/o	life
3.	blast/o	immature form; developing cell
4.	carcin/o	cancer
5.	cancer/o	
6.	caud/o	lower part of the body, tail
7.	cyt/o	cell
8.	dist/o	far
9.	dors/o	back of the body
10.	electr/o	electricity, electric
11.	epitheli/o	epithelium
12.	eti/o	cause
13.	gno/o	knowledge
14.	hist/o	tissue
15.	hom/o	same, like, alike
16.	home/o	sameness, unchanging, constant
17.	iatr/o	physician; medicine
18.	kary/o	nucleus
19.	lei/o	smooth
20.	lip/o	fat
21.	medi/o	middle
22.	my/o	muscle
23.	neur/o	nerve
24.	onc/o	tumor
25.	organ/o	organ
26.	path/o	disease
27.	poster/o	toward the back, behind
28.	proxim/o	near
29.	rhabd/o	rod-shaped
30.	sarc/o	flesh; connective tissue
31.	somat/o	body
32.	super/o	above, excessive, higher than
33.	system/o	system
34.	tax/o	coordination, order
35.	ventr/o	in front, belly side of the body
36.	viscer/o	internal organs; viscera

B. Integumentary System Combining Forms

1. aden/o — gland
2. aut/o — self
3. bi/o — life
4. coni/o — dust
5. crypt/o — hidden
6. cutane/o — skin
   derm/o
   dermat/o
7. fibr/o — fibrous tissue; fiber
8. heter/o — other
9. hidr/o — sweat
10. kerat/o — hard; horny tissue
11. myc/o — fungus
12. necr/o — death
13. onych/o — nail
    ungu/o
14. pachy/o — thick
15. rhytid/o — wrinkle
16. seb/o — sebum (oil)
17. staphyl/o — grapelike clusters
18. strept/o — chainlike
19. trich/o — hair
20. xer/o — dry

C. Musculoskeletal System Combining Forms

1. ankyl/o — stiff
2. aponeur/o — aponeurosis
3. arthr/o — joint
   articul/o
4. burs/o — bursa
5. calcane/o — heel bone, calcaneous
6. calc/i — calcium
7. carp/o — carpals
8. cervic/o — neck
9. chondr/o — cartilage
10. clavic/o — clavicle
    clavicul/o
11. cost/o — rib
12. crani/o — skull
13. disk/o — intervertebral disk
14. femor/o — femur
15. fibul/o — fibula
16. humer/o — humerus
17. ili/o — ilium
18. ischi/o — ischium
19. kinesi/o — movement
20. kyph/o — hump
21. lamin/o — thin, flat layer
22. lord/o — bent forward; abnormal convexity of the spine
23. mandibul/o — mandible
24. maxill/o — maxilla
25. menisc/o — meniscus
26. myel/o — bone marrow; spinal cord
    myelon/o
27. my/o — muscle
    myos/o
28. oste/o — bone
29. patell/o — patella
30. pelv/i, pelv/o — pelvic bone, hip
31. phalang/o — phalanges
32. pub/o — pubis
33. radi/o — radius
34. sacr/o — sacrum
35. scapul/o — scapula

36. scoli/o — bent; curved
37. spin/o — spine, backbone
38. stern/o — sternum
39. synovi/o — synovial fluid; synovial membrane
40. tars/o — tarsals
41. ten/o — tendon
    tend/o
    tendin/o
42. tibi/o — tibia
43. uln/o — ulna
44. vertebr/o — vertebrae; vertebral column
    rachi/o
    spondyl/o

D. Nervous System Combining Forms

1. cerebell/o — cerebellum
2. cerebr/o — cerebrum
3. dur/o — dura mater
4. encephal/o — brain
5. esthesi/o — feeling; sensation; sensitivity
6. gangli/o — ganglion
   ganglion/o
7. gli/o — glue, supportive tissue of the nervous system
8. meningi/o — meninges
   mening/o
9. mon/o — one; single
10. myel/o — spinal cord
11. neur/o — nerve
12. osm/o — sense of smell
13. phas/o — speech
14. poli/o — gray; gray matter
15. psych/o — mind
    ment/o
    phren/o
16. quadr/i — four
17. somn/o — sleep

E. Cardiovascular and Lymphatic Systems Combining Forms

1. angi/o — vessel
2. aort/o — aorta
3. arteri/o — artery
4. ather/o — fatty deposit
5. bacteri/o — bacteria
6. cardi/o — heart
7. ech/o — sound
8. electr/o — electrical activity; electricity
9. hem/o — blood
   hemat/o
10. isch/o — blockage; deficiency
11. lymph/o — lymph
12. phleb/o — vein
    ven/o
13. plasm/o — plasma
14. sphygm/o — pulse
15. splen/o — spleen
16. therm/o — heat
17. thromb/o — clot
18. thym/o — thymus gland
19. valv/o — valve
    valvul/o
20. ventricul/o — ventricle

F. Respiratory System Combining Forms

1. adenoid/o   adenoid
2. alveol/o   alveolus
3. atel/o   incomplete; imperfect
4. bronchi/o   bronchus
   bronch/o
5. bronchiol/o   bronchiole
6. capn/o   carbon dioxide
7. diaphragmat/o   diaphragm
8. epiglott/o   epiglottis
9. laryng/o   larynx
10. lob/o   lobe
11. muc/o   mucus
12. nas/o   nose
    rhin/o
13. orth/o   straight
14. ox/o   oxygen
    ox/i
15. pharyng/o   pharynx
16. pleur/o   pleura
17. pneum/o   lung; air
    pneumat/o
    pneumon/o
18. pulmon/o   lung
19. py/o   pus
20. sinus/o   sinus
    sin/o
21. sept/o   septum; wall off
22. spir/o   breathe; breathing
23. thorac/o   thorax; chest
24. tonsill/o   tonsil
25. trache/o   trachea

G. Digestive System Combining Forms

1. an/o   anus
2. appendic/o   appendix
   append/o
3. cec/o   cecum
4. duoden/o   duodenum
5. chol/e   bile; gall
6. cholecyst/o   gallbladder
7. cholangi/o   bile duct
8. choledoch/o   common bile duct
9. col/o   colon, large intestine
   colon/o
10. dent/i   tooth
11. diverticul/o   diverticulum; blind pouch
                    extending from an organ
12. duoden/o   duodenum
13. enter/o   small intestines
14. esophag/o   esophagus
15. gastr/o   stomach
16. gingiv/o   gum
17. gloss/o   tongue
    lingu/o
18. hepat/o   liver
19. herni/o   hernia
20. ile/o   ileum
21. jejun/o   jejunum
22. lapar/o   abdomen
    abdomin/o
    celi/o
23. palat/o   palate
24. pancreat/o   pancreas
25. peritone/o   peritoneum
26. proct/o   rectum
    rect/o

27. polyp/o   polyp; small growth on a stalk
28. pylor/o   pylorus; pyloric sphincter
29. sial/o   saliva
30. sigmoid/o   sigmoid colon
31. stomat/o   mouth
    or/o
32. uvul/o   uvula

H. Urinary System Combining Forms

1. albumin/o   albumin
2. azot/o   urea; nitrogen
3. cyst/o   bladder; sac
   vesic/o
4. glomerul/o   glomerulus
5. glyc/o   sugar
   glycos/o
   gluc/o
6. hydr/o   water
7. lith/o   stone; calculus
8. meat/o   meatus; opening
9. nephr/o   kidney
   ren/o
10. noct/i   night
11. olig/o   scanty; few
12. pyel/o   renal pelvis
13. son/o   sound
14. ureter/o   ureter
15. urethr/o   urethra
16. urin/o   urine; urinary tract
    ur/o

I. Endocrine System Combining Forms

1. acr/o   extremities
2. adeno/o   gland
3. adren/o   adrenal glands
   adrenal/o
4. calc/i   calcium
5. cortic/o   cortex
6. crin/o   secrete
7. dips/o   thirst
8. endocrin/o   endocrine
9. hormon/o   hormone
10. kal/i   potassium
11. natr/o   sodium
12. parathyroid/o   parathyroid glands
13. thyroid/o   thyroid gland
    thyr/o
14. toxic/o   poison

J. Male Reproductive System Combining Forms

1. andr/o   male; man
2. balan/o   glans penis
3. epididym/o   epididymis
4. orchid/o   testicle; testes
   orchi/o
   orch/o
5. pen/i   penis
   phall/o
6. prostat/o   prostate gland
7. scrot/o   scrotum
8. semin/i   semen, seed, sperm
9. sperm/o   sperm
   spermat/o
10. test/o   testicle; testes
11. vas/o   vessel; duct
12. vesicul/o   seminal vesicles

K. Female Reproductive System Combining Forms

1. arche/o — beginning; first
2. cervic/o — cervix
3. colp/o — vagina
   vagin/o
4. gynec/o — female; woman
   gyn/o
5. hymen/o — hymen
6. hyster/o — uterus
   metr/o
   metri/o
   uter/o
7. lact/o — milk
8. mamm/o — breast
   mast/o
9. men/o — menstruation
10. oophor/o — ovary
11. ov/o — egg; ovum
    ov/i
12. perine/o — perineum
13. salping/o — fallopian tubes
14. vulv/o — vulva
    episi/o

L. Combining Forms Indicating Colors

1. albin/o — white
   leuk/o
2. chlor/o — green
3. cyan/o — blue
4. erythr/o — red
5. melan/o — black
6. xanth/o — yellow

M. Suffixes Used to Indicate Pathological Conditions

1. -algia — pain
   -dynia
2. -cele — hernia
3. -chalasis — relaxation; thickening
4. -cytosis — abnormal increase in cells
5. -ectasis — dilation; swelling
6. -edema — swelling
7. -emesis — vomiting
8. -emia — blood condition
9. -ia — state of; condition
10. -iasis — abnormal condition
11. -ism — condition
12. -itis — inflammation
13. -lapse — to fall; to sag
14. -lepsy — seizure
15. -lith — stone; calculus
16. -lysis — destruction; separation; breakdown
17. -lytic — to destroy; to reduce
18. -malacia — softening
19. -megaly — enlargement
20. -oma — tumor; mass
21. -osis — abnormal increase; abnormal condition
22. -pathy — disease process
23. -penia — decrease; deficiency
24. -phobia — irrational fear
25. -plegia — paralysis
26. -ptosis — drooping; sagging prolapse
27. -ptysis — spitting
28. -rrhage — bursting forth
    -rrhagia

29. -rrhea — flow; discharge
30. -rrhexis — rupture
31. -sclerosis — hardening
32. -spasm — involuntary contraction
33. -stenosis — narrowing
34. -y — process; state; condition

N. Suffixes Used to Indicate Diagnostic and Surgical Procedures

1. -centesis — surgical puncture to remove fluid
2. -clasis — to break
3. -desis — surgical binding; surgical fusion
4. -ectasia — dilation
   -ectasis
5. -ectomy — excision; surgical removal
6. -gram — record; writing
7. -graph — instrument used to record
8. -graphy — process of recording; producing images
9. -meter — instrument used to measure
10. -metry — to measure; measurement
11. -opsy — to view
12. -pexy — surgical fixation
13. -plasty — surgical repair; surgical reconstruction
14. -rrhaphy — suture; sew
15. -scope — instrument used to visually examine
16. -scopy — process of visually examining
17. -stasis — stoppage; stopping; controlling
18. -stomy — new opening
19. -tension — pressure
20. -therapy — treatment
21. -tome — instrument used to cut
22. -tomy — process of cutting; incision into
23. -tripsy — surgical crushing

O. General Suffixes

1. -ase — enzyme
2. -blast — immature form
3. -chezia — defecation
4. -clast — breaking down
5. -cyte — cell
6. -dipsia — thirst
7. -er — specialist; one who
   -or — specializes
   -ician
   -logist
   -ist
8. -gravida — pregnant
9. -ion — process
10. -ium — membrane; structure; tissue
11. -logy — study of
12. -opia — vision
13. -ose — sugar
14. -para — labor; delivery
15. -pepsia — digestion
16. -phagia — to eat; swallow
17. -phasia — speech
18. -plasia — formation; development
19. -pnea — breathing
20. -poiesis — production; formation
21. -ptysis — spitting
22. -tocia — labor and delivery
23. -sis — state of
24. -tion — process of
25. -trophy — development; growth
26. -uria — urine

P. Suffixes Used to Create Adjective Forms

1. -ac   pertaining to
   -al
   -ar
   -ary
   -eal
   -ic
   -ine
   -ior
   -ose
   -ous
   -tic
   -itic
   -an
   -iac
2. -genous   produced by; producing
   -genic
3. -oid   like; resembling
4. -ole   small
   -ule

Q. Prefixes Used to Indicate Direction and Position

1. ab-   away from
2. ad-   toward
3. ante-   before
4. circum- around
5. dia-   complete; through
6. ecto-   outside
7. endo-   within
8. e-   out; outward; outside
   ex-
   exo-
   extra-
9. epi-   upon; on; above
10. eso-   inward; within
11. hyper-   above; excessive
12. hypo-   below; under; deficient
13. in-   in; into; not
14. infra-   below; beneath
15. inter-   between
16. intra-   within
17. ipsi-   same
18. meso-   middle
19. meta-   beyond; change
20. para-   beside; near
21. per-   through
22. peri-   around
23. post-   after
24. pre-   before; in front of
25. pro-   before
26. retro-   back; behind
27. sub-   under; below
28. supra- above
29. trans- across

R. Prefixes Referring to Number or Measurement

1. amphi- both
2. bi-   two
   di-
3. hemi-   half
   semi-
4. mono- one
   uni-
5. multi- many
   poly-
6. nulli-   none
7. primi- first

8. quadri- four
   tetra-
9. tri-   three

S. Miscellaneous Prefixes

1. a-   no; not; lack of; without
   an-
2. acu-   sharp
3. ana-   apart
4. anti-   against
5. apo-   separate; away
6. auto- self
7. brachy- short
8. brady- slow
9. contra- against
10. de-   lack of; removal
11. dis-   apart from
12. dys-   bad; abnormal; difficult; painful
13. echo- sound
14. eu-   good; well; normal; easy
15. in-   not
    ir-
    im-
16. macro- large
17. mal-   bad
18. micro- small
19. neo-   new
20. non-   without
21. pan-   all
22. syn-   together; joined; with
    sym-
23. tachy- fast; rapid
24. ultra- beyond; excessive

T. Plurals

To form a plural, change the:

a as in burs**a**	→	**ae** as in burs**ae**
ax as in thor**ax**	→	**aces** as in thor**aces**
en as in foram**en**	→	**ina** as in foram**ina**
is as in cris**is**	→	**es** as in cris**es**
is as in ir**is**	→	**ides** as in ir**ides**
is as in femor**is**	→	**a** as in femor**a**
ix as in append**ix**	→	**ices** as in append**ices**
nx as in phala**nx**	→	**ges** an in phalan**ges**
on as in spermatozo**on**	→	**a** as in spermatozo**a**
um as in ov**um**	→	**a** as in ov**a**
us as in nucle**us**	→	**i** as in nucle**i**
y as in arter**y**	→	**ies** as in arter**ies**

ABBREVIATIONS

Follow the institution's policies for use of abbreviations. Some institutions do not use abbreviations because of the increased chance of errors. Abbreviations can be written with or without periods.

A. Charting Terms

abd	abdomen
ADL	activities of daily living
approx	approximately
ASAP	as soon as possible
ax	axillary
BE	barium enema
BM	bowel movement

BP, B/P	blood pressure
BSE	breast self-examination
bx	biopsy
CABG	coronary artery bypass graft
CAM	complementary and alternative medicine
cath	catheterization; catheter
CC	chief complaint
chemo	chemotherapy
c/o	complains of
CSF	cerebrospinal fluid
CMA (AAMA)	Certified Medical Assistant (AAMA)
CPAP	continuous positive airway pressure
C-section	cesarean section
cx	cervix
D&C	dilatation (dilation) and curettage
disc, d/c, dc	discontinue
DOB	date of birth
Dr.	doctor
drsg, dsg	dressing
dx	diagnosis
ECP	emergency contraceptive pill
EDC, EDD	estimated date of confinement (due date); estimated date of delivery
EEG	electroencephalogram
EKG, ECG	electrocardiogram
ENT	ear, nose, and throat
ERT	estrogen replacement therapy
ETOH	ethyl alcohol
ER, ED	emergency room, emergency department
FB	foreign body
FH	family history
FHR	fetal heart rate
FU	follow up
fx	fracture
GI	gastrointestinal
GIFT	gamete intrafallopian transfer
GP	general practitioner
grav, gravida	pregnancy
GU	genitourinary
GYN	gynecology
H&P	history and physical
HEENT	head, eye, ear, nose, throat
hr	hour
HRT	hormone replacement therapy
hs	hour of sleep; bedtime
ht	height
hx	history
I&D	incision and drainage
IUD	intrauterine device
Ⓛ	left
LLQ	left lower quadrant
LMP	last menstrual period
LPN	Licensed Practical Nurse
IVF	in vitro fertilization
LUQ	left upper quadrant
MA	Medical Assistant
LVN	Licensed Vocational Nurse
med(s)	medication(s)
mets	metastasis
MRI	magnetic resonance imaging
N&V	nausea and vomiting
NKA	no known allergies
NKDA	no known drug allergies
NP	Nurse Practitioner

NPO	nothing by mouth
NVD	nausea, vomiting, diarrhea
OB	obstetrics
OC	oral contraceptives
OR	operating room
os	opening
P	pulse
PA	Physician Assistant
OCP	oral contraceptive pill
para	live birth
PE, px	physical examination
Peds	pediatrics
PERLA	pupils equally reactive to light and accommodation
PERRLA	pupils equal, round, react to light and accommodation
PH	past history
pt	patient
OB	obstetrics
R	respiration
Ⓡ	right
RLQ	right lower quadrant
RN	Registered Nurse
r/o	rule out
ROM	range of motion
RUQ	right upper quadrant
SOAP	subjective, objective, assessment, plan
stat	immediately
sx	symptoms
T	temperature
T&A	tonsilloadenoidectomy (tonsils and adenoids)
TLC	tender loving care
TSE	testicular-self examination
RMA	Registered Medical Assistant
tx	treatment, therapy
UCHD	usual childhood diseases
vo	verbal order
VS	vital signs
WDWN	well-developed, well-nourished
WNL	within normal limits
wt	weight

B. Diagnostic Terms

AIDS	acquired immune deficiency syndrome
ADD	attention deficit disorder
ADHD	attention deficit hyperactivity disorder
ALL	acute lymphoblastic leukemia
AMI	acute myocardial infarction
AML	acute myelogenous leukemia
ASHD	arteriosclerotic heart disease
BPH	benign prostatic hyperplasia/hypertrophy
CA, Ca	Cancer
CAD	coronary artery disease
CHF	congestive heart failure
COPD	chronic obstructive pulmonary disease
CTS	carpal tunnel syndrome
CVA	cerebral vascular accident
DJD	degenerative joint disease
DLE	discoid lupus erythematosus
DT	delirium tremens
DVT	deep vein thrombosis
FTT	failure to thrive
GAD	generalized anxiety disorder
Gc	gonococcus
GERD	gastroesophageal reflux disease
HAV	hepatitis A virus

HBV	hepatitis B virus
HCV	hepatitis C virus
HIV	human immunodeficiency virus
HPV	human papillomavirus
HSV-1	herpes simplex virus 1
HSV-2	herpes simplex virus 2; herpes genitalis
IBS	irritable bowel syndrome
IDDM	insulin-dependent diabetes mellitus
MI	myocardial infarction
MS	multiple sclerosis
NIDDM	non–insulin-dependent diabetes mellitus
OA	osteoarthritis
OCD	obsessive-compulsive disorder
OM	otitis media
PID	pelvic inflammatory disease
POCS	polycystic ovary syndrome
PMDD	premenstrual dysphoric disorder
PMS	premenstrual syndrome
PTSD	posttraumatic stress disorder
RA	rheumatoid arthritis
RAD	reactive airway disease
RDS	respiratory distress syndrome
RSV	respiratory syncytial virus
SAD	seasonal affective disorder
SARS	severe acute respiratory syndrome
SIDS	sudden infant death syndrome
SLE	systemic lupus erythematosus
SOB	shortness of breath
STD	sexually transmitted disease
STI	sexually transmitted infection
TMJ	temporomandibular joint
TB	tuberculosis
URI	upper respiratory infection
UTI	urinary tract infection

C. Medication Orders And Administration Terms

aa	of each
$\bar{a}$	before
ac	before meals
AD	right ear
ad lib	as desired
AM, am	morning
amp	ampule
amt	amount
aq	water
AS	left ear
ASA	aspirin
ASAP	as soon as possible
AU	both ears
bid	twice daily, two times a day
$\bar{c}$	with
cap	capsule
d	day
elix	elixir
et	and
h, hr	hour
hs, HS	bedtime; hour of sleep
ID	intradermal
IM	intramuscular
inj	by injection
IV	intravenous
noct	night
NSAIDS	nonsteroidal anti-inflammatory drug
OTC	over the counter (drug)

OD	right eye
os	mouth
OS	left eye
OU	both eyes
$\bar{p}$	after
pc	after meals
per	by means of
po	by mouth
PM, pm	afternoon
prn	as needed
$\bar{q}$	every
qd	every day
qh	every hour
qid	four times daily, four times a day
qod	every other day
qoh	every other hour
Rx	take, prescription
$\bar{s}$	without
SC, subq, subcu	subcutaneous
SL	sublingual
$\overline{\overline{ss}}$	half
supp	suppository
tab	tablet
tid	three times daily, three times a day
vag	vaginal

D. Laboratory and Diagnostic Testing Terms

ABO	main blood grouping system
AP	anterior/posterior (x-ray)
BaS	barium swallow
BUN	blood urea nitrogen
CBC	complete blood count
C&S	culture and sensitivity
CT	computed tomography (scan)
CVS	chorionic villus sampling
CXR	chest x-ray
DEXA	dual energy x-ray absorptiometry
diff	differential white blood cell count
ECT	electroconvulsive therapy
ELISA	enzyme-linked immunosorbent assay (used in AIDS diagnosis)
ESR	erythrocyte sedimentation rate; sed rate
ESWL	extracorporeal shock wave lithotripsy
FBS	fasting blood sugar
FOBT	fecal occult blood test
GTT	glucose tolerance test
H&H	hemoglobin and hematocrit
hct	hematocrit
hgb	hemoglobin
HbA1c	glycosylated hemoglobin (A1c)
hCG	human chorionic gonadotropin
HDL	high-density lipoprotein
INR	international normalized ratio
IVP	intravenous pyelogram
KUB	kidney, ureter, bladder
Lap	laparoscopy
LASIK	laser-assisted in-situ keratomileusis
LP	lumbar puncture
lat	lateral (x-ray)
LDL	low-density lipoprotein
O&P	ova and parasites
obl	oblique (x-ray)
Pap	Pap smear
PET	positron emission tomography (scan)

pH	degree of acidity or alkalinity
PKU	phenylketonuria
PSA	prostate-specific antigen
PT	prothrombin time; pro-time
PTT	partial thromboplastin time
qns	quantity not sufficient
RBC	red blood cell
T_3	triiodothyronine
T_4	thyroxine
TENS	transcutaneous electrical nerve stimulation
TURP	transurethral resection of the prostate
RPR	rapid plasma regain test (for syphilis)
UA	urinalysis
US	ultrasound
VBAC	vaginal birth after cesarean section
VDRL	Venereal Disease Research Laboratory (test for syphilis)
WBC	white blood cell

E. Measures

C	centigrade
cc	cubic centimeter
cm	centimeter
dr	dram
F	Fahrenheit
g, gm	gram
gr	grain
gt(t)	drop(s)
kg	kilogram
L	liter
lb, #	pound
mcg, μg	microgram
mg	milligram
mL	milliliter
mn	minum
oz	ounce
pt	pint
qt	quart
tbsp, T	tablespoon
tsp, t	teaspoon
U	unit

F. Compounds and Chemicals

Ba	barium
Ca	calcium
Cl	chloride
CO_2	carbon dioxide
Fe	iron
H	hydrogen
H_2O	water
Hg	mercury
K	potassium
KOH	potassium hydrochloride
Na	sodium
NaCl	sodium chloride
O_2	oxygen

G. Symbols

♂	male
♀	female
>	greater than
<	less than
↑	increase, above
↓	decrease, below
×	times (multiply by)
%	percent
=	equal
+	plus
−	minus
:	ratio
::	proportion
⊕	positive
⊖	negative
	standing
	Sitting
	lying down
Δ	change

2 Anatomy and Physiology

I. INTRODUCTION TO THE BODY

A. General
1. Anatomy: the study of body structures
2. Physiology: the study of body functions

B. Levels of Organization
1. Arranged from smallest to largest
2. Chemical: includes atoms and molecules
3. Cell: basic unit of all life
4. Tissue: group of cells with similar structure and function
5. Organ: group of tissues that work together to perform a function
6. System: group of organs working together to accomplish a set of functions
7. Organism: made up of systems that work together to maintain life

C. Organ Systems
1. Each system has a specific function yet all systems work together
2. Integumentary system
   a. Made up of skin and accessory organs
   b. Provides protection, temperature regulation, chemical synthesis, water balance, and sensory reception
3. Skeletal system
   a. Made up of bones, joints, tendons, and ligaments
   b. Provides protection, provides a framework for the body, assists with movement, stores minerals, hemopoiesis
4. Muscular system
   a. Made up of muscles
   b. Provides movement, body heat, and storage of energy
5. Nervous system
   a. Made up of brain, spinal cord, and nerves
   b. Coordinates all body activities and detects changes in the outside environment
6. Endocrine system
   a. Made up of glands that secrete chemical messengers (hormones)
   b. Coordinates and balances body activities and regulates reproductive systems
7. Cardiovascular system
   a. Made up of heart and blood vessels
   b. Transports substances to the tissues and removes waste products from tissues
8. Lymphatic system
   a. Made up of lymph, lymph vessels, lymph nodes, and lymphoid organs
   b. Removes excess fluid and helps protect the body against disease
9. Digestive system
   a. Made up of mouth, esophagus, stomach, intestines, rectum, liver, gallbladder, and pancreas
   b. Takes in food and processes it into molecules that can be used by the body; eliminates solid waste products
10. Urinary system
    a. Made up of kidneys, ureters, bladder, and urethra
    b. Removes liquid nitrogenous waste products and helps regulate water balance
11. Respiratory system
    a. Made up of nose, pharynx, larynx, trachea, bronchi, and lungs
    b. Brings oxygen (O_2) into the lungs and removes carbon dioxide (CO_2) from the body
12. Reproductive system
    a. Made up of gonads (ovaries and testes), duct systems, accessory glands, and support structures
    b. Produces new individuals

D. Life Processes
1. Characteristics that distinguish a living organism from a nonliving organism
2. Organization: each part has a function and cooperates with all other parts
3. Metabolism: all chemical reactions in the body
4. Responsiveness: ability to detect changes in the internal and external environment and respond to them

5. Movement: all activities accomplished by the muscular system
6. Reproduction: formation of new cells; formation of a new individual
7. Growth: increase in size by an increase in the number of cells
8. Respiration: exchange of O_2 and CO_2
9. Digestion: ability to break down complex foodstuffs into simpler molecules that the body can use
10. Excretion: process of removing waste products from the body
11. Maintaining boundaries: keeping the inside environment separate from the outside

E. Survival Needs
1. Requirements of an organism to sustain life
2. Physical factors that come from the environment
3. Water
   a. Probably more necessary than food
   b. Provides a medium for all chemical reactions
   c. Provides a fluid base for body secretions and excretions
   d. Makes up approximately 60% of body weight
4. Oxygen: necessary for metabolic reactions
5. Nutrients
   a. Taken in from diet
   b. Provide raw materials necessary for growth, replacement, and repair
   c. Provide energy for body processes
6. Temperature
   a. Necessary for chemical reactions to occur
   b. Optimum is 98.6 °F
7. Pressure
   a. Application of a force
   b. Necessary for breathing and blood pressure

F. Homeostasis
1. Body's ability to maintain a constant internal environment, regardless of the external environment
2. When the body is healthy, the internal environment remains stable within limited normal ranges
3. Lack of homeostasis can lead to disease and eventually death

G. Anatomical Terms
1. Universal language
2. Used to describe directions and regions of the body
3. Anatomical position
   a. Beginning position for point of reference
   b. Body is standing erect, face forward, arms at sides with palms facing forward, and toes pointing forward

4. Directions in the body (see Figure 2-1)
   a. Superior: part above another part; toward the head
   b. Inferior: part below another part; toward the feet
   c. Anterior (ventral): toward the front
   d. Posterior (dorsal): toward the back
   e. Medial: toward or near the midline of the body
   f. Lateral: toward or near the side of the body; away from the midline
   g. Proximal: closer to the point of attachment
   h. Distal: farther away from the point of attachment
   i. Superficial: on or near the surface
   j. Deep: away from the surface
5. Planes and sections of the body (see Figure 2-1)
   a. Used to visualize spatial relationships of body parts
   b. Sagittal plane: divides the body into left and right parts
   c. Midsagittal plane: divides the body into equal right and left halves
   d. Transverse plane: divides the body into upper and lower parts; cross-section
   e. Frontal (coronal) plane: divides the body into front and back parts
6. Body cavities (see Figure 2-2): hollow body spaces that contain internal organs
   a. Dorsal cavity: made up of two cavities along the back of the body:
      1) Cranial cavity: contains the brain
      2) Spinal cavity: contains the spinal cord
   b. Ventral cavity: made up of two cavities along the front of the body:
      1) Thoracic cavity: contains heart, lungs, esophagus, and trachea
      2) Abdominopelvic cavity: contains organs below the diaphragm
   c. Diaphragm: separates the thoracic and abdominopelvic cavities
7. Abdominal regions (see Figure 2-3): two methods used to describe locations of body organs or pain
   a. Quadrants: divides abdomen into four regions
      1) Right upper quadrant (RUQ)
      2) Left upper quadrant (LUQ)
      3) Right lower quadrant (RLQ)
      4) Left lower quadrant (LLQ)
   b. Nine regions: more specific
      1) Epigastric
      2) Umbilical
      3) Hypogastric
      4) Right hypochondriac
      5) Left hypochondriac
      6) Right lumbar
      7) Left lumbar
      8) Right iliac
      9) Left iliac

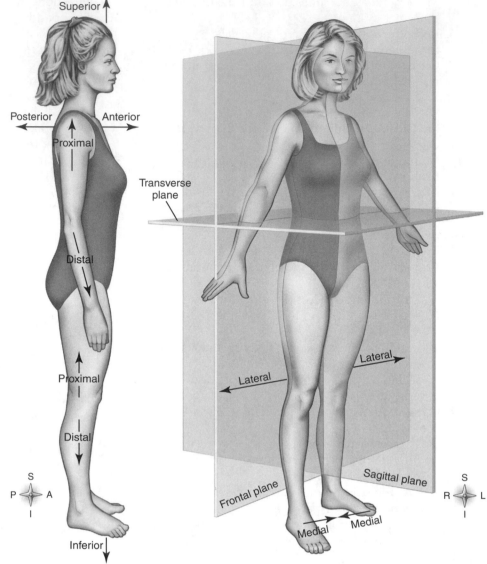

FIGURE 2-1 Directions and planes of the body. (Drawing by Barbara Cousins, from Thibodeau GA, Patton KT: *The human body in health and disease*, ed 5, St Louis, 2009, Mosby.)

8. Body areas
  a. Abdominal: portion of trunk below diaphragm; between thorax and pelvis
  b. Antebrachial: forearm; region between elbow and wrist
  c. Antecubital: space in front of elbow
  d. Axillary: armpit area
  e. Brachial: arm; region between elbow and shoulder
  f. Buccal: cheek area
  g. Carpal: wrist area
  h. Celiac: abdomen
  i. Cephalic: head
  j. Cervical: neck area; cervix
  k. Costal: ribs
  l. Cranial: skull
  m. Cutaneous: skin
  n. Femoral: thigh area; region between the hip and knee
  o. Frontal: forehead
  p. Gluteal: buttock area
  q. Inguinal: groin
  r. Lumbar: lower back area between ribs and pelvis
  s. Mammary: breast
  t. Occipital: lower portion of back of head
  u. Ophthalmic: eyes
  v. Oral: mouth
  w. Otic: ears
  x. Palmar: palm of the hand
  y. Pectoral: chest area
  z. Pedal: foot
  aa. Pelvic: inferior region of abdominal cavity
  bb. Perineal: region between the anus and pubic symphysis; includes region of external reproductive organs
  cc. Plantar: sole of the foot
  dd. Popliteal: area behind the knee
  ee. Sacral: posterior region between hipbones
  ff. Sternal: anterior midline of thorax
  gg. Tarsal: ankle area
  hh. Thoracic: chest
  ii. Umbilical: navel
  jj. Vertebral: backbone

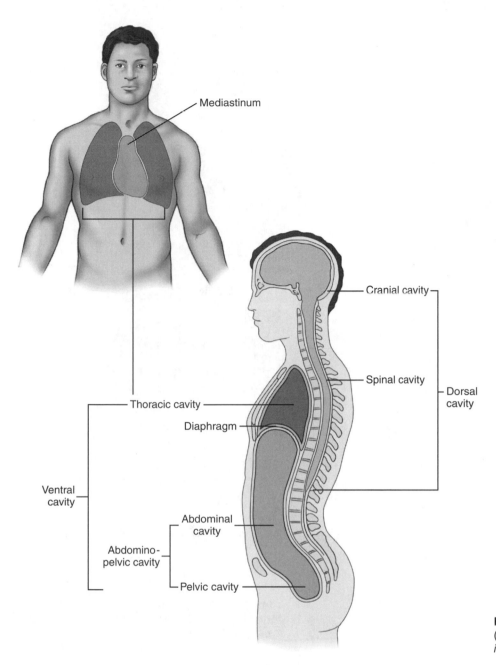

FIGURE 2-2 Major body cavities. (Herlihy B: *The human body in health and illness*, ed 3, St Louis, 2007, Saunders.)

II. CELL

A. General

1. Basic structural and functional unit of the body
2. Vary in size, shape, and function
3. Very well organized in structure

B. Structure (see Figure 2-4)

1. Cell membrane
   a. Thin, flexible, outermost barrier of the cell
   b. Made up of a double layer of phospholipids
   c. Allows water and chemicals to pass in and out
   d. Permeable and selective
2. Cytoplasm
   a. Cytosol
   b. Thick, semisolid substance that contains mostly water
   c. Site of cellular activity
   d. Holds organelles in place
3. Nuclear membrane: encloses the nucleus
4. Nucleus
   a. Controls center of the cell
   b. Contains genetic material (deoxyribonucleic acid [DNA])
5. Nucleolus
   a. Small, dense structure located in the nucleus
   b. Important in the synthesis of ribosomes

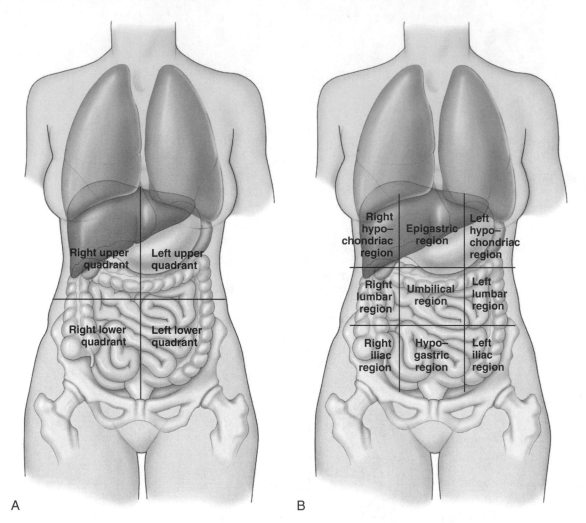

FIGURE 2-3   Areas of the abdomen. **A,** Four quadrants. **B,** Nine regions. (Herlihy B: *The human body in health and illness*, ed 3, St Louis, 2007, Saunders.)

6. Centrioles
   a. Hollow, rod-shaped structures found in the cytoplasm near the nucleus
   b. Play an important role in cell division
7. Endoplasmic reticulum
   a. Complex network of tubular channels
   b. "Transportation system" of the cell
   c. Allows molecules to move from one part of the cell to the other
   d. Two types
      1) Rough: ribosomes attached; transports proteins
      2) Smooth: without ribosomes; manufactures lipids and hormones
8. Golgi apparatus
   a. Stack of flattened sacs
   b. Located near the nucleus
   c. Processes and packages proteins
9. Lysosomes
   a. Sacs of various sizes and shapes
   b. Contain strong chemicals that digest various substances that enter the cytoplasm

10. Mitochondria
   a. Sausage-shaped sacs
   b. Inner layer arranged in folds
   c. "Powerhouse" of the cell
   d. Source of energy for cells and tissues
11. Microtubules
   a. Extremely small, hollow tubes
   b. Crisscross cytoplasm to form a "skeleton"
   c. Give cells strength and shape
12. Peroxisomes
   a. Membranous sacs that resemble lysosomes
   b. Contain enzymes that detoxify harmful substances
13. Ribosomes
   a. Composed of ribonucleic acid (RNA) and protein
   b. Form amino acids into new protein molecules
   c. Some are free floating in the cytoplasm; some are attached to endoplasmic reticulum

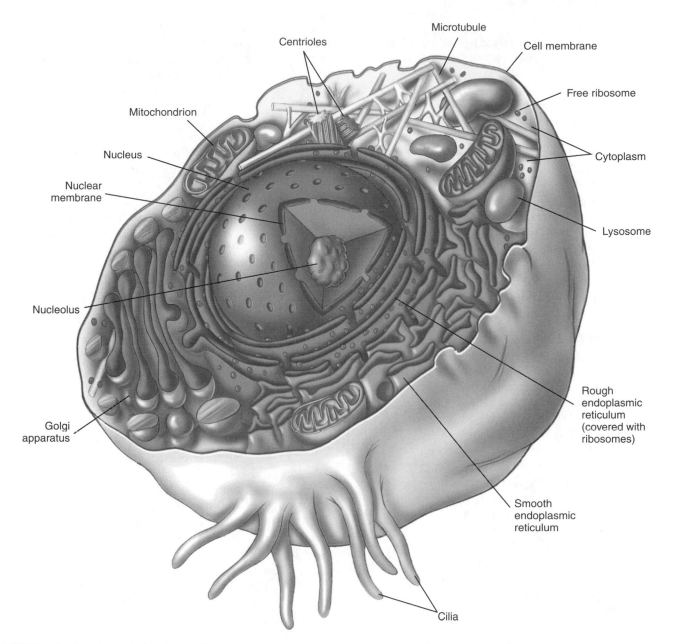

FIGURE 2-4 A typical cell. (Herlihy B: *The human body in health and illness*, ed 3, St Louis, 2007, Saunders.)

14. Vacuoles
   a. Membrane-bound sacs that appear in the cytoplasm when the cell membrane folds inward on itself
   b. Contain fluid or solid substances
   c. Lysosomes can empty their enzymes into the sac
   d. Aid in metabolic activity of the cell
15. Microvilli
   a. Tiny fingerlike extensions that project from the surface of certain cells
   b. Increase absorptive surface of cell
16. Cilia
   a. Hairlike projections on the surface of the cell
   b. Move substances along the cell surface

17. Flagella
   a. Hairlike projection from surface of the cell
   b. Provides movement

C. **Types of Movement Across the Cell Membrane**
   1. Ability of the cell to carry out its function depends on movement or exchange of fluids, particles, and molecules
   2. Movement controlled and facilitated by cell membrane
      a. Diffusion
         1) Movement of solids from an area of higher concentration to an area of lower concentration
         2) Does not require cellular energy

b. Filtration
   1) Movement of a fluid by hydrostatic pressure
   2) Does not require cellular energy
c. Osmosis
   1) Movement of water from an area of higher concentration to an area of lower concentration
   2) Does not require cellular energy
d. Phagocytosis
   1) "Cell eating"; cell engulfs particles
   2) Requires cellular energy
e. Pinocytosis
   1) "Cell drinking"; cell engulfs fluid
   2) Requires cellular energy
f. Active transport
   1) Movement of substances from an area of lower concentration to an area of higher concentration
   2) Requires cellular energy

D. Cell Division
  1. Mitosis
  2. Results in two identical daughter cells
  3. Consists of two separate operations:
     a. Division of the nucleus (karyokinesis)
     b. Division of cytoplasm (cytokinesis)
  4. Entire process has several phases:
     a. Interphase: chromosomes double
     b. Prophase: centrioles move to opposite ends of the cell, trailing a thin, threadlike substance that forms a structure resembling a spindle
     c. Metaphase: chromosomes line up across the spindles and begin to move toward the opposite ends of the cell
     d. Telophase: nuclear area becomes pinched in the middle until two regions have formed; similar change happens in the cell membrane; the cell eventually splits in two
  5. Meiosis: division of gametes producing half the number of chromosomes (23) as in mitosis when fertilization occurs; nuclei of sperm and egg come together to produce a zygote with full number of chromosomes (46)

III. TISSUES AND MEMBRANES

A. General
  1. Group of cells similar in structure and function
  2. Organized into four general types

B. Types of Tissues
  1. Connective tissue
     a. Variety of forms throughout the body
     b. Serves as a framework for other tissues
     c. Combines to form more complex tissues (organs)
     d. Provides support and protection
     e. Serves as storage sites
     f. Fills in spaces between body structures

g. Types include:
   1) Loose (areolar)
      a) Attaches skin to underlying tissues
      b) Surrounds blood and lymph vessels
      c) Fills spaces around muscles and other organs
   2) Dense
      a) Provides great strength
      b) Makes up tendons and ligaments
   3) Elastic: capable of stretching
   4) Adipose
      a) Stores fat
      b) Serves to insulate body and as an energy reserve
   5) Reticular: associated with the formation of blood
   6) Cartilage
      a) Rigid connective tissue
      b) Forms sliding surface for joints
      c) Contains no blood vessels
      d) Three types:
         (1) Hyaline cartilage
         (2) Elastic cartilage
         (3) Fibrocartilage
   7) Bone (osseous)
      a) Compact and rigid
      b) Calcium deposits in fibers give it hardness and strength
  2. Epithelial tissue
     a. Epithelium
     b. Provides covering and lining for surfaces
     c. Classified according to number of cells, arrangement of cells, location of tissue, and shape of cells at the surface of the tissue
  3. Muscle tissue
     a. Makes up muscles
     b. Has ability to contract (shorten)
     c. Basis of and provides for movement
     d. Three kinds:
        1) Skeletal muscle tissue
           a) Attaches to bone and produces movement
           b) Voluntary (under conscious control)
        2) Smooth muscle
           a) Found in internal organs
           b) Involuntary (not under conscious control)
        3) Cardiac muscle tissue
           a) Found in the heart
           b) Complex network of cells
           c) Involuntary
  4. Nervous tissue
     a. Composed of cells that can respond to surroundings
     b. Cells called neurons: supported and nourished by neuroglial cells
     c. Regulates all activities and functions of the body

C. Membranes (see Figure 2-5)

1. Thin sheet of tissue
2. Can cover a surface, serve as a partition, line organs and cavities, or anchor an organ
   a. Serous membrane
      1) Serosa
      2) Lines walls of body cavities that do not open to the outside
      3) Has two layers:
         a) Parietal layer: layer attached to the wall of the cavity or sac
         b) Visceral layer: layer attached to the internal organ
      4) Three main serous membranes
         a) Pleura: lines thoracic cavity and covers the lungs
         b) Pericardium: sac that encloses the heart
         c) Peritoneum: largest serous membrane; lines the wall of the abdominal cavity and covers the abdominal organs
   b. Mucous membrane
      1) Mucosa
      2) Lines the walls of body cavities that open to the outside
      3) Produces a thick, sticky substance (mucus)
   c. Cutaneous membrane: the skin
   d. Synovial membrane
      1) Lines joint cavities
      2) Secretes a lubricating fluid that reduces friction

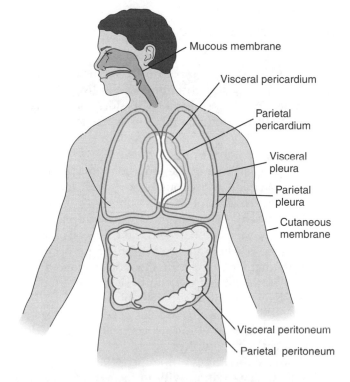

FIGURE 2-5 Epithelial membranes: cutaneous membrane (skin), mucous membranes, and serous membranes (pleura, pericardium, and peritoneum). (Herlihy B: *The human body in health and illness*, ed 3, St Louis, 2007, Saunders.)

IV. INTEGUMENTARY SYSTEM

A. General

1. Considered to be the largest system and organ of the body
2. Made up of skin and its appendages (hair, glands, nails)
3. Forms outer boundary of the body

B. Functions

1. Protection from radiation, water loss, drying, and invasion of microorganisms
2. Control of body temperature
3. Detection of sensation
4. Secretion of waste products
5. Production of vitamin D

C. Structure (see Figure 2-6)

1. Two main layers:
   a. Epidermis
      1) Outer layer
      2) Made up of four to five sublayers (strata)
      3) Innermost layer continuously supplies cells that move up to the next strata
      4) Cells continue to pick up keratin as they pass through the strata
      5) Outermost layer contains lifeless, keratin-filled cells that continually slough off
      6) Contains melanocytes that produce pigment (melanin), which gives skin color
      7) Contains no blood supply
   b. Dermis
      1) Corium; "true skin"
      2) Innermost layer
      3) Contains nerve and blood supply
      4) Also contains appendages of the skin
      5) Provides strength to the skin
      6) Stores water and electrolytes
2. Appendages: special structures that perform a variety of functions
   a. Sudoriferous glands
      1) Sweat glands
      2) Coiled, tubelike structures in the dermis
      3) Produce and transport sweat to the skin surface
      4) Sweat then evaporates and cools the body
   b. Ceruminous glands
      1) Modified sweat glands found in the ear
      2) Secrete cerumen (earwax)
   c. Sebaceous glands
      1) Oil glands
      2) Connected to hair follicle
      3) Secrete sebum that oils the hair and lubricates the skin
   d. Hair
      1) Covers most of the body
      2) Made up of dead, keratinized tissue
      3) Connected to small muscles (erector pili)

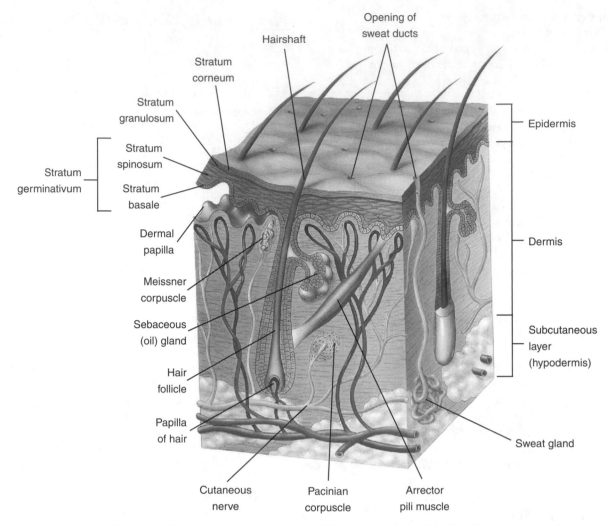

FIGURE 2-6 Normal skin. (Herlihy B: *The human body in health and illness*, ed 3, St Louis, 2007, Saunders.)

e. Nails
1) Hard, keratinized structures found on the fingertips and tips of toes
2) Protective function
3. Subcutaneous tissue
a. Layer of tissue below the dermis
b. Connects dermis to the surface of muscles
c. Made up of adipose tissue, elastic fibers, and fibers
d. Injection site

V. SKELETAL SYSTEM

A. General (see Figure 2-7)
1. Composed of bones, cartilage, and ligaments
2. Adult skeleton composed of 206 bones

B. Functions
1. Provides a framework for the body: shape and support for other structures
2. Provides for movement: places for muscles to attach
3. Provides protection: surrounds body cavities
4. Provides hematopoiesis: blood cell formation in marrow

5. Provides storage: inorganic minerals (calcium [Ca], phosphorus [P], magnesium [Mg], potassium [K], sodium [Na]) stored in matrix and released into circulation as needed

C. Anatomy of Long Bone
1. Diaphysis: shaft of the long bone; made up of compact and cancellous bone
2. Epiphysis: ends of the long bone
3. Epiphyseal cartilage (plate): "growth plate"; layer of cartilage between the diaphysis and epiphysis where the growth in length occurs
4. Articular cartilage: thin sheet of cartilage that covers the end of the epiphysis; provides a cushion and lubrication for joint
5. Periosteum: tough, vascular covering of the bone; made up of fibrous connective tissue; does not cover the epiphysis
6. Endosteum: lining of the medullary cavity
7. Medullary cavity: cavity in the center of long bones; contains marrow
a. Red marrow: produces red blood cells
b. Yellow marrow: made up of fat

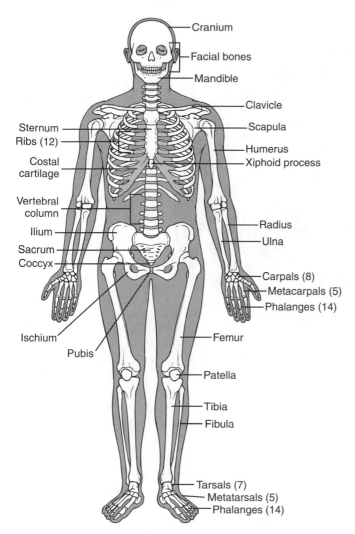

Cranium
Facial bones
Mandible
Clavicle
Sternum
Scapula
Ribs (12)
Humerus
Costal cartilage
Xiphoid process
Vertebral column
Ilium
Radius
Sacrum
Ulna
Coccyx
Carpals (8)
Metacarpals (5)
Phalanges (14)
Ischium
Femur
Pubis
Patella
Tibia
Fibula
Tarsals (7)
Metatarsals (5)
Phalanges (14)

FIGURE 2-7 Normal skeletal system (anterior view). (Frazier MS, Drzymkowski JW: *Essentials of human diseases and conditions*, ed 3, Philadelphia, 2004, Saunders.)

8. Process: bony projection on the surface of a bone
9. Foramen: an opening in a bone
10. Sinus: bony cavity in a bone

D. Bone Classifications
1. Long: length exceeds width
2. Short: smaller than long bone with expanded ends
3. Flat: thin, sheetlike
4. Sesamoid: rounded bones embedded in tendons; round bones
5. Irregular: various shapes

E. Organization of the Skeleton
1. Axial skeleton: consists of bones of the skull, spine, and chest (see Figure 2-8)
   a. Cranium: bones enclose the brain
      1) Frontal: forms forehead
      2) Parietal: forms sides and top
      3) Temporal: forms lower sides and floor; contains ossicles (bones of middle ear):

malleus, incus, and stapes; external auditory meatus (opening into middle ear)
      4) Mastoid process: projection located on temporal bone
      5) Styloid process: sharp projection inferior to external auditory meatus
      6) Zygomatic process: projects anteriorly to form prominence of cheek
      7) Occipital: single bone forming the posterior of cranium; contains foramen magnum where spinal cord exits skull
      8) Sphenoid: butterfly-shaped bone that bridges the temporal regions to form the floor of the cranium; contains sella turcica where the pituitary gland sits
      9) Ethmoid: single bone that forms most of bony area between the nasal cavity and orbits
   b. Facial: forms the basic framework for the face
      1) Nasal: two bones forming the bridge of the nose
      2) Vomer: thin bone that forms the inferior nasal septum
      3) Lacrimal: located in the medial walls of the orbits; contains the lacrimal glands
      4) Zygomatic: forms the arch of the cheekbone
      5) Palatine: forms the posterior of the hard palate
      6) Mandible: lower jawbone (only movable bone in the face)
      7) Hyoid: U-shaped bone that supports the tongue; only bone that does not articulate with another
   c. Spinal column: composed of 26 vertebrae separated by pads of cartilage (intervertebral disks); houses the spinal cord; four distinct curves; common structural pattern (see Figure 2-9)
      1) Cervical vertebrae: first seven, C-1 through C-7; forms the neck
         a) C-1: atlas; supports the skull
         b) C-2: axis; allows for rotation of skull
      2) Thoracic vertebrae: next 12, T-1 through T-12; articulate with the ribs
      3) Lumbar vertebrae: next five, L-1 through L-5; forms the small of the back
      4) Sacrum: triangular-shaped bone; forms the posterior wall of the pelvic cavity
      5) Coccyx: tailbone
   d. Thorax: thoracic cage; protects heart, lungs, and great vessels (see Figure 2-10)
      1) Sternum: breastbone; three parts:
         a) Manubrium: superior, triangular part
         b) Body: middle, slender part
         c) Xiphoid process: projection at end of body; landmark for cardiopulmonary resuscitation (CPR)

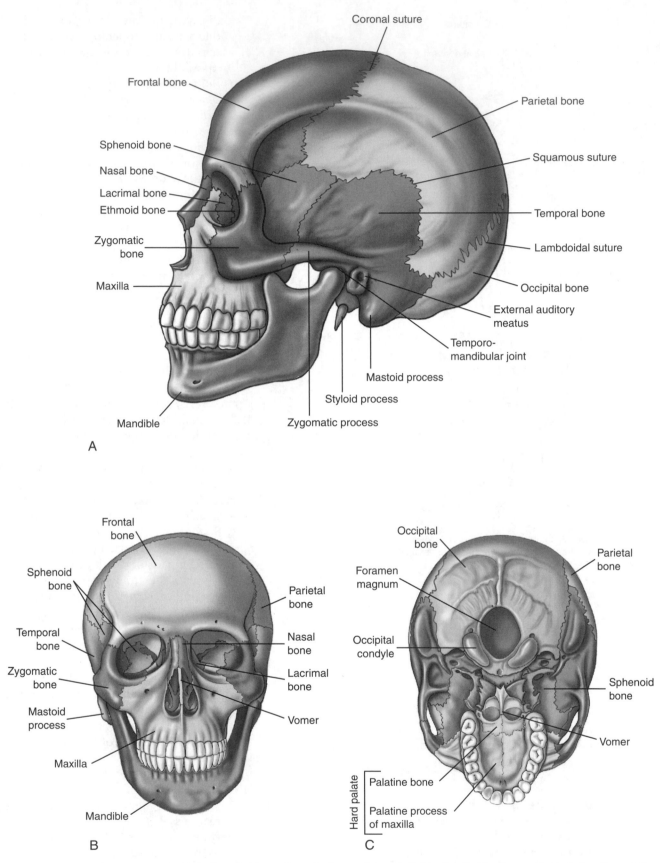

FIGURE 2-8 Bones of the skull. **A,** Side view. **B,** Front view. **C,** Base of the skull. (Herlihy B: *The human body in health and illness*, ed 3, St Louis, 2007, Saunders.)

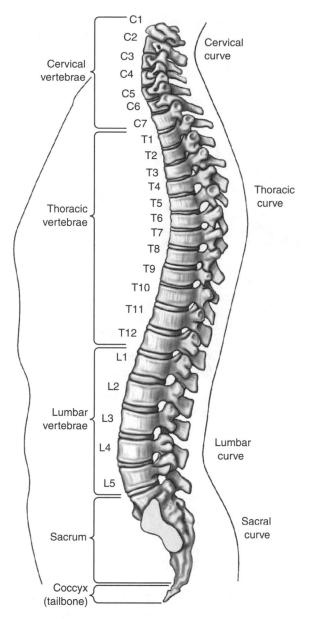

C1
C2
C3
C4
C5
C6
C7

Cervical
vertebrae

Cervical
curve

T1
T2
T3
T4
T5
T6
T7
T8
T9
T10
T11
T12

Thoracic
vertebrae

Thoracic
curve

L1
L2
L3
L4
L5

Lumbar
vertebrae

Lumbar
curve

Sacrum

Sacral
curve

Coccyx
(tailbone)

FIGURE 2-9 The vertebral column. (Herlihy B: *The human body in health and illness*, ed 3, St Louis, 2007, Saunders.)

2) Ribs
   a) Curved, flat bones that form the lateral sides of thorax
   b) 12 pairs
     (1) True ribs; first seven pairs; articulate with the sternum by means of costal cartilage
     (2) False ribs: next three pairs; articulate with the seventh rib by means of costal cartilage
     (3) Floating ribs: last two pairs; do not articulate with the sternum

2. Appendicular skeleton: made up of bones of upper and lower extremities and girdles that are anchored to the axial skeleton (see Figure 2-11)

a. Shoulder girdle
   1) Clavicle: collarbone (two); forms a bridge between shoulder blades and breastbone
   2) Scapula (two): shoulder blade
   3) Humerus: bone of the upper arm
   4) Radius: lateral bone of the forearm (thumb side)
   5) Ulna: medial bone of the forearm (little finger side)
   6) Carpals: two rows of four bones tightly bound by ligaments; make up the wrist
   7) Metacarpals: five bones that make up the hand
   8) Phalanges
     a) Three bones in each finger (proximal, medial, and distal)
     b) Two bones in each thumb (proximal and distal)
b. Pelvic girdle: attaches lower extremities to axial skeleton (see Figure 2-12)
   1) Pelvis: os coxae: basin-shaped bones on floor of trunk; three parts:
     a) Ilium: superior, wing-shaped bones of hips
     b) Ischium: inferior portion; *"sit-down"* bone
     c) Pubis: anterior portion; right and left sides join at symphysis pubis (pad of cartilage)
   2) Femur: thighbone; largest, longest, and strongest bone in the body
   3) Patella: kneecap; triangular-shaped, enclosed in tendon
   4) Tibia: shinbone
     a) Lateral malleolus: bulge on outside of ankle
     b) Medial malleolus: bulge on inside of ankle
   5) Fibula: smaller leg bone lateral to the tibia
   6) Tarsals: seven bones that make up the ankle; largest is the calcaneus (heel bone)
   7) Metatarsals: five bones that make up the instep of the foot
   8) Phalanges: 14 bones that make up the toe
     a) Three in each toe (proximal, medial, and distal)
     b) Two in each great toe (proximal and distal)
c. Articulations: joints; where two bones come together; classified by the amount of movement allowed (see Figure 2-13)
   1) Synarthroses: immovable joints (example: sutures in skull)
   2) Amphiarthroses: slightly movable joints; bones are connected by cartilage (example: symphysis pubis)

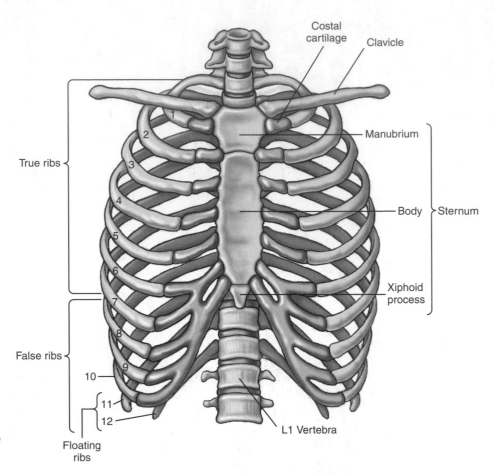

FIGURE 2-10 The thoracic cage. (Herlihy B: *The human body in health and illness*, ed 3, St Louis, 2007, Saunders.)

3) Diarthroses: freely movable joints; ends covered with cartilage; separated by a space containing synovial fluid for lubrication (example: elbow)

VI. MUSCULAR SYSTEM

A. General
1. Approximately 650 muscles in the body
2. Makes up approximately 40% of body weight

B. Functions
1. Movement: contractions (shortening) allows movement of bone
2. Protection: sheets of muscle protect internal organs
3. Posture: provides position and alignment of body parts
4. Heat production: movement produces heat
5. Shape: muscles plus bones give the body shape

C. Types of Muscle Tissue (see Figure 2-14)
1. Skeletal: under conscious control (voluntary); appears striated (striped); provides movement of body
2. Smooth: involuntary muscles (operate automatically); appears nonstriated; helps with metabolic functions
3. Cardiac: found only in the heart; involuntary; causes contraction of heart muscle to maintain blood flow

D. Characteristics of Muscle
1. Excitability: ability to receive and respond to a stimulus
2. Contractility: ability to shorten (contract)
3. Extensibility: ability to stretch
4. Elasticity: ability to return to original shape and length

E. Skeletal Muscle Structure
1. Composed of bundles of fibers held together by fibrous connective tissue
   a. Fiber: skeletal muscle cell
   b. Endomysium: connective tissue membrane that covers a muscle fiber
   c. Fasciculus: bundle of muscle fibers
   d. Perimysium: connective tissue membrane that surrounds the fasciculus
   e. Epimysium: tough tissue membrane that covers the entire muscle
   f. Fascia: connective tissue outside of the epimysium; surrounds and separates the muscles
   g. Tendon: strong, cordlike structure that attaches muscles to bones
   h. Aponeurosis: sheetlike tendon that attaches muscle to muscle

F. Naming of Muscles
1. May be named according to the following:
   a. Size: maximus, medius, longus

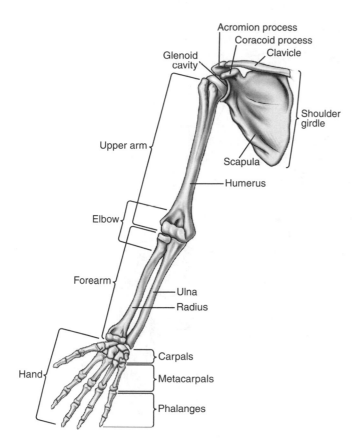

FIGURE 2-11 Bones of the upper limb. (Herlihy B: *The human body in health and illness*, ed 3, St Louis, 2007, Saunders.)

   b. Shape: deltoid, latus
   c. Fiber direction: rectus, oblique
   d. Points of attachment:
      1) Origin: point of attachment that does not move on contraction
      2) Insertion: point of attachment that moves on contraction
   e. Number of attachments: biceps, quadriceps
   f. Action of muscle: adductor, flexor, and levator

G. Muscle Actions
   1. Prime mover: provides movement
   2. Antagonist: opposes prime mover; can cause opposite movement or provide more control and precision to prime mover
   3. Synergist: helps prime mover work more efficiently and effectively
   4. Fixator: stabilizes the origin of the prime mover

H. Movement
   1. Caused by contraction (shortening) of muscle
   2. Complex series of events based on chemical reactions at cellular level
   3. Begins with stimulation by nerve cell and ends when the muscle is relaxed
   4. Requires adenosine triphosphate (ATP) for energy source

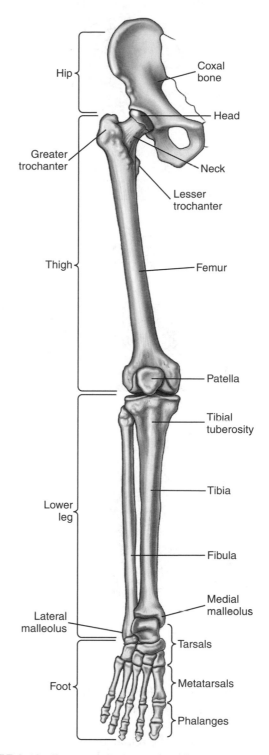

FIGURE 2-12 Bones of the lower limb. (Herlihy B: *The human body in health and illness*, ed 3, St Louis, 2007, Saunders.)

I. Types of Movements (see Figure 2-15)
   1. Flexion: to bend; brings two bones closer together and decreases the angle between them
   2. Extension: to straighten; opposite of flexion; increases the angle between bones
   3. Hyperextension: extension beyond the anatomical position; joint angle in excess of 180 degrees
   4. Abduction: to take away; movement of a bone or limb away from the midline of the body

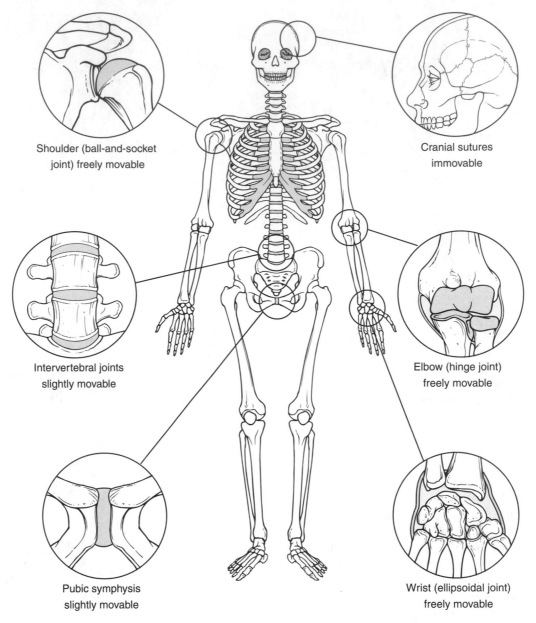

FIGURE 2-13   Examples of types of joints. (Frazier MS, Drzymkowski JW: *Essentials of human diseases and conditions*, ed 3, Philadelphia, 2004, Saunders.)

5. Adduction: to bring together; opposite of abduction; movement of a bone or limb toward the midline of the body
6. Circumduction: circular motion of a body part or segment; the proximal end is stationary, whereas the distal end outlines a large circle
7. Rotation: movement of a bone around its own axis
8. Inversion: turning a body part inward
9. Eversion: opposite of inversion; turning a body part outward
10. Supination: movement of a body part to face upward
11. Pronation: opposite of supination; movement of a body part to face downward

J. **Major Skeletal Muscles (see Figures 2-16 and 2-17)**
  1. Muscles of facial expression
     a. Frontalis: over the frontal bone; raises eyebrows and wrinkles forehead
     b. Orbicularis oris: circular muscle that surrounds mouth; closes mouth, forms words, puckers lips
     c. Orbicularis oculi: circular muscle that surrounds the eye; helps in winking, blinking, and squinting
     d. Buccinator: principal muscle of the cheek; helps in whistling, sucking, and blowing out air
     e. Zygomaticus: extends from the zygomatic arch to corner of mouth; raises the corners of the mouth when smiling

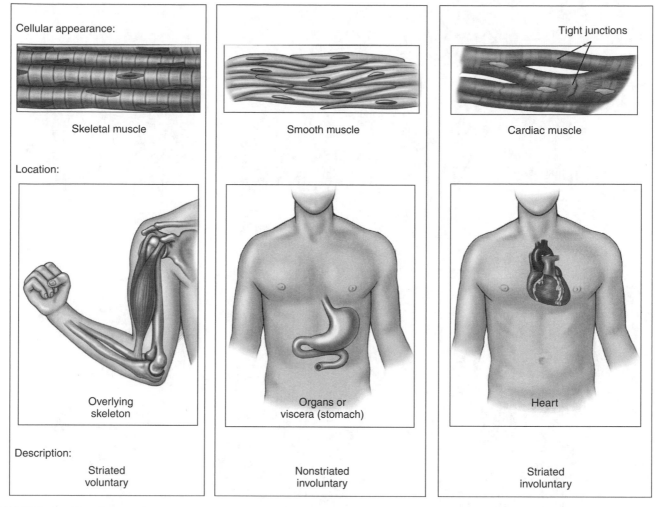

Cellular appearance:

Skeletal muscle   Smooth muscle   Cardiac muscle

Tight junctions

Location:

Overlying skeleton   Organs or viscera (stomach)   Heart

Description:

Striated voluntary   Nonstriated involuntary   Striated involuntary

FIGURE 2-14 Three types of muscle: skeletal, smooth, and cardiac. (Herlihy B: *The human body in health and illness*, ed 3, St Louis, 2007, Saunders.)

2. Muscles of mastication (chewing)
   a. Temporalis: largest; inserts in mandible; responsible for chewing
   b. Masseter: inserts in mandible; used for chewing
3. Neck muscles
   a. Sternocleidomastoid: runs across front of neck from the sternum to clavicle to mastoid process; flexes neck
   b. Trapezius: extends from occipital bone to end of thoracic vertebrae; extends head
4. Vertebral column muscles
   a. Erector spinae: group of muscles on each side of vertebral column from sacrum to skull; keeps vertebral column erect
   b. Quadratus lumborum (deep back muscles): short muscles between vertebrae; responsible for movement of vertebral column
5. Thoracic wall muscles
   a. Intercostal muscles (internal and external): located between ribs; helps with breathing
   b. Diaphragm: dome-shaped muscle located between thorax and abdomen; muscle of respiration

6. Abdominal wall muscles
   a. External oblique: fibers run medially and inferiorally
   b. Internal oblique: fibers run opposite of external obliques
   c. Transversus abdominis: fibers run horizontally
   d. Rectus abdominis: fibers run vertically
7. Muscles that move the shoulder and arm
   a. Trapezius: large, triangular muscle of the back; used to shrug shoulders
   b. Serratus anterior: located on side of chest; used in pushing
   c. Pectoralis major: superficial muscle on anterior chest; adductor; moves arm medially across chest
   d. Latissimus dorsi: large superficial muscle of lower back
   e. Deltoid: large triangular muscle that covers the shoulder; used to abduct arm; injection site
   f. Rotator cuff muscles: infraspinatus, supraspinatus, subscapularis, teres minor; assists with movement of the humerus; form cuff over proximal humerus

FIGURE 2-15 Types of movements at joints. (Herlihy B: *The human body in health and illness*, ed 3, St Louis, 2007, Saunders.)

Temporalis
Orbicularis oculi
Zygomaticus
Buccinator
Orbicularis oris
Deltoid
Biceps brachii
Brachialis
Rectus abdominis
Internal oblique
External oblique
Transversus abdominis
Brachioradialis
Iliopsoas
Adductor longus
Adductor magnus
Rectus femoris
Quadriceps femoris
Vastus lateralis
Vastus medialis
Tibialis anterior
Peroneus longus

Frontalis
Masseter
Sternocleidomastoid
Pectoralis major
Serratus anterior
Linea alba
Sartorius

Anterior view

FIGURE 2-16   Major muscles of the body, anterior view. (Herlihy B: *The human body in health and illness*, ed 3, St Louis, 2007, Saunders.)

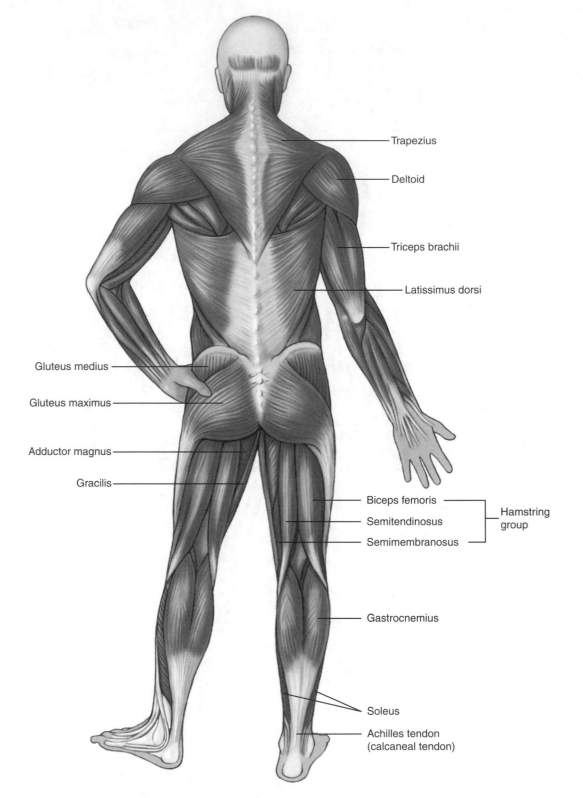

Posterior view

FIGURE 2-17 Major muscles of the body (*posterior view*). (Herlihy B, Maebius N: *The human body in health and illness*, ed 2, Philadelphia, 2003, Saunders.)

8. Muscles that move the forearm and hand
   a. Triceps brachii: posterior of arm; extends the forearm
   b. Biceps brachii: flexes the forearm
   c. Brachialis: flexes the forearm
   d. Brachioradialis: lateral side of forearm; flexes the forearm
9. Muscles that move the thigh
   a. Gluteus maximus: forms the buttocks; extends and straightens the thigh at the hip
   b. Gluteus medius: deep to the gluteus maximus; common injection site; abducts the thigh
   c. Gluteus minimus: deepest of gluteal group; abducts the thigh
   d. Iliopsoas: anterior muscle; flexes the thigh
   e. Adductor longus: medial muscle; adducts the thigh
   f. Adductor brevis: medial muscle; adducts the thigh
   g. Adductor magnus: medial muscle; adducts the thigh
   h. Gracilis: medial muscle; adducts the thigh
10. Muscles that move the leg
    a. Quadriceps femoris: group of muscles located on anterior and lateral sides of thigh; extend the leg and straighten the leg at the knee
       1) Vastus lateralis: injection site for infants and children; extends leg and supports knee joint
       2) Vastus intermedius: extends leg
       3) Vastus medialis: extends leg
       4) Rectus femoris: extends leg
    b. Sartorius: longest muscle in the body; runs obliquely over the quad group; flexes and medially rotates the legs (to sit cross-legged)
    c. Hamstrings: posterior to the thigh; flexes the leg at the knee; strong tendons; includes:
       1) Biceps femoris
       2) Semitendinosus
       3) Semimembranosus
11. Muscles that move the ankle and foot
    a. Tibialis anterior: primary muscle of anterior group; dorsiflexion of foot
    b. Peroneus longus: lateral to the leg; everts the foot
    c. Gastrocnemius: posterior to leg (calf); plantar flexion (*"toe-dancer's"* muscles)
    d. Soleus: posterior to the leg (calf)
    e. Achilles tendon: common tendon for gastrocnemius and soleus; connects muscles to calcaneus; largest tendon in body

VII. NERVOUS SYSTEM

A. **General**
   1. Major controlling, regulating, and communicating system of the body
   2. Works with the endocrine system to regulate and maintain homeostasis

B. **Functions**
   1. Control: regulates internal body functions and processes
   2. Communication: directs processes among body systems
   3. Mental processes: generates thoughts, feelings, perception, sensations, and emotions

C. **Organization (see Figure 2-18)**
   1. Central nervous system (CNS): made up of brain and spinal cord

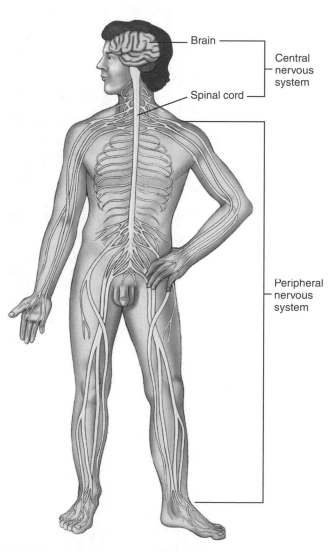

FIGURE 2-18 Divisions of the nervous system: central and peripheral. (Herlihy B: *The human body in health and illness*, ed 3, St Louis, 2007, Saunders.)

2. Peripheral nervous system (PNS): made up of nerves and ganglia; includes
   a. Twelve pairs of cranial nerves originating in the brain
   b. Thirty-one pairs of spinal nerves originating from spinal cord
   c. Afferent (sensory) division: transmits information to brain
   d. Efferent (motor) division: transmits information from brain to organs and body parts
   e. Somatic nervous system: transmits impulses to voluntary muscles
   f. Autonomic nervous system: transmits impulses to involuntary muscles and glands
   g. Sympathetic nervous system: prepares the body for stressful conditions
   h. Parasympathetic nervous system: coordinates the normal resting activities

D. **Organs of the Nervous System (see Figure 2-19)**
   1. Neuron: nerve cell; structural and functional unit of nerve tissue; highly specialized; if destroyed, cannot be replaced (does not go through mitosis)
      a. Cell body: contains nucleus and organelles
      b. Dendrites: one or more branching extensions; receives signals from other neurons and brings them to the cell body
      c. Axon: single extension from the cell body; carries impulses away from the cell body
      d. Myelin sheath: white, segmented, fatty substance that surrounds axons; produced by Schwann cells that cover the axons; serves as an insulator and to speed the conduction of nerve impulses; gives white appearance to fibers (white matter)
      e. Neurilemma: outer membrane of axon
      f. Nodes of Ranvier: gaps in myelin sheath

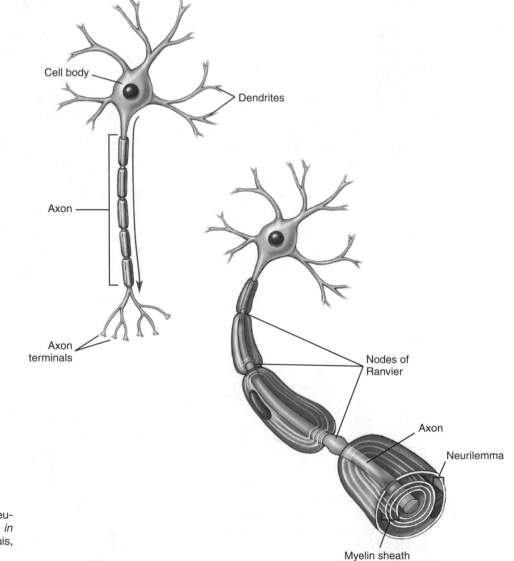

FIGURE 2-19 Structure of a neuron. (Herlihy B: *The human body in health and illness*, ed 3, St Louis, 2007, Saunders.)

g. Neurotransmitter: chemical substance that allows neurons to communicate with each other

2. Neuroglia: "nerve glue"; nonconductive cells of nerve tissue; provides support system (nourishment and protection) for neurons; more numerous than neurons; different types with specialized functions; capable of mitosis

3. Nerves: collection of nerve fibers held together by layers of connective tissue
   a. Afferent (sensory): carry impulses from PNS to CNS
   b. Efferent (motor): carry impulses from CNS to PNS

4. Brain (see Figure 2-20)

a. Cerebrum: largest superior portion; consists of thin layer of gray matter (cerebral cortex) and white matter (bulk of cerebrum)
   1) Cortex: makes us "human"; concerned with memory, language, reasoning, intelligence, personality, and other factors associated with human life
   2) Divided into two halves (hemispheres) by longitudinal fissure
      a) Right hemisphere: controls the left side of the body; responsible for auditory perception, tactile perception, and interpretation of spatial relationships
      b) Left hemisphere: controls the right side of the body; responsible for language and hand movements

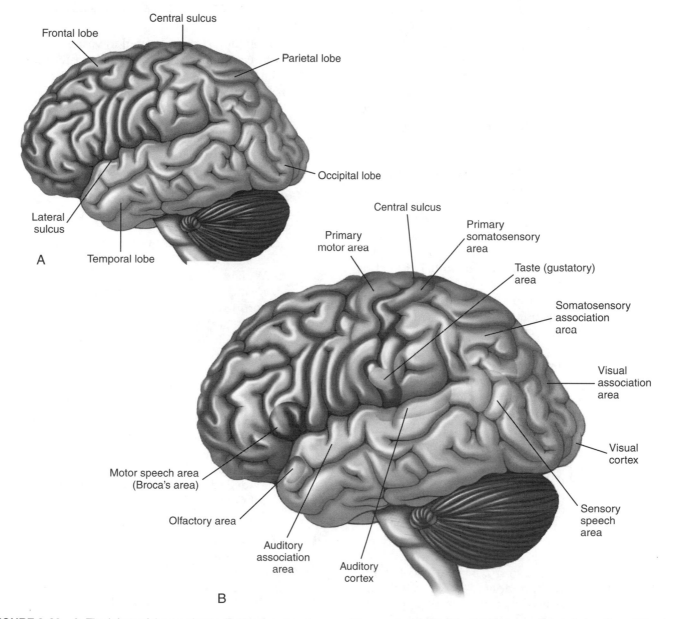

FIGURE 2-20   A, The lobes of the cerebrum. **B,** The functional areas of the cerebrum. (Herlihy B: *The human body in health and illness*, ed 3, St Louis, 2007, Saunders.)

3) Each hemisphere is divided into five lobes named for bones that cover them (except for the insula)
   a) Frontal lobe: controls voluntary muscle movements and speech
   b) Parietal lobe: receives and integrates sensory output
   c) Temporal lobe: interprets sound; involved with personality, emotion, memory, and behavior
   d) Occipital lobe: interprets sight
   e) Insula: visceral effects
4) Ventricles: cavities within each hemisphere that make and store cerebrospinal fluid (CSF)

b. Diencephalon: centrally located; surrounded by cerebral hemispheres
   1) Thalamus: relay station for all sensory input; associated with pain, temperature, and touch sensations; located between cerebrum and midbrain
   2) Hypothalamus: located below thalamus; important role in regulating heart rate, blood pressure, body temperature, water balance, hunger, sleep, and wakefulness

c. Brainstem
   1) Medulla oblongata: lowest portion of brain, connects to spinal cord; contains vital centers for control of heartbeat, respiration, and blood pressure
   2) Pons: bulge at the base of the brain; links the cerebellum to the rest of the nervous system; nerve fibers cross here; one side of the brain controls the other side of the body
   3) Midbrain: upper portion of the brainstem; correlates information about muscle tone and posture; relay center for certain eye and ear reflexes

d. Cerebellum: second largest portion of the brain, located below the cerebrum; responsible for coordination of voluntary movement, posture, and balance

e. Spinal cord: extends from the brainstem through the foramen magnum into the vertebral column to the second lumbar vertebra; approximately 17 inches long; conducts nerve impulses to and from brain; center for spinal reflexes; 31 pairs of spinal nerves connected to cord

f. Meninges: protective membrane covering brain and spinal cord; three layers
   1) Dura mater: strong, fibrous outer layer
   2) Arachnoid: middle, delicate weblike layer that allows for movement of CSF
   3) Pia mater: thin inner layer; contains blood vessels to supply the brain

g. Meningeal spaces
   1) Epidural space: located between dura mater and bone (skull or vertebra); acts as a cushion
   2) Subdural space: located between dura mater and arachnoid; contains serous fluid for lubrication
   3) Subarachnoid space: located between arachnoid and pia mater; contains CSF

h. Cerebrospinal fluid (CSF): clear, colorless, watery fluid found in subarachnoid space and in the ventricles of the brain; is constantly circulating; provides protective cushion for the brain; can detect physiologic changes in the body

VIII. SPECIAL SENSES

A. General
1. Variety of receptors located in various structures
2. Stimulation of a receptor by an appropriate stimulus results in an impulse, which is sent to the CNS, where it is processed
3. Allows the human to be aware of the world around him or her
4. Depends on sensory receptors classified as:
   a. General (widely distributed)
   b. Special (localized in a specific area)

B. General Senses (see Figure 2-21):
1. Somatic senses: found throughout the body
2. Touch and pressure
   a. Mechanoreceptor (responds to a bending, or a change in the shape of, a cell)
   b. Widely distributed in skin
   c. Includes free nerve endings, Meissner's corpuscles (touch), Pacinian corpuscles (pressure)
3. Position and orientation: proprioceptors
4. Temperature
   a. Thermoreceptor (detects change in temperature)
   b. Found immediately under the skin
   c. Ten times more cold receptors than heat receptors
5. Pain
   a. Nociceptors (responds to tissue damage)
   b. Widely distributed in skin and tissues of internal organs
   c. Protective function

B. Special Senses
1. Located within special organs
2. Gustatory sense
   a. Sense of taste
   b. Organs of taste (taste buds) localized on the surface of tongue
   c. Chemoreceptors (sensitive to chemicals in food)

FIGURE 2-21 The general senses. (Herlihy B: *The human body in health and illness*, ed 3, St Louis, 2007, Saunders.)

d. Includes receptors for sensations of salty, sweet, sour, and bitter

3. Olfactory sense
   a. Sense of smell
   b. Receptors found in upper nose
   c. Chemoreceptors
   d. Closely related to sense of taste

4. Visual sense (see Figure 2-22):
   a. Receptors located in the eye
   b. Photoreceptors (detects light)
      1) Eye
         a) Found in protective bony socket (orbit)
         b) Three layers (tunics)
            (1) Sclera
               (a) Outer layer; white of the eye
               (b) Made of tough fibrous tissue
               (c) Anterior portion covered by cornea, which focuses light rays

            (2) Choroid
               (a) Middle layer
               (b) Highly vascular
               (c) Ciliary body; changes shape of the lens
               (d) Suspensory ligament: connects the ciliary body to lens
               (e) Iris: colored portion of the eye
                  (i) Doughnut-shaped muscle with hole in the middle (pupil)
                  (ii) Continually contracts and relaxes to regulate the amount of light entering the eye
            (3) Retina
               (a) Innermost layer
               (b) Posterior portion of the eye
               (c) Contains

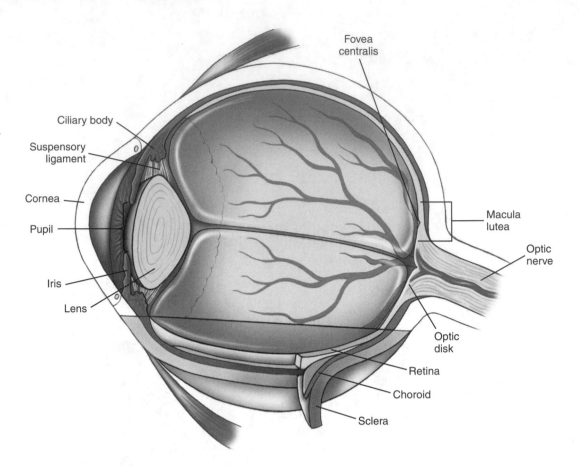

Fovea
centralis

Ciliary body

Suspensory
ligament

Cornea

Pupil

Iris

Lens

Macula
lutea

Optic
nerve

Optic
disk

Retina

Choroid

Sclera

FIGURE 2-22   Structure of the eyeball. (Herlihy B: *The human body in health and illness*, ed 3, St Louis, 2007, Saunders.)

(i) Rods: receptors sensitive to shades of gray

(ii) Cones: receptors sensitive to color

(d) Fovea centralis: area of closely packed cones that function as the area of sharpest vision

(e) Optic disk: area on the retina where the optic nerve exits the eye; the "blind spot"

2) Cavities

a) Anterior cavity: anterior space between the lens and the cornea; filled with aqueous humor (maintains shape and internal pressure)

b) Posterior cavity: between lens and the retina; filled with gel-like substance (vitreous humor); keeps retina against the wall of the eye, supports parts of the eye and helps maintain shape

3) Accessory structures

a) Eyebrows and eyelashes: protects against foreign objects

b) Eyelids: opens and closes eye to keep foreign objects out and to keep eye moist

c) Lacrimal apparatus: lacrimal glands make tears to lubricate, moisten, and cleanse the eye; nasolacrimal duct drains tears into the nasal cavity

d) Conjunctiva: mucous membrane that lines the inner eyelids and anterior eyeball

4) Muscles of the eye

a) Extrinsic muscles: skeletal muscles attached to the orbital bones and outer eye

b) Intrinsic muscles: smooth muscles located in the eye

5) Visual pathway: light ray → cornea → aqueous humor → pupil → lens → vitreous humor → retina (rods and cones) → optic nerve fibers → optic chiasma → thalamus → cerebral cortex

5. Auditory sense: receptors located in the ears; mechanoreceptors (see Figure 2-23)

6. Ear: found on both sides of the head

a. External ear

1) Auricle (pinna): fleshy part visible on sides of head; collects sound waves and directs them toward the auditory meatus

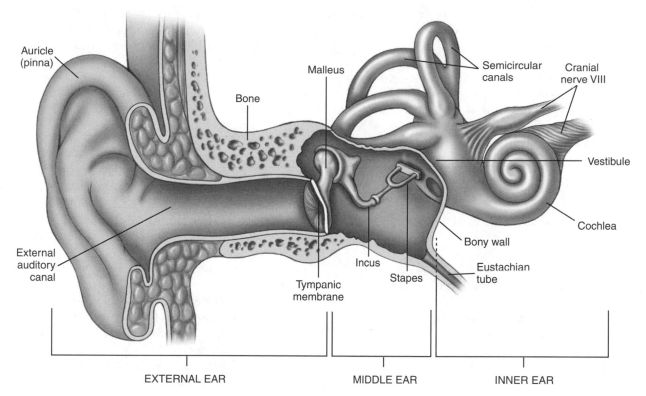

FIGURE 2-23 Structure of the ear and its three divisions. (Herlihy B: *The human body in health and illness*, ed 3, St Louis, 2007, Saunders.)

2) External auditory meatus: short tube that extends from the auricle to the tympanic membrane; lined with glands that produce cerumen (earwax) to protect and lubricate

b. Middle ear: found in the temporal bone
  1) Tympanic membrane: eardrum
  2) Auditory tube: eustachian tube; extends from the middle ear to the throat; equalizes pressure between the outside air and the middle ear cavity
  3) Ossicles: three tiny bones of the middle ear
    a) Malleus: attached to the tympanic membrane
    b) Incus: connects the malleus to the stapes
    c) Stapes: attached to the incus and oval window
  4) Oval window: membrane covering the opening into the vestibule

c. Inner ear
  1) Bony labyrinth
    a) (Series of interconnecting chambers in the temporal bone)
    b) Contains membranous labyrinth filled with fluid (endolymph)
    c) Space between the bony and membranous labyrinth; filled with fluid (perilymph)

d) Divided into three sections:
  (1) Vestibule: involved with balance
  (2) Semicircular canals: involved with equilibrium
  (3) Cochlea: snail-shaped structure involved with hearing; contains the organ of Corti, which contains receptors for sound

2) Auditory pathway: sound wave → pinna → external auditory meatus → tympanic membrane → malleus → incus → stapes → oval window → cochlea → perilymph → auditory nerve fibers → cerebral cortex

IX. BLOOD

A. General
  1. Primary transport medium of the body
  2. Pumped by the heart through a closed system of vessels
  3. Classified as connective tissue (cells and matrix)
  4. Approximately 5 L in adult
  5. 8% of body weight

B. Functions
  1. Transportation
    a. Carries O_2 and nutrients to cells
    b. Carries CO_2 and wastes from the tissues to the lungs and kidneys for removal

c. Carries hormones from the endocrine glands to other parts of the body

2. Regulation
   a. Regulates body temperature by removing heat from active areas and transporting that heat to skin for dissipation
   b. Helps regulate fluid and electrolyte balance
   c. Regulates pH through buffers

3. Protection
   a. Provides clotting mechanism to prevent fluid loss when vessels are damaged
   b. White blood cells engulf and destroy invading microorganisms
   c. Antibodies react with the offending agents

C. Composition of Blood (see Figure 2-24)

1. Plasma
   a. Liquid portion of circulating blood
   b. 55% of total blood volume
   c. 90% water
   d. Continuously changing caused by dissolved solutes

e. Contains plasma proteins
   1) Albumin: maintains osmotic pressure
   2) Globulin: functions in lipid transport and immune reaction
   3) Fibrinogen: formation of blood clots

f. Also contains amino acids, urea, uric acids, nutrients, hormones, O_2, CO_2, antibodies, and electrolytes

2. Formed elements: produced by hemopoiesis (red blood cells in red bone marrow; white blood cells in lymphoid tissue); all types develop from stem cell (hematocytoblast)
   a. Erythrocytes (red blood cells [RBCs])
      1) Most numerous of formed elements
      2) Normal range: 4.5 to 6 million per cubic millimeter of blood
      3) Biconcave disks (thin in the middle and thick around the edge)
      4) Mature cells have no nucleus
      5) Primary function: to carry O_2 to all body cells; O_2 combines with hemoglobin and is transported
      6) Formation regulated by hormone erythropoietin

FIGURE 2-24 Components of blood. (Drawing by Barbara Cousins, from Thibodeau GA, Patton KT: *The human body in health and disease*, ed 5, St Louis, 2009, Mosby.)

7) Iron, vitamin B$_{12}$, and folic acid are essential to RBC production

8) Live approximately 120 days; are then destroyed by spleen and liver

b. Leukocytes (white blood cells [WBCs])

1) Larger in size than RBCs, but fewer in number

2) Normal range: 5000 to 10,000 per cubic millimeter of blood

3) Each contains a nucleus

4) Able to move through capillary walls into tissue

5) Primary function: to provide defense against invading microorganisms and to promote or inhibit inflammatory response

6) Types:

a) Granulocytes: contains granules in cytoplasm

(1) Neutrophil: most common; have multilobed nucleus; responds first to tissue damage; number increases in acute infection

(2) Eosinophil: two-lobed nucleus; large granules in cytoplasm; neutralize histamine; numbers increase during allergic reaction and parasitic infections

(3) Basophil: least numerous of WBCs; has large U-shaped nucleus; can leave blood and enter tissue, where they release histamine and heparin

b) Agranulocytes: granules absent in cytoplasm

(1) Lymphocytes: large round nucleus surrounded by small amount of cytoplasm; role in body's defense system

(a) T-lymphocytes: directly attacks microorganisms

(b) B-lymphocytes: produce antibodies

(2) Monocytes: largest in size of all WBCs; can enter the tissue (macrophage); finish the cleanup process of the neutrophils

c. Thrombocytes (platelets): small fragments of very large cells (megakaryocytes)

1) Normal range: 250,000 to 500,000 per cubic millimeter of blood

2) Initiates formation of blood clots

D. Hemostasis

1. Stoppage of bleeding

2. Can be caused by either an injured vessel or stasis of blood flow

3. Includes three processes (see Figure 2-25):

a. Vascular constriction: reduces flow of blood through torn vessel

b. Platelet plug formation: platelets become sticky and adhere to each other

c. Coagulation: complex series of steps that results in clot formation; requires calcium and vitamin K

E. Blood Typing

1. Based on specific antigens and antibodies related to RBCs; blood type antigens are found on RBCs; antibodies in plasma

2. Main blood groups, ABO blood groups; blood types *must* match in transfusions:

a. Type A: has A antigens on RBCs; has anti-B antibodies

b. Type B: has B antigens on RBCs; has anti-A antibodies

c. Type AB: has A and B antigens on RBCs; has no antibodies

d. Type O: has neither A nor B antigens on RBCs; has both anti-A and anti-B antibodies

3. Rh factor: Rh+ has Rh antigen on RBCs; Rh− has no antigens; neither has anti-Rh in plasma; hemolytic disease of the newborn may develop when Rh− mother has Rh+ fetus

X. LYMPHATIC SYSTEM

A. General

1. Part of the circulatory system

2. Transports a fluid (lymph) through lymphatic vessels and empties it into venous blood

3. Major role in the body's defense system

B. Functions

1. Returns excess interstitial fluid to blood

2. Absorbs fats and fat-soluble vitamins from the digestive system

3. Provides defense against disease

C. Organs of the Lymphatic System (see Figure 2-26)

1. Lymph

a. Similar in composition to blood plasma

b. Picked up from interstitial fluid and returned to blood plasma

2. Lymphatic vessels

a. Found in tissue spaces

b. Carry fluid away from the tissues

c. Vessels empty into the lymphatic ducts

1) Right lymphatic duct: drains lymph from upper right quadrant of the body

2) Thoracic duct: drains the remainder of the body

3. Lymphatic organs

a. Lymph nodes

1) Located along the lymphatic vessels

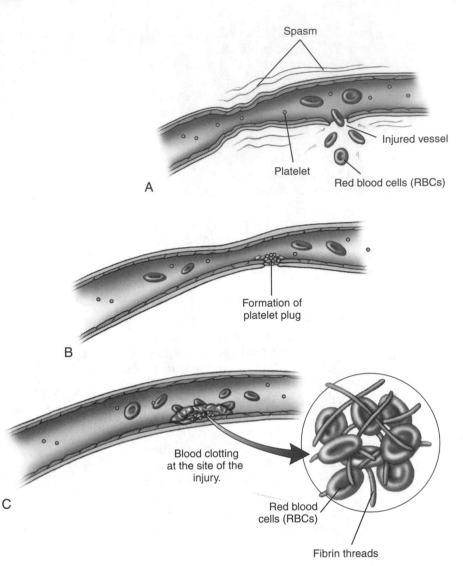

FIGURE 2-25 The steps of hemostasis: **A,** Vascular constriction. **B,** Formation of the platelet plug. **C,** Blood clotting (coagulation). (Herlihy B: *The human body in health and illness*, ed 3, St Louis, 2007, Saunders.)

2) Superficial nodes found in the groin, axilla, and neck
3) Filter and cleanse the lymph before it enters the blood
   b. Tonsils
   1) Provide protection against pathogens that may enter through the mouth or nose
   2) Three groups:
      a) Pharyngeal tonsils: located near the opening of the nose into the pharynx; adenoids
      b) Palatine tonsils: "the tonsils"; located near the opening of the oral cavity into the pharynx
      c) Lingual tonsils: posterior surface of the tongue
   4. Spleen: located in the upper left abdomen beneath the diaphragm, posterior to the stomach; filters blood; acts as a reservoir for the blood

5. Thymus: located posterior to the sternum; large in infants, atrophies after puberty; produces thymosin (stimulates the maturation of lymphocytes in the lymphatic organs)

D. Resistance to Disease
   1. Resistance is the body's ability to counteract pathogens
   2. Susceptibility is the lack of resistance
   3. Resistance is accomplished through defense mechanisms
      a. Nonspecific defense mechanisms: directed against all pathogens and foreign substances; provides first line of defense against invasion (see Figure 2-27)
         1) Barriers
            a) Mechanical (e.g., skin)
            b) Chemical (e.g., hydrochloric acid in stomach)

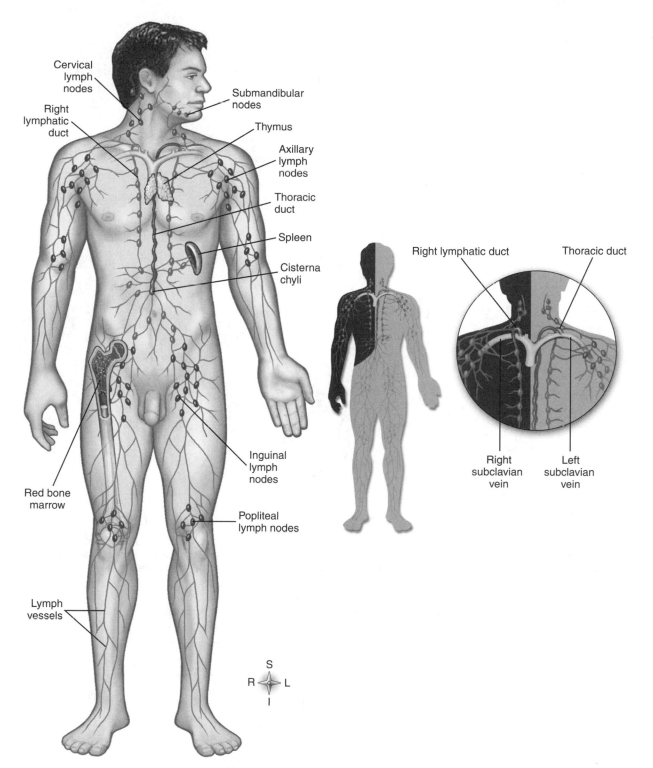

FIGURE 2-26 The lymphatic system. Principal organs and lymph drainage. (Drawing by Barbara Cousins, from Thibodeau GA, Patton KT: *The human body in health and disease*, ed 5, St Louis, 2009, Mosby.)

2) Chemical action
   a) Complement: promotes phagocytosis and inflammation
   b) Interferon: produced by virus-infected cells to provide protection for neighboring cells
3) Phagocytosis: neutrophils and macrophages

4) Inflammation: characterized by redness, warmth, swelling, and pain
b. Specific defense mechanisms: programmed to be selective (specificity); ability to remember invading agent (memory); invading agent called antigen; B-lymphocytes produce antibodies that react with the antigen (see Figure 2-28)

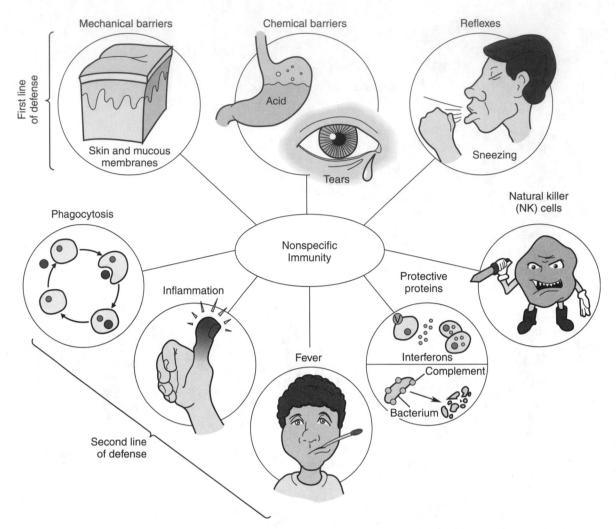

FIGURE 2-27 Nonspecific immunity. The first line of defense includes mechanical barriers, chemical barriers, and reflexes. Processes involved in the second line of defense are phagocytosis, inflammation, fever, protective proteins (complement proteins and interferons) and natural killer cells. (Herlihy B: *The human body in health and illness*, ed 3, St Louis, 2007, Saunders.)

1) Acquired immunity
   a) Active natural immunity: results when a person has a disease
   b) Active artificial immunity: results when a specific antigen is deliberately introduced into a person (immunization)
   c) Passive natural immunity: results when antibodies are transferred from one person to another (as mother to child)
   d) Passive artificial immunity: results when antibodies that developed in another person or animal are injected into a person
2) Natural immunity: acquired through normal activities

XI. CARDIOVASCULAR SYSTEM

A. General
1. Closed, sterile system
2. Consists of heart and blood vessels

B. Functions
1. Transportation: carries important elements throughout the body
2. Temperature regulation: helps with the regulation of body temperature through dilation and constriction of blood vessels
3. Waste removal: assists the lungs, kidneys, and liver
4. Fluid balance: maintains balance between fluid loss and fluid retention

C. Organs
1. Heart (see Figure 2-29)
   a. Hollow, muscular, cone-shaped organ about the size of a fist; located slightly to the left of mid-line in the mediastinum; protected by the sternum and ribs; upper end is base; lower end is pointed and is the apex (apical pulse)
   b. Made up of three layers
      1) Epicardium: outer layer
      2) Myocardium: thick, middle muscular layer
      3) Endocardium: inner layer

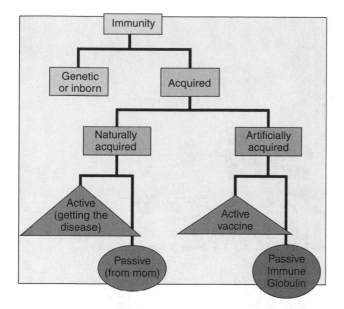

FIGURE 2-28 Immunity is either genetic or acquired. Immunity is acquired either naturally or artificially. Naturally acquired immunity can be either active *(triangles)* or passive *(circles)*. (Herlihy B: *The human body in health and illness*, ed 3, St Louis, 2007, Saunders.)

c. Covered by pericardium (double-layered sac that decreases friction and protects the heart)
d. Contains four chambers
   1) Atria: (singular: *atrium*); two upper chambers; receive blood from veins
   2) Ventricles: two lower chambers; receive blood from atria and pump it into the body
   3) Septum: divides chambers into right and left
   4) Valves: structures that allow one-way flow of blood throughout the heart
     a) Tricuspid valve: permits blood to flow from right atrium to right ventricle; composed of three flaps of tissue
     b) Bicuspid valve: (mitral valve); made up of two flaps of tissue; permits blood to flow from left atrium to left ventricle
     c) Pulmonary valve: located at the entrance of the pulmonary artery; prevents backflow of blood into the right ventricle; semilunar (half-moon shaped)
     d) Aortic valve: located at the entrance of the aorta; prevents backflow of blood into the left ventricle; semilunar:
     e) Blood enters right atrium → right ventricle → pulmonary artery → pulmonary capillaries (exchange of gases) → pulmonary vein → left atrium → left ventricle → aorta → capillaries in body tissues (exchange of gases) → superior and inferior venae cavae → right atrium

e. Electrical conduction system: initiates and maintains the rhythmic heart contractions (see Figure 2-30)
   1) Sinoatrial (SA) node: pacemaker of the heart; located in the right atrial wall near the superior vena cava; initiates heartbeat and sets its pace
   2) Atrioventricular (AV) node: located in lower right atrial septum; causes the atria to contract
   3) Bundle of His: located in ventricular septum
   4) Bundle branches: two branches extending from bundle of His
   5) Purkinje fibers: extend from the bundle branches; causes ventricles to contract
f. Cardiac cycle: complete heartbeat; consists of contraction (systole) and relaxation (diastole) of both atria and ventricles; complete cycle lasts for 0.8 second (75 bpm); sounds associated with heartbeat described as *lubb-dupp*
2. Vessels
  a. Arteries: vessels that carry blood away from the heart
   1) Composed of three layers
     a) Tunica adventitia: outermost layer of tough fibrous connective tissue
     b) Tunica media: middle layer of smooth muscle tissue allowing for contraction and dilation
     c) Tunica intima: innermost layer
   2) Arterioles: small arteries
  b. Veins: vessels that carry blood toward the heart
   1) Same layers as arteries, except tunica adventitia is thicker and tunica intima has valves to prevent backflow
   2) Venules: small veins
  c. Capillaries: microscopic vessels, one cell-layer thick
   1) Connects arterioles and venules
   2) Exchange of substances takes place here

3. Major arteries (see Figure 2-31)
  a. Pulmonary: comes from the right ventricle; transports deoxygenated blood to lungs
  b. Aorta: largest artery in the body; comes from the heart; divided into ascending aorta, aortic arch, descending aorta, and abdominal aorta
  c. Coronary: right and left branches off the ascending aorta; supplies the heart with blood

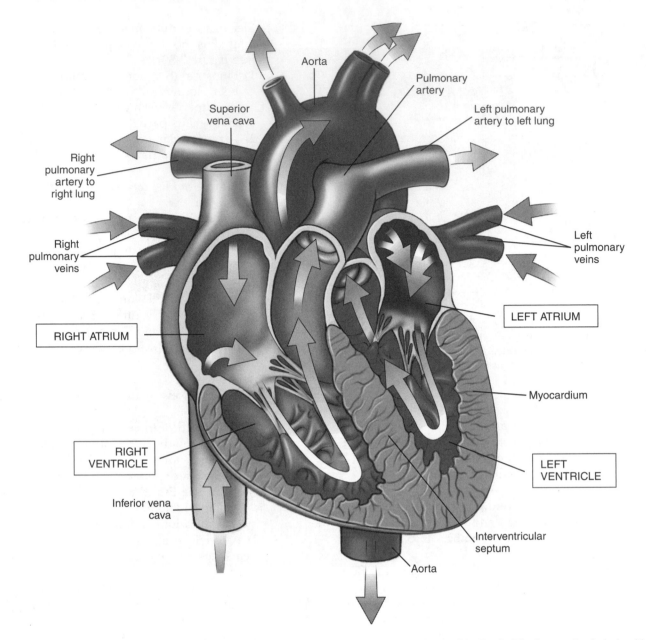

FIGURE 2-29 Chambers of the heart and the large vessels; blood flow through the heart. (Herlihy B: *The human body in health and illness*, ed 3, St Louis, 2007, Saunders.)

d. Brachiocephalic: one of three major branches off the aortic arch; supplies blood to the neck, head, axilla, and upper arm
e. Subclavian: supplies arms and vertebrae
  1) Left subclavian branches from aortic arch
  2) Right subclavian branches from brachiocephalic
f. Carotid: supplies neck and head
  1) Left carotid branches from aortic arch
  2) Right carotid branches from brachiocephalic
g. Facial: branch of carotid; supplies face and cranium
h. Occipital: branch of carotid; supplies neck and cranium

i. Axillary: extension of subclavian; supplies the axilla
j. Brachial: extension of axillary; supplies the upper arm
k. Radial: branch of brachial; supplies forearm, wrist, and hand
l. Ulnar: branch of brachial on little finger side; supplies forearm, wrist, and hand
m. Celiac: branch of abdominal aorta; supplies upper abdomen and organs
n. Splenic: functions similarly to celiac
o. Renal: branch of abdominal aorta; supplies kidneys, ureters, and adrenal glands
p. Mesenteric: branch of abdominal aorta; supplies intestines, colon, and rectum

FIGURE 2-30   Conduction system of the heart. (Herlihy B: *The human body in health and illness*, ed 3, St Louis, 2007, Saunders.)

q. Iliac: extension of abdominal aorta; branches and supplies abdominal and pelvic regions and lower limbs

r. Femoral: extension of iliac; supplies abdominal wall, genitalia, and upper leg

s. Popliteal: extension of femoral; supplies knee and calf

t. Tibial: extension of popliteal
   1) Anterior supplies lower leg, ankle, and foot
   2) Posterior supplies lower leg, foot, and heel

u. Dorsalis pedis: extension of anterior tibial; supplies foot

4. Major veins (see Figure 2-32)

a. Pulmonary: transports blood from lungs to left atrium

b. Coronary: drains blood from the right atrium

c. Vena cava: largest vein in the body; leads from the body into the right atrium
   1) Superior vena cava: drains upper body
   2) Inferior vena cava: drains the lower body

d. Brachiocephalic: left and right branches go into the superior vena cava; drains the head, neck, and upper extremities

e. Jugular: branches go into the brachiocephalic; drains the head and neck

f. Facial: branches go into the jugular; drains the face and cranium

g. Occipital: branches go into the jugular; drains the cranium

h. Axillary: branches go into the brachiocephalic; drains the axillary area and the upper arm

i. Subclavian: branches go into the axillary; drains the upper arm

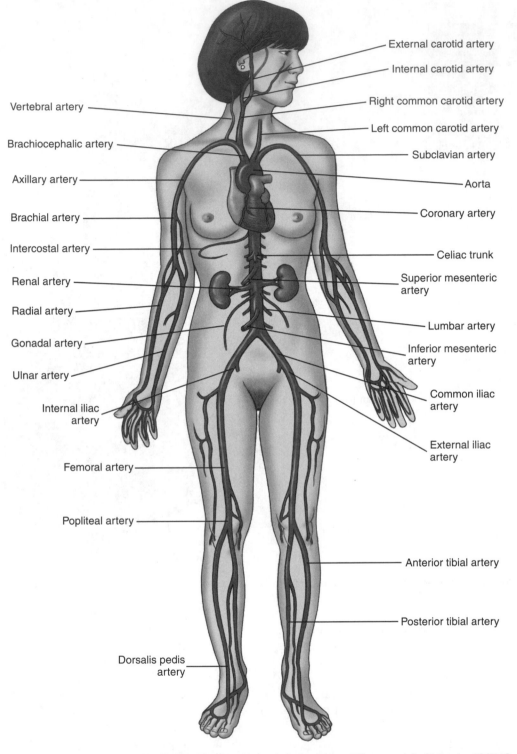

External carotid artery

Internal carotid artery

Right common carotid artery

Left common carotid artery

Subclavian artery

Aorta

Coronary artery

Celiac trunk

Superior mesenteric artery

Lumbar artery

Inferior mesenteric artery

Common iliac artery

External iliac artery

Anterior tibial artery

Posterior tibial artery

Vertebral artery

Brachiocephalic artery

Axillary artery

Brachial artery

Intercostal artery

Renal artery

Radial artery

Gonadal artery

Ulnar artery

Internal iliac artery

Femoral artery

Popliteal artery

Dorsalis pedis artery

FIGURE 2-31   Major arteries of the body. (Herlihy B: *The human body in health and illness*, ed 3, St Louis, 2007, Saunders.)

j. Cephalic: goes into the axillary; drains the upper and lower arm

k. Radial: goes into the axillary; drains the thumb side of the forearm and wrist

l. Basilic: goes into axillary on little finger side; drains the upper and lower arm

m. Ulnar: goes into the axillary; drains the little finger side of the forearm and wrist

n. Gastric, cholecystic, and splenic: goes into portal hepatic vein; drains the stomach, gallbladder, and spleen

o. Mesenteric: goes into the hepatic portal vein; drains the intestines, colon, and rectum

p. Hepatic: goes into the inferior vena cava; drains the liver

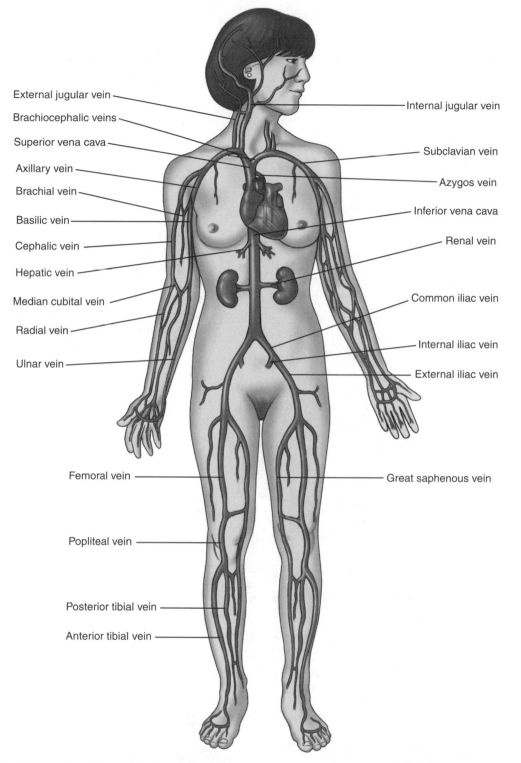

External jugular vein

Brachiocephalic veins

Superior vena cava

Axillary vein

Brachial vein

Basilic vein

Cephalic vein

Hepatic vein

Median cubital vein

Radial vein

Ulnar vein

Internal jugular vein

Subclavian vein

Azygos vein

Inferior vena cava

Renal vein

Common iliac vein

Internal iliac vein

External iliac vein

Femoral vein

Great saphenous vein

Popliteal vein

Posterior tibial vein

Anterior tibial vein

FIGURE 2-32 Major veins of the body. (Herlihy B: *The human body in health and illness*, ed 3, St Louis, 2007, Saunders.)

q. Renal: goes into the inferior vena cava; drains the kidneys and gonads

r. Iliac: extension of the inferior vena cava; drains the abdominal, pelvic, and lower limb regions

s. Femoral: extension of right and left iliac; drains the upper leg

t. Popliteal: extension of femoral; drains the knee and calf

u. Saphenous: longest vein in the body
   1) Great saphenous goes into femoral; drains the medial leg
   2) Small saphenous goes into popliteal; drains the lower leg

v. Tibial: goes into popliteal; drains the lower leg

XII. RESPIRATORY SYSTEM

A. General
1. Supplies continuous supply of O_2 to the body
2. Works with the circulatory system to bring O_2 to the entire body and to remove waste products

B. Functions
1. Air exchange and distribution: O_2 carried to tissues and CO_2 carried away
2. Filtration: small hairs in nasal cavity trap substances before air enters the trachea
3. Sound production: enhances sounds produced during speech
4. Sense of smell: located in the nose
5. pH regulation: regulates the pH of blood

C. Organs: Divided into Two Sections (see Figure 2-33):
1. Upper respiratory tract: organs outside of thoracic cavity
   a. Nose
   1) External nose: nasal bones and cartilage; forms nostrils (nares)
   2) Internal nose: nasal cavity; found over roof of mouth; divided into two halves by the nasal septum; functions to warm, filter, and humidify air
   b. Pharynx
   1) Throat
   2) Has three divisions
      a) Nasopharynx: nearest to nasal cavity; contains adenoids
      b) Oropharynx: behind the mouth; contains the tonsils
      c) Laryngopharynx: leads to trachea and esophagus
   c. Larynx: voice box; made up of cartilage with ciliated mucous membrane; contains vocal cords; carries air from pharynx to trachea
2. Lower respiratory tract: organs within the thorax
   a. Trachea: windpipe; made up of 16 to 20 C-shaped rings of cartilage that extend from larynx to the bronchi

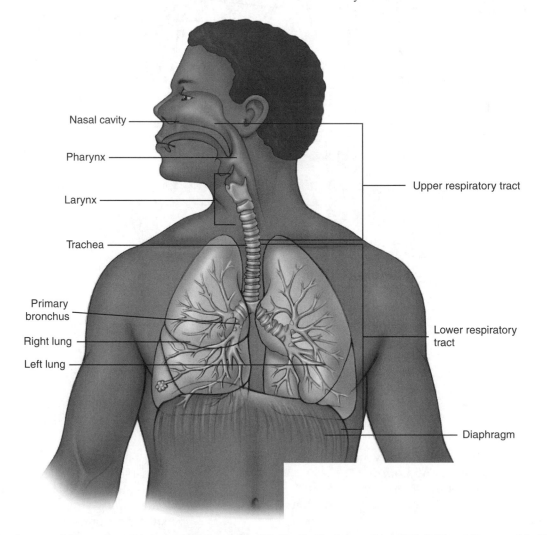

FIGURE 2-33 Organs of the upper and lower respiratory tract. (Herlihy B: *The human body in health and illness*, ed 3, St Louis, 2007, Saunders.)

b. Bronchi: end of the trachea; divided into right and left bronchi; enters lungs and further divides into secondary bronchi that further branch into bronchioles; branches end in alveolar ducts

c. Alveoli: air sacs; functional units of respiration; resemble clusters of grapes; these form the terminal end of bronchioles; composed of single layers of epithelium surrounded by capillaries; gases exchanged here

d. Lungs: cone-shaped organs located in thoracic cavity; each contains approximately 300 million alveoli; responsible for air distribution and exchange; bottom portion (base) rests on diaphragm

   1) Left lung divided into two lobes (eight segments)

   2) Right lung divided into three lobes (10 segments)

      a. Covered by double-layered membrane (pleura); fluid between layers (pleural fluid) lubricates and reduces friction during respiration

D. Respiration

1. Controlled by respiratory control center of medulla

2. Medulla controls rhythm and depth of inspiration and expiration

3. Monitors O_2, CO_2, and pH of blood, which triggers breathing

4. Involves two processes

   a. Pulmonary ventilation: carries out breathing by means of pressure gradient; has two phases

      1) Inspiration: air drawn into lungs by contraction of diaphragm (makes thoracic cavity larger)

      2) Expiration: air expelled from lungs by relaxation of diaphragm

   b. Cellular respiration; has two phases:

      1) External: exchange of gases between alveoli and capillaries

      2) Internal: exchange of gases between capillaries and body cells

XIII. DIGESTIVE SYSTEM

A. General

1. Includes the digestive tract (gastrointestinal [GI] tract, alimentary canal) and accessory organs

2. Digestive tract: long, continuous tube that starts at the mouth and ends at the anus

3. Processes food into molecules small enough to be utilized by the body

B. Functions

1. Digestion: physical and chemical breakdown of complex foodstuffs into simple nutrients

2. Absorption: passage of simple nutrients through the walls of the small intestine into the blood or lymph

3. Elimination: excretion of indigestible waste from the body in the form of feces

C. Organs (see Figure 2-34)

1. Mouth (oral cavity)

   a. Receives food by ingestion

   b. Breaks down food into small particles by mastication (chewing)

   c. Mixes food with saliva

   d. Lips and cheeks help hold food in place for chewing

   e. Also helps with speech

      1) Palate: separates oral cavity from nasal cavity

         a) Anterior portion (hard palate): supported by bone

         b) Posterior portion (soft palate): made of muscle and connective tissue; ends in fingerlike projection (uvula); uvula and soft palate move upward during swallowing to keep food from entering the nasal cavity

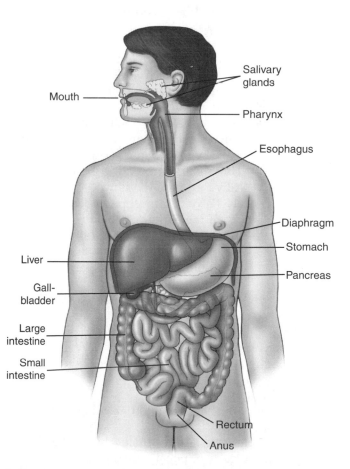

FIGURE 2-34 The digestive system. (Herlihy B: *The human body in health and illness*, ed 3, St Louis, 2007, Saunders.)

2) Tongue: moves food around in mouth; helps with speech; covered by papillae; papillae provide friction and contain taste buds

3) Teeth: used for mastication
   a) Two different sets develop:
      (1) Deciduous (baby teeth): first 20 teeth, which eventually fall out
      (2) Permanent: set of 32 adult teeth, which replace deciduous teeth
   b) Shape of tooth corresponds to the way it handles food
      (1) Incisors: chisel-shaped and sharp edges for biting foods
      (2) Cuspids (canines): conical-shaped with points for grasping and tearing foods
      (3) Bicuspids: flat surfaces for crushing and grinding
      (4) Molars: also have flat surfaces for crushing and grinding
   c) Tooth is divided into:
      (1) Crown: exposed portion; covered with enamel (hardest surface in the body)
      (2) Neck: narrow portion below crown, protected by gums
      (3) Root: end portion of neck that fits into socket in mandible and maxilla
      (4) Pulp cavity: central core of tooth; contains pulp, which consists of connective tissue, blood vessels, and nerves; surrounded by dentin

4) Salivary glands
   a) Produce saliva, which contains water, mucus, and enzyme amylase; moistens food; begins chemical digestion
   b) Three pairs of exocrine glands secrete saliva into the mouth:
      (1) Parotid: largest pair; located in front of the ears (mumps)
      (2) Submandibular: located in the floor of the mouth
      (3) Sublingual: smallest pair; located under the tongue

2. Pharynx (throat): passageway that transports food to esophagus
3. Esophagus: muscular tube that carries food from pharynx to stomach
4. Stomach: located in the left upper quadrant of abdomen
   a. Can hold up to 1.5 L
   b. Temporarily stores and partially breaks down food
   c. Secretes substances (mucus, hydrochloric acid (HCl), gastrin, pepsinogen) that aid in digestion
   d. Destroys bacteria that enter the digestive tract
   e. Three regions:
      1) Superior region (fundus); opening guarded by the cardiac sphincter
      2) Main portion (body)
      3) Lower portion (pylorus); connects to small intestines; opening to the small intestines guarded by the pyloric sphincter
   f. Wall of the stomach has three layers made up of smooth muscle; the innermost layer has folds (rugae), which allow for expansion

5. Small intestines
   a. Coiled tubular structure approximately 6 meters in length and approximately 2.5 cm in diameter
   b. Fills most of the abdominal cavity
   c. Completes chemical digestion
   d. Primary site for absorption of nutrients
   e. Has three divisions:
      1) Duodenum: upper portion
      2) Jejunum: middle portion
      3) Ileum: end portion
   f. Suspended from the abdominal wall by a fold of peritoneum (mesentery)
   g. Lining contains fingerlike projections (villi); villi contain capillaries and lacteals, which rise off of the surface area and absorb nutrients

6. Large intestines
   a. Folded tube approximately 1.5 meters in length and 6 cm in diameter
   b. Absorbs fluid and electrolytes; eliminates waste products
   c. Produces vitamin K (necessary for blood clotting)
   d. Divided into:
      1) Cecum: first division connected to ileum of small intestine; contains ileocecal valve; vermiform appendix attached to cecum
      2) Ascending colon: vertical length of colon that runs along the right side of the abdominal cavity
      3) Transverse colon: horizontal length of colon that runs across the abdominal cavity
      4) Descending colon: vertical length of colon that runs along the left side of the abdominal cavity
      5) Sigmoid colon: S-shaped length of colon that connects to the rectum
      6) Rectum: continues to the anal canal; thick muscular wall
      7) Anal canal: continues from the rectum to outside (anus); guarded by two sphincter muscles

7. Peritoneum: serous membrane that covers most of the abdominal organs and holds them in place
   a. Mesentery: holds intestines in coils
   b. Transverse mesocolon: binds transverse colon to posterior abdominal wall
   c. Omentum: sheet of serous membrane that contains fat; protects the abdominal organs

8. Accessory organs
   a. Liver
      1) Accessory organ of digestion
      2) "Can't live without a liver"
      3) Largest gland in the body
      4) Located in the right upper quadrant
      5) Divided into right and left lobes
      6) Filters and destroys wastes and toxic substances
      7) Produces bile, which breaks down (emulsifies) fats
      8) Stores iron, glycogen, and vitamins A, B_{12}, D, E, and K
      9) Produces clotting factors
      10) Recycles iron and hemoglobin from worn-out red blood cells
      11) Controls carbohydrate and lipid metabolism
   b. Gallbladder
      1) Pear-shaped sac attached to inferior surface of liver by cystic duct
      2) Stores, concentrates, and sends bile into the duodenum through the common bile duct (the cystic duct joins the hepatic duct from the liver to form the common bile duct)
   c. Pancreas
      1) Located behind stomach
      2) Endocrine and exocrine functions
         a) Endocrine: beta cells of the islets of Langerhans secrete insulin, which lowers blood glucose levels; alpha cells of the islets of Langerhans secrete glucagon (which raises blood glucose levels)
         b) Exocrine: acinar cells secrete digestive enzymes (amylase, trypsin, peptidase, and lipase)

D. Digestion
   1. Breakdown of foodstuffs; has two processes:
   a. Mechanical digestion: breaks down food, moves it along the canal, and eliminates the waste from the body;
      1) Begins with mastication (chewing), which reduces the size of food and mixes the food with saliva to form a bolus
      2) Bolus is swallowed (deglutition)
      3) Wavelike motion of GI tract (peristalsis) moves food along the digestive tract
      4) Food is churned in stomach to mix with gastric juices to form chyme
      5) Chyme is pushed into the duodenum approximately every 20 seconds until empty
      6) Chyme mixes with pancreatic liver and intestinal juices
      7) Chyme leaves the jejunum approximately 5 hours after entering the small intestine

      8) Residue not absorbed enters the large intestine, where excess water is absorbed and waste (feces) is formed and expelled from the body
   b. Chemical digestion: breaks down large complex molecules into smaller molecules for absorption; accomplished by hydrolysis and enzymes
      1) Carbohydrates: initially broken down by amylase; final breakdown by sucrase, lactase, and maltase
      2) Proteins: broken down into amino acids by proteases: pepsin (stomach), trypsin (pancreas), and peptidase (intestines)
      3) Fats: first emulsified by bile in small intestine; finally digested by pancreatic lipase

E. Absorption
   1. Process of transporting nutrients from small intestinal mucosa to blood or lymph
   2. Most absorption occurs in small intestine
   3. Nutrients travel to the liver through portal system

F. Elimination
   1. Solid waste expelled from body by process of defecation
   2. Defecation is triggered by stimulation of receptors caused by full rectum
   3. Controlled by internal sphincter (involuntary) and external sphincter (voluntary)

XIV. URINARY SYSTEM

A. General
   1. Produces and excretes urine from the body
   2. Kidneys clean blood of waste products
   3. Plays vital role in electrolyte, water, and acid-base balance

B. Functions
   1. Waste elimination: excretes nitrogen-containing liquid waste (urine) from the body
   2. Regulation of blood volume: balances water loss and gain
   3. Regulation of pH: balances gain and loss of bicarbonate and hydrogen ions
   4. Regulations of electrolytes: balances levels through excretion and reabsorption
   5. Detoxification: assists liver in neutralizing substances

C. Organs (see Figure 2-35)
   1. Kidney: two bean-shaped organs located retroperitoneal; surrounded by a cushion of fat; two layers
      a. Cortex: outer layer

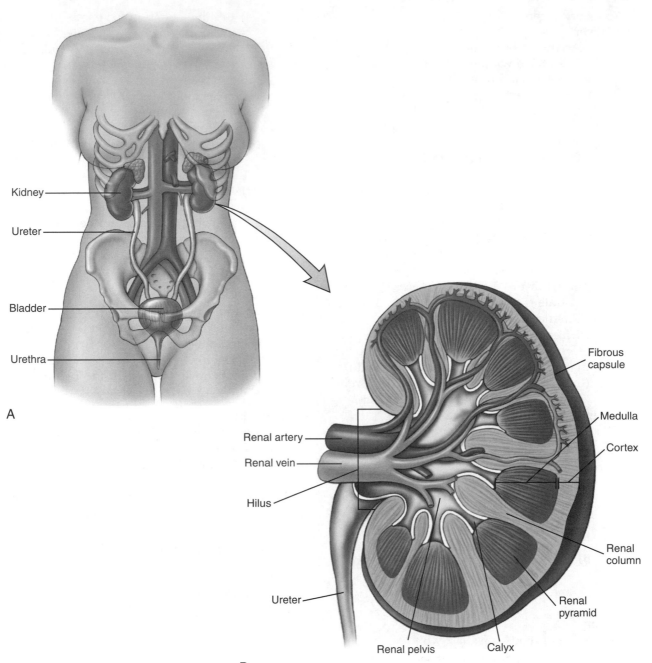

A

B

FIGURE 2-35 The urinary system. **A,** The major organs. **B,** Internal structure of a kidney. (Herlihy B: *The human body in health and illness,* ed 3, St Louis, 2007, Saunders.)

b. Medulla: inner layer; contains renal pyramids
   1) Triangle-shaped wedges that contain the nephron
   2) Points of pyramids come together into a cuplike structure (calyx [singular])
   3) Calyces (plural) join together to form renal pelvis where urine is collected
   4) Nephron: microscopic functional unit of kidneys; filters blood and produces urine; made up of:
      a) Bowman's capsule: cup-shaped structure in renal cortex; holds the glomerulus

   b) Glomerulus: ball-shaped cluster of capillaries that sits in Bowman's capsule; Bowman's capsule and glomerulus make up the renal corpuscle
   c) Proximal convoluted tubule: extension of Bowman's capsule; makes up first part of the renal tubule
   d) Loop of Henle: extends from proximal convoluted tubule
   e) Distal convoluted tubule: extends from the loop of Henle

f) Collecting tubule: tubule formed by union of distal convoluted tubules; convoluted tubules join to form one renal pyramid; pyramids join to form calyx

2. Ureter
   a. Tube that runs from kidneys into urinary bladder
   b. Renal pelvis narrows as it leaves kidney to form ureter
3. Urinary bladder
   a. Muscular sac located behind symphysis pubis
   b. Capable of great expansion caused by folds (rugae) in its inner lining
   c. Serves as temporary storage place for urine
4. Urethra
   a. Tube that carries urine from the bladder to the outside of the body
   b. Opening to outside is urinary meatus

D. Blood Flow to Kidneys

1. Renal artery: enters kidney at hilum
2. Afferent arteriole: enters Bowman's capsule
3. Glomerulus: network of capillaries
4. Efferent arteriole: comes from glomerulus and exits Bowman's capsule
5. Peritubular capillaries: extend from efferent arteriole; surrounds renal tubule
6. Renal venule: extends from peritubular capillaries
7. Renal vein: extends from renal venule; exits kidney at hilum; joins inferior vena cava

E. Urine

1. Formation
   a. Series of three processes:
      1) Filtration: continuous process; glomerular blood pressure causes water and dissolved substances to filter out of the glomeruli and into Bowman's capsule
      2) Reabsorption: movement of substances out of renal tubules into blood in peritubular capillaries; water, nutrients, and electrolytes reabsorbed
      3) Secretion: movement of substances not reabsorbed into urine into collecting tubules
2. Composition
   a. Water: 95% of urine
   b. Nitrogenous waste products: urea, ammonia, uric acid, and creatinine (end products of protein metabolism)
   c. Electrolytes: sodium, potassium, phosphate, sulfates, ammonium, bicarbonate, and chloride
   d. Toxins
   e. Pigment: urochrome

XV. ENDOCRINE SYSTEM

A. General

1. Body's slower-acting control system
2. Made up of glands that secrete substances (hormones)
3. Hormones travel through the bloodstream to target organs and cells

B. Functions

1. Control: regulates internal body functions and processes
2. Communication: complements the nervous system; directs communication among the body systems for optimum functioning

C. Hormones: Chemical Substances Secreted from Endocrine Glands

1. Tropic hormones: stimulate other endocrine glands to secrete their hormones
2. Sex hormones: stimulate reproductive tissue
3. Anabolic hormones: stimulate cells to grow and repair
4. Prostaglandins: tissue hormones that regulate cellular activity

D. Glands (see Figure 2-36)

1. Pituitary gland: master gland; hypophysis
   a. Located on inferior surface of the brain
   b. Connected to hypothalamus by stalk (infundibulum)
   c. Divided into two sections:
      1) Anterior hypophysis (adenohypophysis) (see Figure 2-37); secretes:
         a) Growth hormone (GH): promotes tissue growth; stimulates fat metabolism; helps maintain blood glucose levels
         b) Prolactin (PRL): promotes development of breast and milk secretion; works with luteinizing hormone during menstrual cycle
         c) Thyroid-stimulating hormone (TSH): stimulates development and hormone production of thyroid gland
         d) Adrenocorticotropic hormone (ACTH): stimulates development and hormone production of adrenal cortex
         e) Follicle-stimulating hormone (FSH)
            (1) In female: stimulates follicle development and secretion of estrogen
            (2) In male: stimulates sperm production
         f) Luteinizing hormone (LH)
            (1) In female: stimulates secretion of estrogen and progesterone
            (2) In male: stimulates secretion of testosterone

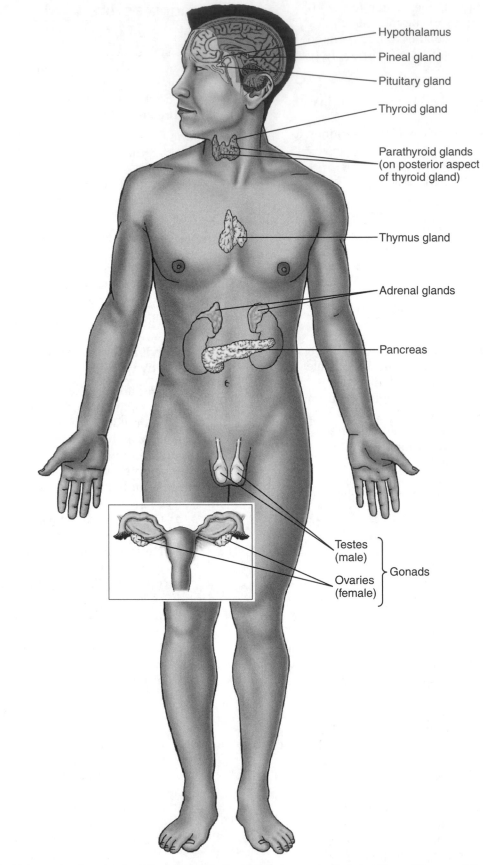

Hypothalamus

Pineal gland

Pituitary gland

Thyroid gland

Parathyroid glands
(on posterior aspect
of thyroid gland)

Thymus gland

Adrenal glands

Pancreas

Testes
(male)

Ovaries
(female)

Gonads

FIGURE 2-36   Major endocrine glands of the body. (Herlihy B: *The human body in health and illness*, ed 3, St Louis, 2007, Saunders.)

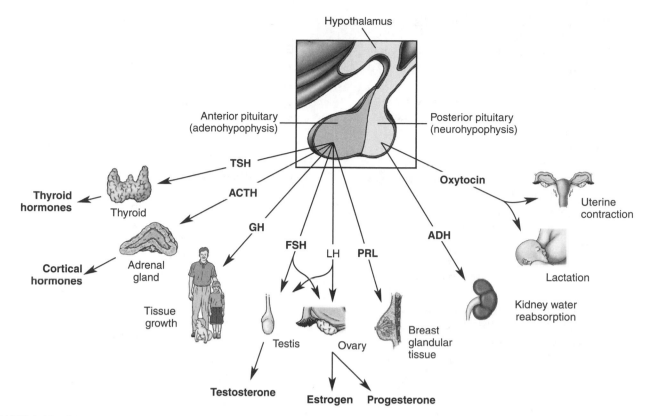

FIGURE 2-37 Pituitary gland. Hormones secreted by the anterior and posterior pituitary glands; also shows the target organs. (Herlihy B: *The human body in health and illness*, ed 3, St Louis, 2007, Saunders.)

  g) Melanocyte-stimulating hormone (MSH): regulates normal color of skin; helps regulate adrenal gland's response to ACTH

 2) Posterior pituitary (neurohypophysis):

  a) Does not manufacture hormones

  b) Stores and releases hormones made in hypothalamus

   (1) Antidiuretic hormone (ADH): prevents excessive formation of urine

   (2) Oxytocin: stimulates the uterus to contract during childbirth; causes letdown of milk

2. Pineal gland

 a. Pinecone-shaped gland located behind the hypothalamus

 b. Produces melatonin that regulates the body's *"biological clock"*

3. Thyroid gland

 a. Butterfly-shaped gland located in the neck, lateral and anterior to the trachea

 b. Secretes two hormones:

  1) Thyroxine (tetraiodothyronine [T_4]) and triiodothyronine (T_3); regulate metabolism of the body; needs iodine for synthesis

  2) Calcitonin: stimulates movement of calcium from the blood to the bone

4. Parathyroid gland

 a. Four pea-shaped glands embedded in the thyroid gland

 b. Secretes parathormone (PTH), which causes calcium to leave bone and enter the bloodstream

5. Adrenal glands

 a. Located on top of each kidney

 b. Composed of two regions:

  1) Adrenal cortex: outer region: secretes corticosteroids

   a) Aldosterone: regulates mineral salts

   b) Cortisol: regulates blood pressure

   c) Androgen and estrogen: minor sex hormones

  2) Adrenal medulla: inner region: secretes hormones that are important in the sympathetic and parasympathetic nervous systems

   a) Epinephrine

   b) Norepinephrine

6. Pancreas

 a. Elongated gland that extends posterior to stomach

 b. Produces glucagon; from alpha cells; stimulates conversion of glycogen to glucose in liver

c. Produces insulin; from beta cells; decreases glucose levels in blood

d. Produces somatostatin; from delta cells; regulates other pancreatic cells

7. Gonads
   a. Testes in male: secrete testosterone, which stimulates the development of male sex characteristics
   b. Ovaries in female
      1) Secrete estrogen: from follicles; stimulates development of female sex characteristics
      2) Secrete progesterone: from corpus luteum; maintains a pregnancy

8. Thymus
   a. Located in mediastinum below sternum
   b. Largest in children; atrophies during adolescence
   c. Produces thymosin; stimulates T-lymphocytes for immunity

9. Placenta: produces human chorionic gonadotropin (HCG) during pregnancy

XVI. REPRODUCTIVE SYSTEM

A. **General**
   1. Produces offspring for the survival of the species

B. **Functions**
   1. Production of egg and sperm cells
   2. Nurturing of developing offspring
   3. Production of hormones

C. **Organs and Structures of the Male System (see Figure 2-38)**
   1. Testes
      a. Essential organs (gonads)
      b. Produces sperm (male gamete)
      c. Glandular structures located outside of the body in the scrotum
      d. Made up of seminiferous tubules (sperm development) and interstitial cells (produces testosterone)
   2. Epididymis
      a. Continuation of seminiferous tubules
      b. Lies on the superior surface of the testes
      c. Secretes part of seminal fluid

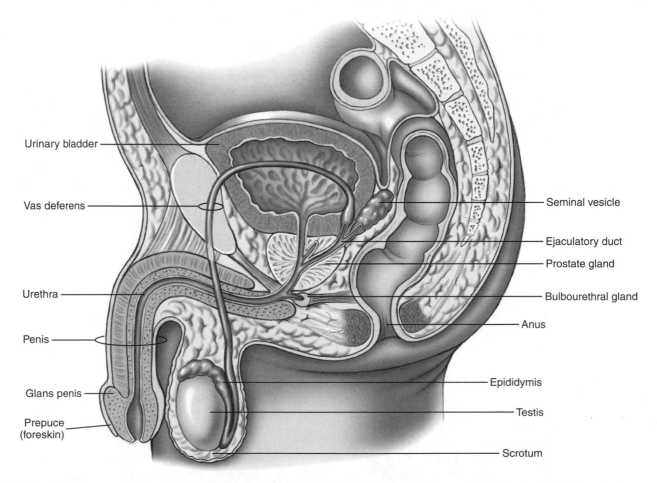

FIGURE 2-38 Male reproductive organs. (Herlihy B: *The human body in health and illness*, ed 3, St Louis, 2007, Saunders.)

3. Vas deferens
   a. Extension of the epididymis
   b. Passes through the inguinal canal into the abdominal cavity; arches over the bladder and joins the seminal vesicles
   c. Site of male sterilization (vasectomy)
4. Seminal vesicles
   a. Bilateral pouches behind the urinary bladder
   b. Secrete a nutrient-rich fluid that nourishes sperm
5. Ejaculatory duct
   a. Formed by the union of the vas deferens and seminal vesicles
   b. Passes through the prostate gland and enters the urethra
   c. Propels sperm and seminal fluid into the urethra during orgasm
6. Prostate gland
   a. Doughnut-shaped gland that encircles the base of the urethra on the posterior surface of the bladder
   b. Secretes an alkaline fluid that protects the sperm from the acidity of the vagina
7. Bulbourethral gland (Cowper's gland)
   a. Pea-shaped glands located on both sides of the urethra
   b. Secretes lubrication during intercourse
8. Scrotum
   a. Pouch of skin suspended from the perineal area
   b. Holds the testes and epididymis
   c. Keeps the testes away from the body; body temperature is too high for sperm production
9. Penis
   a. External male genitalia
   b. Composed of three cylinders of erectile tissue
   c. During sexual arousal, erectile tissue fills with blood and becomes erect
   d. Contains the urethra
   e. Distal end covered by the prepuce (foreskin), which is removed by circumcision

D. **Organs and Structures of the Female System (see Figure 2-39)**
1. Ovaries
   a. Essential organs (gonads)
   b. Produce ova (female gamete)
   c. Almond-shaped glands located in the pelvic cavity
   d. Contain ovarian (Graafian) follicles where ova develop
   e. Produce estrogen and progesterone
2. Uterus
   a. Pear-shaped muscular organ located in the pelvic cavity between the bladder and rectum

   b. Three divisions:
      1) Fundus: upper region
      2) Body: large central region
      3) Cervix: lower neck region; opens to vagina
   c. Three layers:
      1) Endometrium: inner layer; the fertilized ovum implants and grows here; shed monthly (menstruation; menses)
      2) Myometrium: middle muscular layer
      3) Perimetrium (epimetrium): outer layer
   d. Contracts to deliver the fetus
3. Fallopian tubes (oviducts)
   a. Attached to the upper, outer sides of uterus
   b. Serve as the site of fertilization; the fertilized ovum travels through the tube into the uterus for implantation
   c. Distal ends contain fingerlike structures (fimbriae); gentle movement of fimbriae draws the ovum into the tube after release from the ovary
   d. Site of female sterilization (tubal ligation)
4. Vagina
   a. Tubular structure that extends from cervix to the outside
   b. Located between the rectum and urethra
   c. Capable of great expansion
   d. Serves as the birth canal and means of shedding menstrual tissues
5. Vulva
   a. External genitalia
   b. Includes:
      1) Mons pubis: fat pad that covers the symphysis pubis
      2) Labia majora: two large folds of skin extending from the mons pubis to the anus
      3) Labia minora: two small folds of skin medial to the labia majora
      4) Clitoris: small nodule of erectile tissue superior to the labia majora; plays a role in sexual arousal
      5) Bartholin glands: located at the entrance to the vagina; secretes lubricating fluid during intercourse
6. Perineum: region between the vaginal opening and the rectum; may be cut or torn during childbirth (episiotomy)
7. Breasts
   a. Mammary glands
   b. Fatty tissue and milk glands that overlie the pectoral muscles
   c. Produces milk (lactation) for offspring
   d. Nipple is protrusion for delivery of milk
   e. Areola is dark area that surrounds nipple

E. **Reproductive Cycle**
1. Ovarian cycle: ovum develops and matures in the ovary

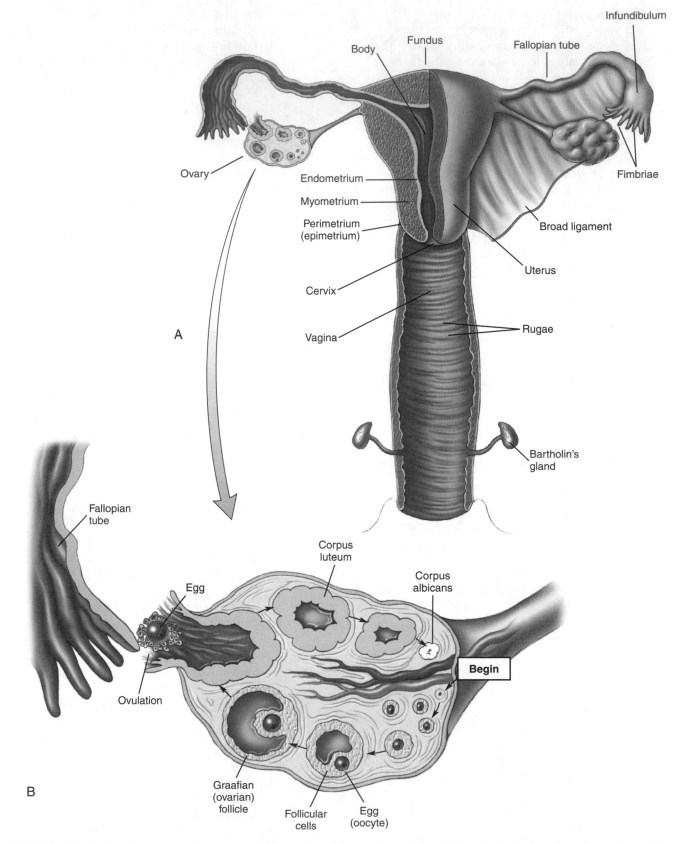

FIGURE 2-39   A, Female reproductive organs. **B,** Maturation of the ovarian follicle. (Herlihy B: *The human body in health and illness,* ed 3, St Louis, 2007, Saunders.)

2. Menstrual cycle
   a. Menses: days 1 to 5; if the ovum is not fertilized, the endometrium is shed
   b. Postmenstrual: days 6 to 13; the endometrium thickens as the ovum matures in the ovary; estrogen levels increase
   c. Ovulation: day 14; the mature ovum is released from the ovary
   d. Premenstrual: days 15 to 28; the corpus luteum develops on the ovary where the ovum was released and secretes progesterone; endometrium thickens in preparation for a fertilized ovum

F. Pregnancy
   1. Ovulation: release of ovum
   2. Insemination: sperm are released into the vagina and travel through the cervix and uterus into the Fallopian tube
   3. Conception: union of sperm and egg; occurs in the Fallopian tube; results in a zygote with 46 chromosomes (23 from ovum, 23 from sperm)
   4. Zygote divides and implants in the uterine wall; becomes an embryo at the third week of development until the end of the eighth week; becomes a fetus at the ninth week until birth
   5. Placenta: highly vascular disk-shaped organ; develops from embryonic and maternal tissues; attaches the developing fetus to the uterus; performs nutrition, excretory, and respiratory functions; excretes HCG for continued pregnancy
   6. Gestation: lasts approximately 40 weeks; three 3-month trimesters
   7. Parturition: childbirth; occurs in three stages:
      a. Onset of contractions to cervical dilation (10 cm)
      b. Dilation to birth of the fetus
      c. Expulsion of the placenta

XVII. COMMON DISEASES AND DISORDERS OF THE BODY SYSTEMS

A. Disease Terminology
   1. Acute: signs and symptoms appear suddenly, persist for a short time, then disappear
   2. Anomaly: a deviation from normal
   3. Chronic: diseases that develop slowly, last for a long time
   4. Communicable: can be transmitted from one person to another
   5. Congenital disorder: abnormal condition that exists at birth
   6. Disease: abnormality in body function that threatens health
   7. Endemic: disease that is native to a local region
   8. Epidemic: disease spreads to many individuals at the same time

9. Etiology: study of the cause of disease
10. Functional: disease with no detectable physical changes to explain the symptoms being experienced by the patient
11. Health: physical, mental and social well-being; disturbance in homeostasis
12. Hereditary disorder: condition caused by a defective gene
13. Idiopathic: diseases with underlying causes
14. Nosocomial: hospital-acquired infection that was not present on admission
15. Organic: disorder in which there are physical changes that explain symptoms being experienced by the patient
16. Pandemic: epidemics that affect large geographic regions
17. Pathogen: microorganism that causes disease
18. Pathology: study of disease
19. Sign: objective abnormalities seen by someone besides the patient
20. Somatoform: presence of physical symptoms that suggest general medical conditions but are not explained by the patient's actual condition
21. Symptom: subjective abnormality felt by the patient
22. Syndrome: collection of different signs and symptoms

B. Mechanisms of Disease (Disturbances to Homeostasis and How the Body Responds)
   1. Genetic mechanism
   2. Pathogenic organisms
   3. Tumors and cancer
   4. Physical and chemical agents
   5. Malnutrition
   6. Autoimmunity
   7. Inflammation
   8. Degeneration

C. Risk Factors (Predisposing Conditions)
   1. Genetic factors
   2. Age
   3. Lifestyle
   4. Stress
   5. Environmental factors
   6. Preexisting conditions

D. Diseases and Disorders of the Integumentary System
   1. Abrasion: scrape
   2. Abscess: localized collection of pus within a circumscribed area; associated with tissue destruction
   3. Acne vulgaris: inflammation of a sebaceous gland; characterized by papules, pustules, and comedos
   4. Actinic keratosis: premalignant lesion of the skin caused by excess exposure to sunlight

5. Albinism: whiteness of skin caused by lack of melanin
6. Alopecia: baldness
   a. alopecia areata: characterized by well-defined bald areas usually on the scalp and face
   b. alopecia capitas totalis: characterized by the loss of all the hair on the scalp
   c. alopecia universalis: total loss of hair on all parts of the body
7. Avulsion: torn-away tissue
8. Bulla: large vesicle
9. Burn: tissue injury resulting from thermal, chemical, electrical, or radioactive agents
   a. First degree: superficial involvement of epidermis; characterized by erythema, tenderness, and pain
   b. Second degree: involves epidermis and dermis; characterized by vesicles
   c. Third degree: involves epidermis, dermis, and injury to underlying tissues; characterized by charring, tissue damage, and loss of fluid
   d. Rule of Nines: method of determining percentage of body surface area affected:
      1) Head and neck = 9%
      2) Torso = 36%
      3) Arms = 18%
      4) Legs = 36%
      5) Genitals = 1%
10. Callus: thickened area of epidermis caused by pressure or friction
11. Carcinoma: skin cancer: caused by exposure to ultraviolet (UV) rays and radiation; types include:
    a. Basal cell: malignant tumor of the basal cell layer of epidermis
    b. Squamous cell: malignant tumor of the squamous epithelial cells of the epidermis
    c. Malignant melanoma: cancerous growth of melanocytes
12. Cellulitis: infection of connective tissue with severe inflammation within the skin layers
13. Cloasma: pigmentation disorder characterized by brownish spots on the face; mask of pregnancy
14. Comedo: papule having a small, dark central region (blackhead) or pale region (whitehead)
15. Contusion: injury that does not break the skin; characterized by swelling, pain and discoloration
16. Cyanosis: blue coloration of the skin due to lack of O_2
17. Cyst: raised or flat fluid-filled or solid-filled sac
18. Decubitus ulcer: bedsore; open lesion caused by poor or no circulation to the area resulting from pressure against the tissue
19. Dermatitis: inflammation of the skin; characterized by pruritus, various lesions, and erythema
    a. Seborrheic dermatitis: chronic dermatitis; caused by an increase in sebaceous secretions; characterized by greasy scales, pruritus, dandruff
    b. Atopic dermatitis: inflammation with rash
    c. Contact dermatitis: inflammation caused by irritant
20. Eczema: dry, leathery vesicles in adults; characteristic pattern on face, neck, elbows, and knees
21. Dermatophytosis: superficial fungal infection; caused by *Tinea* species: lesions are round, scaly, or ring-shaped
    a. *Tinea corporis:* ringworm; involves exposed skin
    b. *Tinea unguium:* involves toenail
    c. *Tinea pedis:* athlete's foot
    d. *Tinea cruris:* jock itch
22. Diaphoresis: excessive sweating
23. Ecchymosis: purplish area caused by bleeding within the skin; a bruise
24. Eczema: an acute or chronic skin inflammation characterized by redness, scales, crusts, and itching
25. Erythema: redness caused by local inflammation or irritation
26. Excoriation: scratch
27. Fissure: crack, groove, or crevice
28. Furuncle: boil
29. Hematoma: bruise; caused by collection of blood under the tissue from a blood vessel injury
30. Hemangioma: benign tumor made up of blood vessels
31. Herpes simplex: cold sore or fever blister; small painful vesicles that erupt around the mouth, lips, nose, or mucous membranes; caused by herpes simplex virus type I
32. Herpes zoster: shingles; acute inflammatory eruption of painful vesicles along the course of a peripheral nerve; caused by herpes zoster virus
33. Hirsutism: excessive hairiness
34. Impetigo: infectious bacterial infection caused by staphylococci or streptococci; vesicles dry to form crusts especially around the mouth and nose
35. Infestation: parasite found on an external surface
36. Jaundice: yellowing of the skin; can be caused by liver, blood, or gallbladder disorders
37. Keloid: abnormal scar formation
38. Lesion: any injury, wound, or area of disease
39. Lipoma: benign fatty deposit under the skin
40. Macule: flat lesion (freckle)

41. Nevus (pl. *nevi*): mole
42. Nodule: raised lesion made of a solid tissue mass
43. Onychocryptosis: ingrown toenail
44. Onychomycosis: fungal infection of the nail
45. Papule: firm, raised lesion (pimple)
46. Pediculosis: infestation by lice (genus: *Pediculus*)
    a. Pediculosis capitas: head lice
    b. Pediculosis corporis: body lice
    c. Pediculosis palpebrarum: infestation of eyebrows and lashes
    d. Pediculosis pubis: "crabs" (genital lice)
47. Petechiae: small pinpoint hemorrhages; smaller versions of bruises
48. Polyp: cyst on a stalk
49. Port-wine stain: large, reddish purple discoloration of the face or neck; present at birth and does not resolve without treatment
50. Pruritus: itching
51. Psoriasis: chronic disease characterized by red lesions and silvery scales; may be autoimmune
52. Pustule: pus-filled vesicle
53. Rosacea: chronic condition of unknown cause that produces redness, tiny pimples and broken blood vessels
54. Scabies: skin infection caused by an infestation with the itch mite
55. Scleroderma: thick, dense, fibrous skin
56. Sebaceous cyst: cyst of a sebaceous gland containing yellow, fatty material
57. Skin tags: small, flesh-colored or light brown growths that hang from the body by fine stalks
58. Ulcer: open sore
59. Urticaria: hives; usually caused by allergic reaction
60. Verruca (pl. *verrucae*): warts; caused by papilloma virus
61. Vesicle: fluid-filled lesion (blister)
62. Vitiligo: white patches on skin caused by lack of melanin production
63. Wheal: circular, raised lesion having central pallor and circumscribed redness
64. Xeroderma: excessively dry skin

E. Diseases and Disorders of the Skeletal System
1. Abnormal spinal curvatures
   a. Scoliosis: abnormal lateral curvature of the spine
   b. Kyphosis: humpback; abnormal outward curvature of the spine
   c. Lordosis: swayback; abnormal inward curvature of the spine
2. Arthralgia: pain in a joint or joints
3. Arthritis: inflammation of the joints
   a. Osteoarthritis: chronic inflammation of joint; results in degeneration of cartilage, which causes hypertrophy of bone
   b. Rheumatoid arthritis: chronic, systemic inflammatory disease of joint; causes erosion of cartilage
   c. Juvenile rheumatoid arthritis: affects children; characterized by pain and swelling in joints, skin rash, fever, slowed growth and fatigue
   d. Gouty arthritis: associated with the formation of uric acid crystals in the joint; gout
4. Ankylosing spondylitis: rheumatoid arthritis of the spine
5. Bursitis: inflammation of the bursa (thin sac that helps tendons and muscles move over bones)
6. Crepitation: crackling sensation that is felt and heard when the ends of a broken bone move together; crepitus
7. Ewing's sarcoma: cancer usually occurring in the diaphyses of the long bones in the arms and legs of children and adolescents
8. Fractures: crack or break in a bone
   a. Simple (closed): fracture with no external wound
   b. Compound (open): fracture with external break in the skin
   c. Greenstick: incomplete break
   d. Comminuted: shattering of the bone (bone fragments)
   e. Impacted: one broken end is forced into the other
9. Lumbago: pain in the lumbar region; low back pain
10. Neoplasms
    a. Osteosarcoma: malignant tumor of connective tissue arising from the bone
    b. Osteochondroma: tumor of bone and cartilage
    c. Chondrosarcoma: tumor of cartilage
11. Osteomalacia: condition of softening of bones; caused by low level of vitamin D
12. Osteomyelitis: inflammation of bone, usually following compound fracture or symptoms
13. Osteoporosis: condition of porous, brittle bones, especially in menopausal and post-menopausal women; caused by low levels of calcium and potassium
14. Paget's disease: osteitis deformans; chronic metabolic disease causing bones to thicken and soften
15. Spina bifida: congenital abnormality characterized by failure of vertebrae to close around the spinal cord
16. Subluxation: partial displacement of a bone from its joint
17. Talipes: club foot

F. Diseases and Disorders of the Muscular System

1. Carpal tunnel syndrome: inflammation of the tendons passing through the carpal tunnel of the wrist
2. Contracture: abnormal shortening of muscle tissues making the muscle resistant to stretching
3. Fasciitis: inflammation of a fascia
4. Intermittent claudication: complex of symptoms including cramplike pain of the leg muscles caused by poor circulation
5. Muscular dystrophy: congenital disorder; characterized by progressive wasting of muscle tissue
   a. Becker's muscular dystrophy: less severe form that does not appear until early adolescence or adulthood
   b. Duchenne's muscular dystrophy: severe form that appears between ages 2 and 6 years of age
6. Myalgia: muscle pain or tenderness
7. Myasthenia gravis: chronic, progressive neuromuscular disease; may be autoimmune; characterized by muscle weakness, dysphagia, and blepharoptosis
8. Rotator cuff tendinitis: inflammation of the tendons of the rotator cuff
9. Shin splint: pain caused by the muscle tearing away from the tibia
10. Spasm: sudden, violent involuntary contraction of a muscle or a group of muscles; cramp
11. Sprain: acute partial tear of a muscle, tendon, or ligament
12. Strain: result of overuse, overstretching, or excessive forcible stretching of a muscle
13. Tendinitis (sometimes spelled *tendonitis*): inflammation of tendon

G. Diseases and Disorders of the Brain and Nervous System and Psychiatric Disorders

1. Addiction: compulsive, uncontrollable dependence on a substance, habit or action to the degree that stopping causes severe emotional, mental or physiologic reactions
2. Alcoholism: chronic dependence or abuse of alcohol with specific signs and symptoms of withdrawal
3. Alzheimer's disease: senile dementia; chronic organic brain syndrome; characterized by degeneration of nervous tissue resulting in lowered intellectual functioning and untimely death
4. Amnesia: disturbance in memory marked by total or partial inability to recall past experiences
5. Amyotrophic lateral sclerosis (ALS); also known as Lou Gehrig's disease; affects motor neurons; characterized by muscle atrophy and weakness

6. Anxiety state: feeling of apprehension, tension or uneasiness that stems from the anticipation of danger, largely unknown or unrecognized
7. Aphasia: inability to speak, write or comprehend speech or the spoken word; often follows a stroke
8. Ataxia: inability to coordinate muscles for voluntary movement
9. Attention deficit disorder: characterized by a child having a short attention span and impulsiveness that are inappropriate for the child's developmental age
10. Attention deficit hyperactivity disorder: characterized by a pattern of inattention and hyperactivity that are inappropriate for the child's developmental age
11. Autism: characterized by a young child's inability to develop normal social relationships, behaves in compulsive and ritualistic ways, and frequently has poor communication skills; autistic disorder
12. Cephalalgia: pain in the head; headache
13. Cerebral palsy: caused by congenital brain defects or injury at birth; characterized by loss of sensation or control of muscle movements
14. Concussion: violent shaking or jarring of the brain
15. Conscious: state of being awake, aware and responding appropriately
16. Convulsion: sudden, violent, involuntary contraction of muscles caused by a disturbance in brain function; seizure
    a. Clonic: state marked by alternate contraction and relaxation of muscles resulting in jerking movements of the face, trunk, and extremities
    b. Tonic: state of continuous muscular contraction that results in rigidity and violent spasms
17. Dementia: slowly progressive decline in mental abilities including impaired memory, thinking and judgment
18. Dyslexia: learning disability characterized by difficulty using and interpreting written forms of communication
19. Encephalitis: inflammation of the brain
20. Epilepsy: abnormal electrical activity of the brain; characterized by random, intense electrical discharges that result in seizure activity
    a. Grand mal: more severe form; characterized by generalized tonic-clonic seizures
    b. Petit mal: milder form; characterized by a sudden, temporary loss of consciousness lasting only seconds
21. Guillain-Barré syndrome: acute rapidly progressive disease of the spinal nerves

22. Hallucination: sense perception that has no basis in external stimulation
23. Hydrocephalus: excessive amount of CSF causing macroencephaly
24. Insomnia: abnormal inability to sleep
25. Lethargy: lowered level of consciousness characterized by listlessness, drowsiness and apathy
26. Major depressive episode: prolonged period during which there is either a depressed mood or the loss of interest or pleasure in activities
27. Manic episode: distinct period during which there is an abnormally, and persistently elevated, expansive and irritable mood
28. Meningitis: inflammation of meninges; can be caused by virus or bacteria
29. Mental retardation: significantly below average general intellectual functioning accompanied by a significant limitation in adaptive functioning
30. Migraine: periodic severe headaches; accompanied by nausea and vomiting, auras, and throbbing pain
31. Multiple sclerosis (MS): chronic inflammation of CNS; attacks myelin sheath causing sensory and motor abnormalities
32. Munchausen syndrome: characterized by the "patient" repeatedly making up clinically convincing simulations of disease for the purpose of gaining attention
    a. Munchausen syndrome by proxy: parent falsifies an illness in a child by making up or creating symptoms and then seeking medical care; form of child abuse
33. Narcolepsy: syndrome characterized by recurrent uncontrollable drowsiness and sleep
34. Neuralgia: pain in a nerve or nerves
35. Neuritis: inflammation of peripheral nerves
36. Obsessive-compulsive disorder: pattern of specific behaviors that are caused by obsessions and compulsions
37. Paralysis: loss of voluntary muscular control and sensation to a body part or organ
    a. Hemiplegia: paralysis of one side of body, often caused by stroke (cerebrovascular accident [CVA])
    b. Paraplegia: paralysis of trunk and lower extremities, caused by spinal cord injury; the area below the injury is paralyzed
    c. Quadriplegia: paralysis of all four extremities
    d. Bell's palsy: paralysis of muscles on one side of face
38. Panic attack: mental state that includes intense feelings of apprehension, fearfulness, terror and impending doom and physical symptoms that include shortness of breath and heart palpitations

39. Parkinson's disease: chronic disease; characterized by tremors and muscle rigidity
40. Poliomyelitis: viral infection of the gray matter of the spinal cord that may result in paralysis
41. Post-polio syndrome: recurrence later in life of some polio symptoms in individuals who have had polio and recovered from it
42. Posttraumatic stress disorder: development of symptoms such as sleep disorders and anxiety after a psychologically traumatic event
43. Schizophrenia: psychotic disorder characterized by delusions, hallucinations, incoherent disorganized speech and disruptive or catatonic behavior
44. Sciatica: inflammation of the sciatic nerve; results in pain along the course of the nerve through the thigh and leg
45. Stroke: CVA; "brain attack"; caused by occlusion or hemorrhage of blood vessels supplying the brain; results in impairment and paralysis of the affected side
    a. Hemorrhagic stroke: damage to brain tissue caused by the rupture of blood vessel within the brain; brain bleed
    b. Ischemic stroke: damage to the brain caused by narrowing or blockage of the carotid artery; CVA
46. Syncope: fainting
47. Tic douloureux: inflammation of the trigeminal nerve characterized by sudden, intense, sharp pain on one side of the face; trigeminal neuralgia
48. Transient ischemic attack (TIA): "mini" stroke; temporary, recurrent episodes of impaired neurological activity; caused by lack of blood flow to the brain

H. Diseases and Disorders of the Eye

1. Amblyopia : dimness of vision or the partial loss of sight without detectable disease of the eye
2. Astigmatism: irregular focusing of light rays caused by a nonspheroid cornea
3. Blepharitis: inflammation of the eyelids
4. Blepharoptosis: drooping of the eyelid
5. Blindness: inability to see
6. Cataract: opaqueness, cloudiness of the lens of the eye
7. Chalazion: a localized swelling of the eyelid resulting from obstruction of one of the oil-producing glands of the eyelid
8. Conjunctivitis: "pinkeye"; inflammation of the conjunctiva
9. Corneal abrasion: an injury, such as a scratch or irritation, to the outer layers of the cornea
10. Detached retina: retina is pulled away from its normal position of being attached to the choroid in the back of the eye
11. Diplopia: double vision

12. Exophthalmos: abnormal protrusion of the eye
13. Glaucoma: accumulation of fluid in the eye: increases pressure that can cause damage to the retina and the optic nerve
14. Hordeolum: "stye"; infection of the sebaceous gland of eye
15. Hyperopia: farsightedness; ability to clearly see far objects but not near objects
16. Keratitis: inflammation of the eyelids
17. Macular degeneration: degenerative disease in the center of the field of vision (macula lutea); affects central vision, not peripheral
18. Myopia: nearsightedness; ability to clearly see near objects but not far objects
19. Nyctalopia: difficulty seeing at night
20. Nystagmus: repetitive involuntary movement of the eye
21. Presbyopia: inability to focus quickly; caused by age-related loss of lens elasticity
22. Refractive disorder: the lens of the eye and cornea do not bend light so they do not focus properly on the retina
23. Retinal detachment: partial or complete separation of the retina from the choroid; results in blindness
24. Retinopathy: any condition of the retina
25. Strabismus: "lazy eye"; inability of both eyes to focus on the same thing
26. Xerophthalmia: drying of the eye surfaces; can result in the loss of the conjunctiva and cornea

I. **Diseases and Disorders of the Ear**
1. Deafness: inability to hear
   a. Conductive: outer or middle ear does not conduct sound vibrations to the inner ear
   b. Noise-induced: damage to the sensitive hairlike cells of the inner ear caused by repeated exposure to intense noise
   c. Sensorineural: caused by problems affecting the inner ear; nerve deafness
2. Impacted cerumen: solidified earwax compacted within the ear canal
3. Meniere's disease: chronic disease of the inner ear; characterized by vertigo, tinnitus, progressive hearing loss, and sensation of fullness, pressure, in the ear
4. Myringitis: inflammation of the tympanic membrane
5. Otalgia: pain in the ear; earache
6. Otitis: inflammation of the ear
   a. Otitis externa: inflammation of the outer ear
   b. Otitis media: inflammation of the middle ear
7. Otosclerosis: bone formation around the oval window and stapes; causes partial to complete deafness
8. Presbycusis: progressive age-related hearing loss

9. Ruptured tympanic membrane: an opening in the eardrum caused by middle ear inflammation caused by sharp objects in the canal or a blow to the ear; major risk is infection developing in the middle ear
10. Tinnitus: ringing in ears
11. Vertigo: dizziness

J. **Diseases and Disorders of the Blood**
1. Anemia: abnormal decrease in hemoglobin, RBC count, or hematocrit
   a. Aplastic: marked absence of all formed elements
   b. Cooley's: group of genetic disorders characterized by short-lived RBCs that lack the normal ability to produce hemoglobin; thalassemia
   c. Hemolytic: RBCs are destroyed faster than they can be replaced
   d. Megaloblastic: bone marrow produces large, abnormal RBCs with a reduced capacity to carry oxygen
   e. Pernicious: autoimmune disorder that results in the ability of the body to absorb vitamin B_{12}
   f. Sickle cell: genetic disorder that causes abnormal hemoglobin that results in the RBCs assuming an abnormal sickle shape
2. Dyscrasia: any abnormal or pathological condition of blood
3. Erythrocytosis: an abnormal increase in the number of circulating RBCs
4. Hemophilia: hereditary bleeding disorders in which one of the factors to clot the blood is missing
5. Hemorrhage: loss of a large amount of blood in a short time
6. Leukemia: malignant neoplasm of blood-forming organs; usually involves one specific type of blood cell
7. Leukopenia: abnormal decrease in the number of WBCs
8. Polycythemia: abnormal increase in hemoglobin, RBC count, or hematocrit
9. Septicemia: presence of pathogenic microorganisms or their toxins in the blood; blood poisoning
10. Thrombocytopenia: decrease in thrombocytes; results in decrease in clotting capabilities

K. **Diseases and Disorders of the Lymphatic System and Immunity**
1. Acquired immunodeficiency syndrome (AIDS): suppression or deficiency of immune system caused by the human immunodeficiency virus (HIV)
2. Anaphylaxis: severe response to a foreign substance

3. Autoimmune disorder: disorder of the immune system in which the body attacks itself
4. Hodgkin's lymphoma: malignant condition of lymphatic tissue in spleen and nodes
5. Inflammation: localized response to tissue injury or destruction
6. Lymphadenitis: inflammation of the lymph nodes; swollen glands
7. Lymphedema: abnormal accumulation of lymph caused by obstruction of vessels; occurs in the extremities
8. Lymphoma: malignancy that develops in the lymphatic system
9. Mononucleosis: acute infectious disease caused by Epstein-Barr virus by direct oral contact
10. Non-Hodgkin's lymphoma: all lymphomas other than Hodgkin's lymphoma

L. Diseases and Disorders of the Cardiovascular System

1. Angina pectoris: chest pain; usually caused by a lack of blood supply to the heart
2. Arrhythmia: irregularity or loss of normal rhythm of the heartbeat; dysrhythmia
3. Aneurysm: abnormal ballooning of a vessel wall
4. Atherosclerosis: formation of fatty plaques along the vessel walls, causing them to narrow; can be the cause of arteriosclerosis
5. Arteriosclerosis: hardening of the arteries; walls of vessels become thick and lose elasticity
6. Bradycardia: abnormally slow heart rate (<60 bpm)
7. Cardiac arrest: unexpected stoppage of the heart function; may follow myocardial infarction (MI)
8. Carditis: inflammation of the heart
9. Congestive heart failure (CHF): characterized by the inability of the heart to keep blood circulating; results in generalized edema
10. Coronary artery disease: atherosclerosis of the coronary arteries that may cause angina, myocardial infarction and sudden death
11. Coronary thrombosis: thrombus blocking a coronary artery
12. Embolism: a blood clot, air, fat globule, or piece of tissue that has broken loose and entered the circulation
13. Endocarditis: inflammation of endocardium, including valves
14. Fibrillation: rapid, random and ineffective contractions of the heart
   a. Atrial fibrillation: atria beat faster than the ventricles
   b. Ventricular fibrillation: irregular contractions of the ventricles; can be fatal if not reversed by electrical defibrillation
15. Flutter: cardiac arrhythmia in which the atrial contractions are rapid but regular
16. Infarct: localized area of tissue death caused by an interruption of the blood supply
17. Hypertension (HTN): high blood pressure (>140/90 mm Hg)
18. Mitral stenosis: narrowing of mitral valve that prevents normal flow of blood from the atrium to the ventricle
19. Mitral valve prolapse: abnormal narrowing of the opening of the mitral valve
20. Myocardial infarction (MI): heart attack; caused by occlusion of coronary vessels that decreases the blood supply to the heart; tissue without blood supply necroses
21. Myocarditis: inflammation of the myocardium
22. Palpitation: pounding or racing heart
23. Patent ductus arteriosus: abnormal opening between the aorta and the pulmonary artery
24. Pericarditis: inflammation of the pericardium
25. Phlebitis: inflammation of a vein
26. Rheumatic heart disease: can be caused by streptococci; causes inflammation of the heart and scarring of the valves; can be the result of rheumatic fever or MI
27. Tachycardia: abnormally rapid heart rate (>100 bpm)
28. Tetralogy of Fallot: congenital heart abnormality; characterized by four abnormalities: ventricular septal defect, pulmonary stenosis, displacement of the aorta to the right, ventricular enlargement
29. Thrombophlebitis: inflammation of a vein accompanied by clot formation
30. Thrombus: blood clot
31. Varicosity (varicose veins): large, twisted, superficial vein; can occur in lower legs, rectum, esophagus

M. Diseases and Disorders of the Respiratory System

1. Acute respiratory distress syndrome (ARDS): type of lung failure resulting from many different disorders that cause pulmonary edema
2. Allergic rhinitis: allergic reaction to airborns allergens that causes an increased flow of mucus
3. Allergy: overreaction by the body to a particular antigen
4. Anoxia: lack of O_2
5. Apnea: lack of breathing
6. Asphyxia: decrease in O_2 intake
7. Asthma: spasms of bronchus; results in dyspnea and wheezing
8. Atelectasis: partial or complete collapse of alveoli
9. Bronchitis: inflammation of bronchi; may be chronic or acute

10. Bradypnea: abnormally slow rate of respiration (<10 breaths per minute)
11. Bronchiectasis: chronic dilation of bronchi or bronchioles
12. Bronchitis: inflammation of the bronchial walls
13. Bruit: an abnormal sound or murmur heard on auscultation
14. Carcinoma: malignant tumor of lung or respiratory system
15. Cheyne-Stokes respiration: alternating episodes of tachypnea and apnea; usually precedes death
16. Chronic obstructive pulmonary disease (COPD) and chronic obstructive lung disease (COLD): a group of disorders characterized by progressive, irreversible obstruction of airflow; major disorders observed include chronic bronchitis, emphysema, and asthma
17. Croup: acute viral infection characterized by barklike cough
18. Cystic fibrosis: genetic disorder in which the lungs are clogged with large quantities of abnormally thick mucus
19. Dyspnea: painful or difficult breathing
20. Emphysema: loss of elasticity and enlargement of alveoli
21. Epistaxis: nosebleed
22. Eupnea: easy, normal breathing
23. Hemoptysis: spitting of blood or blood-stained sputum
24. Hyperpnea: increase in the volume of breathing
25. Hypoxia: decrease in O_2
26. Infectious mononucleosis: mono; acute viral infection caused by Epstein-Barr virus; may include upper respiratory symptoms
27. Influenza: acute, highly contagious viral respiratory infection; spread by respiratory droplets
28. Laryngitis: inflammation of larynx, causes loss of voice
29. Mycoplasma pneumonia: milder but longer lasting form of pneumonia caused by the fungus *Mycoplasma pneumoniae;* walking pneumonia
30. Orthopnea: breathing facilitated by an upright position
31. Pertussis: whooping cough; lung disease caused by *Bordetella pertussis* bacterium; characterized by "whoop"-sounding cough
32. Pharyngitis: inflammation of throat
33. Pleurisy: inflammation of the pleural membranes
34. Pneumonia: inflammation of bronchioles and alveoli; can be viral or bacterial; air sacs fill with pus and other liquid
35. Pneumonitis: inflammation of the lungs
36. Pneumothorax: collection of air in the pleural cavity; may cause the lung to collapse
37. Pulmonary edema: accumulation of fluid in lung tissue
38. Pulmonary embolism: clot located in the pulmonary artery or one of its branches; restricts blood flow to the lungs
39. Rales: crackling sounds on inspiration
40. Respiratory acidosis: decreased pH level of body caused by inadequate removal of CO_2 by the lungs; can progress to tissues outside of the lungs
41. Respiratory alkalosis: increased pH levels caused by excessive removal of CO_2 by the lungs
42. Rhinitis: inflammation of the nose
43. Rhinorrhea: excessive flow of mucus from the nose; runny nose
44. Rhonchus: added lung sound with a musical pitch occurring on inspiration; wheezing
45. Sinusitis: inflammation of paranasal sinuses
46. Smoker's respiratory syndrome: group of symptoms seen in smokers that include a cough, wheezing, vocal hoarseness, pharyngitis, difficult breathing and susceptibility to respiratory infections
47. Stridor: high-pitched sounds on inspiration caused by obstruction
48. Suffocation: prevention of breathing by external causes
49. Tachypnea: abnormal, rapid breathing
50. Tonsillitis: inflammation of the tonsils
51. Tuberculosis (TB): communicable lung disease caused by *Mycobacterium tuberculosis;* characterized by tubercles in the tissue
52. Upper respiratory infection (URI): acute inflammatory process affecting mucous membranes that line the upper respiratory tract

N. Diseases and Disorders of the Digestive System
1. Amebic dysentery: intestinal infection caused by the amoeba *Entamoeba histolytica*
2. Anorexia: lack of appetite
3. Anorexia nervosa: eating disorder characterized by a refusal to maintain a minimally normal body weight and an intense fear of gaining weight
4. Appendicitis: inflammation of appendix
5. Bruxism: involuntary grinding or clenching of the teeth; usually occurs during sleep; is associated with stress and tension
6. Bulimia: eating disorder characterized by episodes of binge-eating followed by self-induced vomiting
7. Celiac sprue: malabsorption syndrome; characterized by intolerance to gluten and damage to intestinal mucosa
8. Cholecystitis: inflammation of the gallbladder

9. Cholelithiasis (gallstones): caused by collection of solid cholesterol or calcium in the gallbladder or bile ducts
10. Cirrhosis: degenerative disease of the liver
11. Colitis: inflammation of the colon
12. Constipation: hard stools resulting in difficulty in defecating
13. Crohn's disease: common chronic inflammatory disease of the GI tract; walls of the bowel become edematous and inflamed
14. Dehydration: condition in which fluid loss exceeds fluid intake; disrupts the body's normal electrolyte balance
15. Dental calculus: hardened dental plaque on the teeth that irritates the surrounding tissues
16. Dental caries: disease process that destroys the enamel and dentin of the tooth; tooth decay; cavities
17. Dental plaque: soft deposit consisting of bacteria and bacterial byproducts that build up on the teeth; major cause of dental caries and periodontal disease
18. Diarrhea: loose, watery stools
19. Diverticulitis: inflammation of pouches (diverticula) in the colon
20. Dyspepsia: indigestion
21. Dysphagia: difficulty in swallowing
22. *E. coli*: intestinal infection caused by *Escherichia coli*; characterized by fever, diarrhea, vomiting and dehydration
23. Emaciated: abnormally thin
24. Emesis: vomiting
25. Eructation: belching
26. Esophageal reflux: upward flow of stomach acid into the esophagus; gastroesophageal reflux disease (GERD)
27. Esophageal varices: enlarged and swollen veins at the lower end of the esophagus
28. Gallstone: hard deposit that forms in the gallbladder and bile ducts
29. Gastritis: inflammation of the stomach
30. Gastroenteritis: inflammation of stomach and intestines
31. Gingivitis: inflammation of the gums
32. Halitosis: unpleasant breath odor; bad breath
33. Hematemesis: vomiting blood
34. Hemorrhoids: inflammation and dilation of surface veins in the rectum and anus
35. Hepatitis: inflammation of the liver; can be acute or chronic
36. Hernia: protrusion of a part of the intestine into an adjacent area or cavity
    a. Hiatal hernia: protrusion of part of the stomach through the esophageal sphincter in the diaphragm
    b. Inguinal hernia: protrusion of a small loop of bowel through a weak place in the lower abdominal wall or groin
37. Intussusception: telescoping of one part of the intestine onto another part just below it
38. Irritable bowel syndrome (IBS): collection of symptoms with no organic cause; characterized by abdominal pain, constipation, and diarrhea
39. Jaundice: yellow discoloration of the skin and tissues caused by greater than normal amounts of bilirubin in the blood
40. Malabsorption syndrome: disease process that inhibits absorption of nutrients
41. Malnutrition: lack of proper food or nutrients; can be due to shortage of food, improper absorption, or distribution of nutrients
42. Melena: black stools containing digested blood
43. Mumps: inflammation of parotid salivary glands
44. Nausea: sensation that leads to the urge to vomit
45. Obesity: an excessive accumulation of fat in the body
46. Pancreatitis: inflammation of the pancreas
47. Periodontal disease: inflammation of the tissues that surround and support teeth
48. Phenylketonuria: genetic disorder in which an essential digestive enzyme is missing
49. Pica: eating disorder characterized by persistent eating of nonnutritional substances
50. Regurgitation: return of swallowed food into the mouth
51. Stomatitis: inflammation of mouth
52. Thrush: yeast infection of the mouth; caused by *Candida albicans*
53. Ulcer: lesion in the mucosa of the stomach or intestine
    a. Duodenal ulcers: peptic ulcers occurring in the upper part of the small intestine
    b. Peptic ulcer: lesion of the mucous membranes of the digestive system caused by the bacterium *Helcobacter pylori*
54. Vincent's angina: (trench mouth); ulcerations of the mucosa of the mouth
55. Volvulus: twisting of the intestine on itself that causes an obstruction

O. Diseases and Disorders of the Urinary System

1. Albuminuria: protein in the urine
2. Anuria: no urine produced
3. Bacteriuria: bacteria in the urine
4. Cystitis: inflammation of the bladder
5. Diuresis: increased excretion of urine
6. Dysuria: difficult or painful urination
7. Enuresis: involuntary discharge of urine
8. Glycosuria: glucose in the urine
9. Hematuria: blood in the urine
10. Incontinence: voiding urine involuntarily
11. Ketonuria: ketones in the urine
12. Nephrolithiasis (renal calculi): kidney stones
13. Nocturia: excessive urination at night
14. Oliguria: scanty urine output

15. Polycystic kidney disease: collecting tubular disease characterized by swollen, fluid-filled sacs; tubules are unable to empty into the renal pelvis
16. Polyuria: excessive urination
17. Proteinuria: protein in the urine
18. Pyuria: pus in the urine
19. Renal failure: kidneys fail to function; may be chronic or acute
20. Urethritis: inflammation of the urethra
21. Urinary tract infection (UTI): mostly caused by gram-negative bacteria; can occur in any organ in the tract

P. Diseases and Disorders of the Endocrine System

1. Acromegaly: hypersecretion of GH after puberty
2. Addison's disease: hyposecretion of cortisol; characterized by hypotension and increased skin pigmentation
3. Adenitis: inflammation of a gland
4. Adenoma: benign tumor of a gland
5. Cretinism: hypothyroidism caused by hyposecretion of thyroxine during infancy; characterized by slow growth, impaired intelligence, and delayed development of secondary sex characteristics
6. Cushing's syndrome: hypersecretion of cortisol; characterized by "moon face," acne, fatty deposits on upper back
7. Diabetes insipidus: hyposecretion of ADH; characterized by polyuria and polydipsia
8. Diabetes mellitus: hyperglycemia; hyposecretion of insulin; characterized by polyuria, polyphagia, and polydipsia
    a. Gestational: occurs during pregnancy and usually disappears after delivery
    b. Type 1: insulin deficiency disorder; insulin-dependent diabetes mellitus
    c. Type 2: insulin resistance disorder; non-insulin-dependent diabetes mellitus
9. Dwarfism: hyposecretion of GH; characterized by abnormally small size
10. Giantism: hypersecretion of GH; characterized by abnormally large size
11. Goiter: enlargement of thyroid gland; caused by iodine deficiency
12. Graves' disease: hyperthyroidism caused by hypersecretion of thyroxine; characterized by weight loss, exophthalmia, nervousness, diaphoresis, and heat intolerance
13. Myxedema: hyposecretion of thyroxine later in life; characterized by fatigue, weight gain, and cold intolerance
14. Polydipsia: excessive thirst

Q. Diseases and Disorders of the Female Reproductive System

1. Amenorrhea: absence of menstruation
2. Anteversion: abnormal tipping, tilting or turning forward of the entire uterus
3. Bacterial vaginosis: bacterial infection of the vagina
4. Breast augmentation: mammoplasty to increase breast size
5. Cervical dysplasia: abnormal growth of cells of the cervix; can be precancerous
6. Cervicitis: inflammation of the cervix
7. Ductal carcinoma in situ: breast cancer at the earliest stage before the cancer has broken through the walls of the duct
8. Dysmenorrhea: painful menstruation
9. Dyspareunia: painful intercourse
10. Endometriosis: growth of endometrial tissue outside of the uterus, usually within the pelvic cavity
11. Fibrocystic breast disease: presence of single or multiple cysts in the breast
12. Fibroid: benign tumor that is found in the muscle of the uterus
13. Infertility: inability of a couple to achieve pregnancy after 1 year of regular, unprotected intercourse
14. Invasive ductal carcinoma: form of cancer that starts in the milk duct, breaks through the duct wall, and invades the fatty tissue of the breast
15. Invasive lobular carcinoma: form of cancer that starts in the milk glands, breaks through the wall of the gland and invades the fatty tissue of the breast
16. Leukorrhea: profuse white discharge from the uterus and vagina
17. Mastitis: inflammation of the breast
18. Menorrhagia: excessive amount of menstrual flow over a longer duration than a normal period
19. Mittelschmerz: pain experienced at the time of ovulation
20. Oligomenorrhea: markedly reduced menstrual flow and abnormally infrequent menstruation
21. Oophoritis: inflammation of the ovary
22. Ovarian cyst: solid or fluid-filled cyst found on the ovary
23. Pelvic inflammatory disease (PID): acute or chronic infection of the female reproductive tract
24. Premenstrual syndrome (PMS): various symptoms that occur before the menstrual period; can include fatigue, irritability, depression, swollen and tender breasts, edema, or cramping
25. Polycystic ovary syndrome: enlargement of the ovaries caused by the presence of many cysts

26. Retroflexion: abnormal tipping of the uterus with the body bent, forming an angle with the cervix
27. Sexually transmitted disease (STD); sexually transmitted infection (STI)
    a. Trichomonas: parasitic infection caused by *Trichomonas vaginalis*
    b. Gonorrhea: highly contagious bacterial infection caused by *Neisseria gonorrhoeae*
    c. Syphilis: highly contagious infection caused by the spirochete *Treponema pallidum*
    d. Genital herpes: highly contagious viral infection caused by herpes simplex virus type 2
    e. Genital warts: highly contagious growths caused by human papillomavirus
    f. Chlamydia: highly contagious bacterial infection caused by *Chlamydia trachomatis*
28. Uterine prolapse: falling or sinking of the uterus until it protrudes through the vaginal opening
29. Vaginal candidiasis: vaginal yeast infection caused by *Candida albicans*
30. Vaginitis: inflammation of the vagina

R. Diseases and Disorders of Pregnancy and Childbirth
1. Abortion: termination of a pregnancy; can be spontaneous (miscarriage) or therapeutic
2. Abruptio placentae: placenta prematurely separates from uterine wall
3. Breech presentation: abnormal birth position in which the buttocks or feet are presented first
4. Eclampsia (toxemia): serious condition of pregnancy characterized by hypertension, edema, and proteinuria; if untreated, may result in seizures and coma
5. Ectopic pregnancy: implantation of fertilized ovum outside of uterus; usually in the fallopian tube
6. Hyperemesis gravidarum: excessive vomiting during pregnancy
7. Lochia: vaginal discharge during the first week or two after childbirth
8. Nulligravida: a woman who has never been pregnant
9. Placenta previa: placenta implants over the cervix
10. Stillbirth: fetus that dies before delivery
11. Twins: two fetuses developing within the uterus at the same time
    a. Fraternal: two embryos resulting from the fertilization of separate ova by separate sperm
    b. Identical: two embryos resulting from the fertilization of a single ovum by a single sperm that has been separated into two separate parts

S. Diseases and Disorders of the Male Reproductive System
1. Anorchism: congenital absence of one or both testicles
2. Azoospermia: absence of sperm in the semen
3. Balanitis: inflammation of the glans penis
4. Benign prostatic hypertrophy (BPH): abnormal growth of prostatic cells causing enlargement of gland
5. Cryptorchism: undescended testes; testes remain in abdomen
6. Epispadias: congenital abnormality in which the opening of the urethra is on the upper surface of the penis
7. Gynecomastia: excessive mammary development in the male
8. Hydrocele: accumulation of fluid in the scrotum
9. Hypospadias: abnormal congenital opening of the urethra on the underside of the penis
10. Impotence: inability to develop or sustain an erection
11. Oligospermia: abnormally low number of sperm in the ejaculate; low sperm count
12. Orchitis: inflammation of the testes
13. Phimosis: narrowing at the opening of the foreskin so it cannot be retracted to expose the glans
14. Prostatitis: inflammation of the prostate
15. Varicocele: varicose vein of the testicles; may cause infertility

T. Tumors and Cancer
1. Benign: tumors that remain localized within the tissues from which they arose
    a. Papilloma: type of tumor that forms fingerlike projections (wart)
    b. Adenoma: tumors of glandular epithelium
    c. Nevus: small, pigmented tumors of the skin (mole)
    d. Lipoma: tumors from adipose tissue
    e. Osteoma: tumor from bone tissue
    f. Chondroma: tumor from cartilage
2. Carcinoma: malignant tumors that come from epithelial tissues
3. Malignant: tumors that spread to other regions of the body; cancer
    a. Melanoma: cancer that involves melanocytes
    b. Adenocarcinoma: malignant tumors of glandular tissue
    c. Lymphoma: cancer of the lymphatic tissue
    d. Osteosarcoma: cancer of bone tissue
4. Metastasis: spreading of malignant cells
5. Neoplasm: "new growth"; abnormal growth of cells
6. Sarcoma: malignant tumor that arises from connective tissue

U. Diseases and Disorders Caused by Pathogens
1. Tuberculosis
   a. Cause: *Mycobacterium tuberculosis*
   b. Transmission: inhalation
   c. Symptoms/signs: cough, hemoptysis, sweats, weight loss
   d. Tests/specimens: sputum culture, radiographs, skin tests
   e. Prevention/immunization: BCG vaccine
2. Urinary tract infection
   a. Cause: *Escherichia coli, Proteus, Pseudomonas aeruginosa*
   b. Transmission: ascends the urethra from contaminated area
   c. Symptoms/signs: frequency, burning, blood in urine, flank pain, fever
   d. Tests/specimens: clean-catch urine for culture
   e. Prevention/immunization: good personal hygiene
3. Legionnaires' disease
   a. Cause: *Legionella pneumophila*
   b. Transmission: grows in water (air conditioning systems)
   c. Symptoms/signs: pneumonia-like symptoms
   d. Tests/specimens: sputum, blood
   e. Prevention/immunization: isolation
4. Tetanus (lockjaw)
   a. Cause: *Clostridium tetani*
   b. Transmission: open wounds, fractures, punctures
   c. Symptoms/signs: toxins affects motor nerves; muscle spasms, convulsions, rigidity
   d. Tests/specimens: blood
   e. Prevention/immunization: DPaP vaccine in childhood; Td every 10 years
5. Gangrene
   a. Cause: *Clostridium botulinum*
   b. Transmission: wounds
   c. Symptoms/signs: gas and watery exudates from wound; blackened tissue
   d. Tests/specimens: swab; aspirate of wound for culture
   e. Prevention/immunization: proper wound care
6. Botulism
   a. Cause: *Clostridium botulinum*
   b. Transmission: improperly cooked canned foods
   c. Symptoms/signs: neurotoxin affects speech, swallowing, vision; paralysis of respiratory muscles; death
   d. Tests/specimens: contaminated food, blood
   e. Prevention/immunization: botulinum antitoxin; boiling canned goods before eating
7. Diphtheria
   a. Cause: *Corynebacterium diphtheriae*
   b. Transmission: respiratory secretions
   c. Symptoms/signs: sore throat, fever, headache, gray membrane in back of throat
   d. Tests/specimens: swabs; Gram stain; culture; Schick test
   e. Prevention/immunization: DTaP in childhood, TaP for adults
8. Whooping cough (pertussis)
   a. Cause: *Bordetella pertussis*
   b. Transmission: respiratory secretions
   c. Symptoms/signs: upper respiratory tract symptoms; high-pitched crowing "whoop"
   d. Tests/specimens: swabs for culture
   e. Prevention/immunization: DTaP in childhood, TaP for adults
9. Pneumonia
   a. Cause: *Streptococcus pneumoniae*
   b. Transmission: direct contact, droplets
   c. Symptoms/signs: productive cause, fever, chest pain
   d. Tests/specimens: culture; Gram stain
   e. Prevention/immunization: vaccine
10. Strep throat
    a. Cause: *Streptococcus pyogenes* (group A strep)
    b. Transmission: direct contact, droplets, fomites
    c. Symptoms/signs: severe sore throat, fever, malaise
    d. Tests/specimens: direct swab; rapid strep tests
    e. Prevention/immunization: none
11. Wound infection, abscesses, boils
    a. Cause: *Staphylococcus aureus*
    b. Transmission: direct contact with carriers, fomites, poor hand washing
    c. Symptoms/signs: area red, warm swollen; pus; pain; ulceration
    d. Tests/specimens: deep swab; aspirate of drainage
    e. Prevention/immunization: none
12. Food poisoning
    a. Cause: *Staphylococcus aureus*
    b. Transmission: poor hygiene, improper refrigeration of foods
    c. Symptoms/signs: vomiting, abdominal cramps, diarrhea
    d. Tests/prevention: suspected foods, stool
    e. Prevention/immunization: refrigerate food to prevent toxin production
13. Toxic shock
    a. Cause: *Staphylococcus aureus*
    b. Transmission: use of absorbent pack material (tampons, nasal packs)
    c. Symptoms/signs: fever, headache, vomiting, delirium, low blood pressure
    d. Tests/prevention: swab, blood
    e. Prevention/immunization: change tampons and packing materials often

14. Gonorrhea
    a. Cause: *Neisseria gonorrhoeae*
    b. Transmission: sexually transmitted
    c. Symptoms/signs: women: pelvic pain, discharge; may be asymptomatic in men: urethral discharge, pain on urination
    d. Tests/specimens: swab of cervix, urethra; rectal and pharyngeal swabs
    e. Prevention/immunization: avoid unprotected sex; abstinence
15. Meningococcal meningitis
    a. Cause: *Neisseria meningitidis*
    b. Transmission: respiratory secretions
    c. Symptoms/signs: high fever, headache, projectile vomiting, delirium, neck and back rigidity
    d. Tests/specimens: nasopharyngeal swabs, CSF culture, blood
    e. Prevention/immunization: vaccine; prophylactic antibiotics
16. Syphilis
    a. Cause: *Treponema pallidum* (spirochete)
    b. Transmission: sexually transmitted
    c. Symptoms/signs: painless sore (chancre), generalized rash
    d. Tests/specimens: blood for VDRL, RPR, FTA-ABS
    e. Prevention/immunization: avoid unprotected sex; abstinence
17. Lyme disease
    a. Cause: *Borrelia burgdorferi* (spirochete)
    b. Transmission: tick bite
    c. Symptoms/signs: fever, joint pain, red bull's-eye rash
    d. Tests/specimens: swab for culture
    e. Prevention/immunization: avoid tick-infected areas
18. Pyloric ulcers
    a. Cause: *Helicobacter pylori*
    b. Transmission: unknown
    c. Symptoms/signs: burning pain in stomach especially between meals
    d. Tests/specimens: blood, stool
    e. Prevention/immunization: unknown
19. Rocky Mountain spotted fever
    a. Cause: *Rickettsia rickettsii*
    b. Transmission: tick bite
    c. Symptoms/signs: headache, fever, chills, characteristic rash on trunk and extremities
    d. Tests/specimens: blood, skin biopsy
20. Atypical pneumonia (walking pneumonia)
    a. Cause: *Mycoplasma pneumoniae*
    b. Transmission: respiratory secretions
    c. Symptoms/signs: fever, cough, chest pain
    d. Tests/specimens: blood, sputum culture
21. Nongonococcal urethritis and vaginitis
    a. Cause: *Chlamydia trachomatis*
    b. Transmission: sexual
    c. Symptoms/signs: may be asymptomatic
    d. Tests/specimens: swabs for DNA probe, serologic testing
22. Inclusion conjunctivitis, pneumonia
    a. Cause: *Chlamydia trachomatis*
    b. Transmission: infected mother during birth
    c. Symptoms/signs: severe conjunctivitis in newborns; afebrile pneumonia in newborns
    d. Tests/specimens: swabs for DNA probe, serological testing
23. Thrush (oral yeast), vulvovaginal candidiasis or monilia (vaginal yeast)
    a. Cause: *Candida* species (yeast)
    b. Transmission: oral: during birth; other: following antibiotic therapy, oral birth control, diabetes
    c. Symptoms/signs: white, cheesy growth
    d. Tests/specimens: swab for KOH prep; cultures
24. Pinworm
    a. *Enterobius vermicularis* (roundworm)
    b. Transmission: fecal-oral
    c. Symptoms/signs: severe rectal itching
    d. Tests/specimens: clear tape applied to perianal area
25. Scabies
    a. Cause: *Sarcoptes scabiei* (itch mite)
    b. Transmission: direct contact, clothing, bedding
    c. Symptoms/signs: nocturnal itching; skin lesions
    d. Tests/specimens: skin scrapings for parasite
26. Lice
    a. Cause: *Pediculus* species
    b. Transmission: direct contact, clothing, bedding
    c. Symptoms/signs: intense itching; skin lesions
    d. Tests/specimens: finding adult lice or eggs (nits) on body or hair
27. Smallpox
    a. Cause: variola major virus
    b. Transmission: direct contact, fomites
    c. Symptoms/signs: vesicles on entire body including soles and palms
    d. Tests/specimens: none
    e. Prevention/immunization: eradicated; vaccine still available
28. Infectious mononucleosis
    a. Cause: Epstein-Barr virus
    b. Transmission: direct, airborne
    c. Symptoms/signs: sore throat, malaise, lymph gland involvement
    d. Tests/specimens: serology for heterophile antibodies; CBC
    e. Prevention/immunization: avoid direct contact

29. Influenza
    a. Cause: myxovirus influenza A and B
    b. Transmission: droplets, fomites
    c. Symptoms/signs: fever, body aches, cough
    d. Tests/specimens: nasopharyngeal swab, nasal wash
    e. Prevention/immunization: immunization for the old, young, and debilitated
30. Warts (veruccae)
    a. Cause: human papillomavirus
    b. Transmission: direct and indirect contact
    c. Symptoms/signs: circumscribed outgrowths on skin
    d. Tests/specimens: scrapings
    e. Prevention/immunization: none
31. Rabies
    a. Cause: rhabdovirus
    b. Transmission: contact with saliva on infected animal
    c. Symptoms/signs.: fever, uncontrollable excitement, spasms of the throat, profuse salivation
    d. Tests/specimens: DFA from brain or hair follicle
    e. Prevention/immunization: vaccine available; vaccinate pets
32. Mumps
    a. Cause: paramyxovirus
    b. Transmission: direct contact
    c. Symptoms/signs: pain and swelling of salivary glands, fever
    d. Tests/specimens: serum titers
    e. Prevention/immunization: MMR vaccine
33. Measles (variola)
    a. Cause: paramyxovirus
    b. Transmission: direct contact, droplets
    c. Symptoms/signs: fever, nasal discharge, red eyes, Koplik's spots, rash
    d. Tests/specimens: serum titers
    e. Prevention/immunization: MMR vaccine
34. German measles (rubella)
    a. Cause: rubella virus
    b. Transmission: direct contact, droplets
    c. Symptoms/signs: rash, swollen lymph glands; can cause severe birth defects
    d. Tests/specimens: serum titer
    e. Prevention/immunization: MMR vaccine
35. Chickenpox (varicella)
    a. Cause: herpesvirus varicella-zoster
    b. Transmission: direct contact
    c. Symptoms/signs: slight fever, malaise, clear vesicles
    d. Tests/specimens: clinical signs
    e. Prevention/immunization: varicella vaccine
36. Common cold
    a. Cause: rhinovirus
    b. Transmission: direct, droplets
    c. Symptoms/signs: headache, fever, runny nose, congestion
    d. Tests/specimens: none
    e. Prevention/immunization: good hygiene
37. Polio
    a. Cause: poliovirus
    b. Transmission: direct contact
    c. Symptoms/signs: fever, headache, stiff neck and back, paralysis of muscles
    d. Tests/specimens: none
    e. Prevention/immunization: IPV vaccine

Psychology and Stages of Human Growth and Development

I. MAJOR THEORISTS

A. Sigmund Freud

1. Provided the foundation from which all other psychological theories developed
2. Believed that infancy and childhood are the critical periods for psychological development
3. Psychoanalytical theory: theory of personality development that includes:
   a. Levels of awareness
      1) Conscious: experiences within one's immediate awareness; reality-based
      2) Subconscious: stores memories, thoughts, and feelings
      3) Unconscious: closed to one's awareness
   b. Components of the personality
      1) Id: body's basic primitive urges
      2) Ego: closely related to reality
      3) Superego: further development of ego; makes judgments; controls and punishes
   c. Psychosexual stages of development
      1) Oral stage: birth to end of first year of life; mouth is the source of all comfort and pleasure
      2) Anal stage: end of first year of life to third year; elimination gives pleasure and satisfaction
      3) Phallic stage: ages 3 to 6; associates pleasure and conflict with genital organs; Oedipus complex (boy's unconscious sexual attraction to his mother) and Electra complex (girl's unconscious sexual attraction to her father) develop
      4) Latency stage: ages 6 through 12; sexual urges are dormant; peer relationships develop with the same sex
      5) Genital stage: begins at puberty; body is preparing for reproduction; sexual attraction and heterosexual relationships begin

B. Erik Erikson

1. Broadened Freud's theory of personality development

2. Psychosocial theory: eight stages
   a. Trust versus mistrust: birth to 18 months; to develop a basic trust in the mothering figure and to be able to generalize it to others
   b. Autonomy versus shame and doubt: 18 months to 3 years; to gain self-control and independence within the environment
   c. Initiative versus guilt: 3 to 6 years; to develop a sense of purpose and the ability to initiate and direct the individual's own activities
   d. Industry versus inferiority: 6 to 11 years; to achieve a sense of self-confidence by learning, competing, performing successfully, and receiving recognition from others
   e. Identity versus role confusion: 12 to 20 years; to integrate the tasks mastered in the previous stages into a secure sense of self
   f. Intimacy versus isolation: 20 to 30 years; to form an intense, lasting relationship or a commitment to another person, cause, institution, or creative effort
   g. Generativity versus stagnation: age 30 to 65; to achieve the life goals established for oneself while considering the welfare of future generations
   h. Ego integrity versus despair: age 65 to death; to review the individual's life and derive meaning from both positive and negative events while achieving a positive sense of self-worth

C. Jean Piaget

1. Cognitive development
2. Concerned with acquisition of intellect and development of thought processes
3. Believed that the child's cognitive abilities progress through four stages:
   a. Sensorimotor stage: birth to 2 years; acquires knowledge through exploration of the environment; attaches meaning and recognition of things
   b. Preoperational stage: 2 to 6 years; develops language; child sees him or herself as the center of the universe

   c. Concrete operational stage: 6 to 12 years; begins to solve problems and to think logically; becomes less egocentric and more social

   d. Formal operational stage: 12 to 15 years; ability to think logically in hypothetical and abstract terms; cognitive maturity achieved

D. Abraham Maslow

1. Described human behavior as being motivated by needs that are ordered in a hierarchy
2. Believed people must meet their most basic needs before they can move up the hierarchy to any higher level
3. Hierarchy begins at the bottom with basic survival needs and moves to the top with more complex needs
   a. Physiologic needs: basic fundamental needs; includes food, water, elimination, air, sleep, exercise, shelter, and sexual expression
   b. Safety and security: these needs are for avoiding harm and maintaining comfort, order, structure, physical safety, protection, and freedom from fear
   c. Love and belonging: needs for giving and receiving affection, companionship, satisfactory interpersonal relationships, and identification with a group
   d. Self-esteem: seeks self-respect and respect from others, works to achieve success and recognition within the group, and desires prestige from accomplishments
   e. Self-actualization: possesses a feeling of self-fulfillment and the realization of the person's highest potential

E. Lawrence Kohlberg

1. Introduced a theory of moral development
2. Expanded on Piaget's theory
3. Believed that the child progressively develops moral reasoning as he or she gains the ability to think logically
4. Identified three levels of moral development, subdivided into six stages of acquired moral reasoning:
   a. Level 1: preconventional thinking; ages 4 to 10; the child learns reasoning through parents' demands for obedience; begins to recognize right from wrong
      1) Stage 1: obedience and punishment orientation
      2) Stage 2: instrumental relativist orientation
   b. Level 2: conventional thinking; ages 10 to 13; the child begins to seek approval from society; influenced by external forces such as peers and environment
      1) Stage 3: interpersonal concordance orientation
      2) Stage 4: law and order orientation

   c. Level 3: postconventional thinking; postadolescence; develops own moral code based on adult principles
     1) Stage 5: social contract legalistic orientation
     2) Stage 6: universal ethical principle orientation

F. Elisabeth Kübler-Ross

1. Identified stages of dying
2. Can also apply to the grieving process
3. Stages:
   a. Denial: direct denial or periods of disbelief
   b. Anger: realization of what is happening; may display rage
   c. Bargaining: attempts to make deals with a deity
   d. Depression: may show signs and symptoms such as withdrawal, lethargy, and periods of crying
   e. Acceptance: comes to accept the facts and fate

G. Carl Jung

1. Understanding of psyche through examination of dreams, art, mythology, religion, and philosophy
2. Pioneer in field of dream analysis; studied with Freud
3. Concepts:
   a. Archetype: reconciliation between the individual and the broader world through symbolic language (art, dreams, drama, and religion)
   b. Collective unconscious: humans have a shared psychological predisposition; revealed through examination of symbolic communication (art, dreams, religion, and myth)
   c. Anima (female) and animus (male): components of both sexes
   d. Introvert (finding meaning within) and extrovert (finding meaning in the outside world)
   e. Family systems theory: family members who are type-alike form allies; persons who are unlike are naturally in conflict; children who have preference different from parents may be coerced into a false personality; the child may resist, and conflict may occur

II. STAGES OF LIFE CYCLE

A. Basic Principles of Growth and Development

1. Each person is unique from the time of conception
2. Growth is continuous
3. Skills increase as physical size increases
4. Development depends on a balance among physical, mental and psychosocial changes
5. If basic needs are not met, growth pattern is altered

B. Basic Categories of Growth and Development through the Lifespan
1. Physical growth
   a. Physical size
   b. Motor and sensory skills
2. Mental growth
   a. Cognitive development
   b. Thinking
   c. Understanding
3. Psychosocial growth
   a. Emotional development
   b. Social development

C. Newborn to 1 Year
1. Physical characteristics:
   a. Head is larger in proportion to the rest of the body at birth; fontanelles close between 12 and 18 months
   b. Birth weight doubles by 5 to 6 months and triples by the first year
   c. Teething begins at approximately 5 to 6 months
   d. Senses are present at birth and develop more fully during the first year
   e. Blood pressure increases, and pulse and respiration decrease as the child ages
2. Developmental milestones:
   a. Gross motor skills (involve large muscles of the arms and legs)
      1) 2 months: controls head
      2) 3 months: sits without support
      3) 7 months: sits alone
      4) 10 months: creeps
      5) 9 to 11 months: stands without support
      6) 12 to 15 months: walks alone
   b. Fine motor skills (refined use of hands and fingers)
   c. Psychosocial (Erikson's stages of growth and development)
   d. Cognitive (mostly sensorimotor; heightened use of touch, taste, sight, hearing, and smell)

D. Toddlerhood (1 to 3 Years)
1. Physical characteristics:
   a. Grows up to 3 inches each year
   b. Gains 4 to 6 pounds each year
   c. Extremities grow faster than the trunk
   d. Face and jaw grow bigger to permit room for more teeth
   e. Bones begin to ossify
   f. Visual acuity developing; hearing is fully developed
2. Developmental milestones:
   a. Gross motor skills
      1) Depends on growth and maturation of muscles, bones, and nerves
      2) Can usually run, and walk up steps using both feet

   b. Fine motor skills
      1) Puts simple puzzles together
      2) Can turn knobs and open jar lids
   c. Psychosocial
      1) Attached to mother; tolerates short separation
      2) Dresses and undresses self
      3) Nearly toilet trained
   d. Cognitive
      1) Searches for and finds toys
      2) Locates body parts
      3) Gives full name on request
   e. Language
      1) Uses words and gestures to indicate needs
      2) Uses two-word sentences
      3) Initiates sounds and words
      4) Can sing simple songs
      5) Vocabulary of approximately 1000 words

E. Preschool (3 to 6 Years)
1. Physical characteristics:
   a. Trunk and body lengthen in proportion to rest of body
   b. Gains 5 to 7 pounds each year
   c. Grows 2½ to 3 inches each year
   d. Deciduous teeth may begin to fall out; dental health is important
   e. Visual acuity improves to 20/20; frequent ear infections
2. Developmental milestones:
   a. Gross motor skills
      1) Able to walk and run on tiptoes
      2) Able to hop and to balance on one foot
      3) May begin certain sports such as soccer, baseball, skating, and dance
   b. Fine motor skills
      1) Manages self-care activities
      2) Manipulates clothing and clothing fasteners with ease
      3) Handles eating utensils; can begin to learn table manners
      4) Can draw faces, copy letters, and print own name
   c. Psychosocial
      1) Learns to trust
      2) Aware of genital organs and sexual identity
      3) Needs discipline and limits
   d. Cognitive
      1) Longer attention span than as toddler
      2) Develops memory
      3) Can pretend
   e. Language
      1) Becomes talkative
      2) May show some difficulty with pronunciation
      3) Can recite full name, address, and telephone number
      4) Imitates others

F. School Age (6 to 11 Years)
  1. Physical characteristics:
     a. Growth is steady but slows
     b. Permanent teeth appear
     c. Weight increases by 4½ to 6½ pounds each year
     d. Height increases by 2 to 3 inches each year
     e. Visual maturity achieved; peripheral vision and depth perception improve
     f. Immune system matures
  2. Developmental milestones:
     a. Gross motor skills
        1) Increase in muscle mass improves skills
        2) Gender differences exist in motor skills
     b. Fine motor skills
        1) Can print and begins to master script writing
        2) Can throw and catch
        3) Can begin to learn to play musical instruments
     c. Psychosocial
        1) Outgoing, talkative, and enthusiastic
        2) Fearlessness puts child at risk for injury
        3) Sexual curiosity continues
        4) Initiates a task and able to see it through to completion
        5) Sibling rivalry can occur
        6) Peers are more important than family
        7) Privacy becomes important
        8) Emotions have wide range of expression
     d. Cognitive
        1) Has collections of stickers, books, and sports cards
        2) Breaks things down into small parts and reassembles them
        3) Takes views of others into consideration
        4) Understands concepts of time, space, and dimension
        5) Starts and continues formal education
     e. Language
        1) Use of language and communication techniques improve
        2) Language becomes important for socialization
        3) Can use proper parts of speech, proper tense of words

G. Adolescence (11 to 19 Years)
  1. Puberty (ages 11 to 14); puberty ends and adolescence begins with the onset of menses (menarche) in girls and sperm production in boys
     a. Rapid physical growth
     b. Changes in body proportions; trunk and limbs grow swiftly
     c. Development of primary sexual characteristics
     d. Development of secondary sexual characteristics

  2. Physical characteristics:
     a. Puberty is the period of the greatest amount of rapid growth; growth slows after puberty
     b. Muscular strength increases greatly
     c. Epiphyseal line closes in long bones; growth nearly complete
     d. Trunk broadens at the hips and shoulders
     e. Posture may be poor from the fast growth; slouching
     f. Sexual growth and development are completed
     g. Shows great concern about one's changing body
     h. Sebaceous glands produce more oil and become larger
     i. Changes in fat distribution
  3. Developmental milestones:
     a. Motor development
        1) Comparable to adult
        2) Hand-eye coordination improves
     b. Sexual development
        1) Heightened emotions
        2) Increased worries
        3) Lack of self-confidence
        4) Sex is given high priority; girls set limits on interactions
        5) Good sex education enables responsible choices
     c. Psychosocial
        1) Rebelliousness, argumentative, or rude
        2) Egocentric
        3) Need for privacy
        4) Dishonesty
        5) Responsibility
        6) Curfews
        7) Friends
        8) Self-absorbed
        9) Society places many demands
        10) Discipline is important
     d. Cognitive
        1) Maturation of central nervous system leads to formal operational thought processes (logical thought)
        2) School is at the center of development
        3) Moral reasoning and spiritual awareness develop
     e. Communication
        1) Vocabulary increases
        2) Verbal communication allows thoughts and beliefs to be known
        3) Development of common language typical to a group, time, and culture (slang)

H. Early Adulthood (20 to 40 Years)
  1. Physical characteristics:
     a. Physical growth is completed
     b. Men usually have more muscle mass
     c. Wisdom teeth erupt; may need to be removed
     d. Other body systems begin to decline at the end of this period

2. Developmental milestones:
   a. Major milestones include choosing and establishing a career, fulfilling sexual needs, establishing a family and a home, expanding social circles, and developing maturity
      1) Motor development
         a) Peak physical efficiency reached
         b) Physical efficiency declines toward the end of this period
      2) Sexual development
         a) Sexuality established
         b) Ability to experience and share love
      3) Psychosocial development
         a) Strong sense of identity
         b) Sharing of innermost thoughts
         c) Career and work roles understood
      4) Cognitive development
         a) No longer egocentric, as a rule
         b) Can solve problems and process information
         c) Attends college or vocational school
      5) Health concerns
         a) Pap smear
         b) Mammography and breast self-examination
         c) Testicular self-examination
         d) Cholesterol
         e) Obesity
         f) Stress
         g) Family planning

I. Middle Adulthood (Mid-40s to Early 60s)
   1. Physical characteristics:
      a. May lose height
      b. Body contour changes; higher percentage of body fat
      c. Visual and aural acuity decline
      d. Skin becomes less elastic; wrinkles form
      e. Gradual loss of taste
   2. Developmental milestones:
      a. Sexual development
         1) Menopause and loss of reproductive capacity
         2) Options, opportunities, and means of sexual expression may change
      b. Psychosocial development
         1) Achievement of goals
         2) Desire to serve the larger community
         3) Family roles may change from child-centered to couple-centered roles
         4) Grandparenting
         5) Change in relationship with parents
         6) Peak earning capacity
      c. Cognitive development: capable of thinking in a concrete manner

J. Late Adulthood (Age 65 to Death)
   1. Physical characteristics:
      a. Quality of life depends on the person's ability to perform activities of daily living (ADL)

   b. Formation and composition of body changes
   c. Body systems begin to decline
   d. Sensory systems become less efficient
   e. Problems with memory loss and learning difficulty develop
   2. Developmental milestones:
      a. Motor development
         1) Movement slows
         2) Fine motor skills affected by stiffening of the joints
      b. Sexual development: capable of enjoying a satisfying sexual relationship
      c. Psychosocial development
         1) Ego integrity achieved
         2) Life review reassures about accomplishments and worth
         3) Body image changes
         4) Fear of loss of independence
         5) Death of a spouse produces change of roles
         6) Work and leisure activities change
         7) Concept of death takes on a different meaning
      d. Cognitive development
         1) Healthy persons retain cognitive abilities
         2) Memory changes; short-term stores less than long-term

III. THE SICK ROLE

A. General
   1. Illness or injury forces the patient to adopt the sick role; includes duties and rights
   2. Duties include:
      a. To make every effort to get well
      b. To seek professional help, and cooperate to get well
   3. Rights include:
      a. Exemption from responsibility for injury or illness
      b. Exemption from normal social obligations

B. Sick Role May Bring Benefits
   1. Financial protection: disability, workers' compensation
   2. Social gain: sympathy and attention

C. Sick Role May Bring Detriment
   1. Uncertainty about the future
   2. Creation of social stigmas
   3. Loss of independence
   4. Loss of privacy
   5. Loss of income
   6. Loss of body image and self-esteem
   7. Loss of social role

D. Terminally Ill or Dying Patient Has Special Needs
   1. Kübler-Ross' stages of dying
   2. Excessive stress

IV. THE PROVIDER ROLE

A. Empower the Patient

B. Do Not Undermine the Patient's Participation in His or Her Care

C. Provider-Patient Relationship Is Unequal
1. Provider is responsible for:
   a. Concern for the patient's well-being
   b. Carrying out ethical duties
   c. Respect for each patient as an individual
   d. Knowing what is important to the patient
   e. Assisting patient in adapting to the sick role
   f. Assuming cooperation from the patient
   g. Displaying confidence
   h. Promoting and encouraging proper patient behavior

D. Issues in the Provider-Patient Relationship May Occur
1. May be the result of:
   a. Personal bias: describes a person's feelings toward a patient or a thing
   b. Prejudice: strong adverse attitude toward a patient because of that patient's association with a particular group
   c. Overidentification: "I know how you feel"; difficulty seeing the patient as an individual
   d. Countertransference: response to the patient in a personal manner, such as a child or sibling
   e. Transference: overdependence by the patient on the provider

E. Cultural Differences Are Important In Provider-Patient Relationship
1. The medical assistant needs to be aware of various cultural norms for optimum care and optimal patient comfort

I. COMMUNICATION

A. Definition of Communication
1. The process of sharing meaning

B. Communication Process
1. Source
   a. Sender of the message
   b. Can be a person, a group, or a company
   c. What is sent varies and is affected by the sender's experiences
2. Message
   a. What is sent by the source
   b. Message has three parts:
      1) Meaning: usually ideas or feelings
      2) Symbols: words or actions that represent the meaning; the process of turning words or actions into symbols is *encoding*
      3) Organization or form: syntax and grammar of the message; putting the symbols in order
3. Channel
   a. Which symbols are given
   b. Can be visual, audio, print, or touch
4. Receiver
   a. Where the message is being sent
   b. Receiver processes into meaning (*decoding*)
5. Feedback
   a. Response of the receiver
   b. Can be verbal or nonverbal
   c. Tells the source if the message was heard, seen, or understood
6. Noise
   a. Anything that interferes with the communication process
   b. Can be:
      1) External: stimuli that draws attention away from the message
      2) Internal: personal thoughts and feelings that draw a person away from the message
      3) Semantic: message symbols that prevent the meaning from being understood (accents, dialect, grammar)

C. Therapeutic Communication
1. Process of relaying information from health care provider to patient
2. Can be through verbal disclosure, touch, or gesture
3. Techniques include:
   a. Acknowledgment: emphasizes the importance of the patient in the communication process
   b. Establishing guidelines: helps the patient know what is expected of him or her
   c. Focusing: directs the communication toward important topics
   d. Listening: communicates interest in the topics raised by the patient
   e. Open-ended comments: helps the patient to decide what is relevant; encourages discussion ("Describe what you think is going to happen.")
   f. Reflecting: shows the importance of the patient's ideas and feelings
   g. Restating: lets the patient know how the health care provider interpreted the message the patient sent ("I hear you saying...")
   h. Clarification: demonstrates the desire to understand what the patient is communicating (may ask who, what, where, when)
   i. Silence: communicates acceptance
4. Ineffective techniques include:
   a. Advising: telling what the patient should do
   b. Minimizing: health care provider making light of the patient's situation
   c. Defending: health care provider protecting self from criticism
   d. Stereotyping: health care provider using clichés when responding
   e. Probing: health care provider discussing, or trying to discuss, topics the patient does not want to discuss
   f. Approval and disapproval: health care provider overly approving or disapproving of the patient's behavior
   g. Agreeing and disagreeing: health care provider overly agreeing or disagreeing with the patient's perceptions, thoughts, or feelings

5. Barriers to communication
   a. Embarrassment: patient may be in awe of the health care provider, thereby being embarrassed to ask questions of the health care provider
   b. Discomfort: patient may be uncomfortable or ashamed to discuss patient's private body parts or symptoms
   c. Communication difficulties: patient can see disabilities as making the patient intellectually inferior
   d. Withdrawal: patient does not respond to health care provider's communication
   e. Ineffective techniques (see number 4) by health care provider may raise barriers
   f. Physical impairment: physical impairments that may limit the ability to communicate
   g. Language: non-English speaking patients may require more gestures and body language
   h. Prejudice: unfair treatment of a person because of race, age, gender, religion, handicap, or any other reason
   i. Stereotyping: application of a standardized mental picture
   j. Perception: capacity for comprehension

D. **Nonverbal Communication**
   1. Messages conveyed without the use of words
   2. Body language
   3. Involves the health care provider's grooming, dress, eye contact, facial expressions, hand gestures, space, tone of voice, and posture

II. PATIENT RELATIONSHIPS

A. **General**
   1. Medical assistant needs to understand the patient's concerns, needs, and reactions
   2. Stress and anxiety are common patient responses
   3. First impressions are lasting impressions

B. **Unconscious Defense Mechanisms**
   1. Compensation: overemphasizing a trait to make up for a failure
   2. Denial: avoiding reality
   3. Displacement: shifting an impulse from a threatening to a nonthreatening one
   4. Dissociation: disconnecting the significance from an event
   5. Identification: mimicking the behavior of another
   6. Introjection: adopting the feelings of others
   7. Projection: assigning the person's own feelings to another as if these feelings had originated with the other person
   8. Rationalization: justifying the person's thoughts, feelings, or behavior

9. Regression: returning to a former behavior or more immature behavior
10. Repression: putting unpleasant thoughts or events out of the person's mind
11. Sarcasm: biting edge added to words that are said; can be hostile and cruel
12. Sublimation: diverting unacceptable thoughts or feelings into acceptable behaviors
13. Substitution: making up for a deficiency by concentrating on another
14. Suppression: deliberately forgetting or avoiding dealing with an unpleasantness
15. Verbal aggression: attacking another without addressing the original complaint or disregarding it; loudly lashes out verbally

C. **Interaction with Patients**
   1. Interaction is a therapeutic relationship
   2. Assists patients to resolve problems and achieve goals
   3. Maximizes patient comfort
      a. Children
         1) Establish a friendly relationship
         2) Be aware of your own feelings toward children in general
         3) Speak in quiet tones; speak at the child's physical level (not looking down at the child)
         4) Use language appropriate for the child's age
         5) Allow the child to assist in his or her treatment
         6) Keep the child patient from experiencing long waits
         7) Understand that the child may regress when ill
         8) Be truthful with the child, which fosters trust
         9) Offer rewards for proper behavior
         10) Allow the child to play with the health care provider's equipment if doing so is safe and appropriate
         11) Infants should be held and comforted before any treatment procedures
      b. Adolescents
         1) Patient demands independence yet requires comfort
         2) Permit patient's privacy
         3) Health care provider must allow examinations with the patient's parent present
         4) Treat the patient with respect and dignity
         5) Set fair limits for the patient
         6) Answer the patient's questions openly and honestly
         7) Explain the procedures to the patient in terms he or she will understand

c. Elderly patient
   1) Allow additional time with the patient; this circumstance may be a social interaction for a lonely patient
   2) Keep the patient physically and environmentally comfortable
   3) Patient may find comfort in a health care provider's routine
   4) Allow as much independence as possible
   5) Do not overprotect or be overattentive
   6) Speak slowly and precisely, but do not patronize
d. Terminally ill patient
   1) Help both the patient and the patient's family adjust to the patient's loss in strength, sensation, mobility, and endurance
   2) Give support to the patient's family members
   3) Be willing to listen
   4) Patient will likely experience some, or all, of the stages of dying
e. Angry patient
   1) Patient's anger may be caused by the patient's medical condition
   2) Health care provider's goal is to calm the patient
   3) Health care provider must remain calm, firm, and direct
   4) Health care provider must not take the anger personally
   5) Health care provider must listen closely to the patient's concerns
   6) Health care provider must keep speaking tone calm and in control
   7) Keep the angry patient out of public areas of the office; escort the angry patient to a private room
f. Sensory-impaired patient
   1) Patient may need an interpreter (if hearing impaired or if speaks only a foreign language) to assist in communication
   2) Health care provider should be positioned directly in front of the patient and should speak slowly
   3) For the sight-impaired patient, the health care provider should ask how best to assist the patient
   4) Health care provider should be flexible, open, and supportive
g. Frightened patient
   1) A frightened patient may be uncooperative
   2) Health care provider should recognize fear and assist the patient in dealing with the fright
   3) Health care provider should maintain control of the situation

h. Depressed patient
   1) The depressed patient will experience feelings of gloom, hopelessness, and dread and may have feelings of no self-worth
   2) Health care provider should provide sympathy, support, and a friendly ear
   3) Health care provider should demonstrate an interest in the patient's needs
   4) Health care provider should keep the environment secure and nonthreatening
i. Suicidal patient
   1) Suicidal feelings can be the patient's final response to his or her depression
   2) Suicidal patient may disclose intentions to the health care provider
   3) All suicidal threats or attempts must be taken seriously
   4) Health care provider must listen closely to the suicidal patient
   5) Health care provider should demonstrate empathy
   6) Health care provider should seek professional advice or actions for the suicidal patient
j. Mentally impaired patient
   1) Patient may be confused and disoriented
   2) By correcting the patient's confusion, the health care provider may make the patient less frightened
   3) Health care provider must treat the patient kindly but must not be condescending
k. Abused patient
   1) Health care provider must treat the abused patient's physical injuries first
   2) Health care provider must focus on the patient as a victim; health care provider should express assurances of the patient's self-worth
   3) Refer the abused patient to existing social agencies
l. Drug-dependent patient
   1) Health care provider should not belittle the patient for the patient's behavior
   2) Health care provider should be compassionate, empathetic, and patient
   3) Health care provider should involve the patient's family in the patient's treatment
m. Significant others
   1) Part of the patient's emotional support group
   2) Health care provider should respect the wishes of the patient concerning the patient's loved ones
   3) Health care provider should keep any waiting relatives notified of progress and keep them informed of any delays

4) Health care provider should address the concerns of the patient's family and friends

5) Health care provider must be aware of confidentiality issues

D. Multicultural Issues
1. Causes of illness
2. Treatment and traditional practices
3. Behavioral requirements

Law, Ethics, and HIPAA   5

I. INTRODUCTION TO THE LAW

A. Definition of Law
1. System by which society gives order to our lives

B. Functions of Law
1. Regulate: controls rules and standards
2. Punish: enforce penalties for infractions of rules and standards
3. Remedy: make wrongs that are committed right
4. Benefit: help society

C. Sources of Law
1. Common law: derived from the customs of society and court decisions
2. Administrative law: derived from agencies that enact state and federal law
3. Constitutional law: derived from the U.S. Constitution
4. Statutory law: derived from state and federal legislation

D. Types of Law
1. Civil law: a wrong, or perceived wrong, committed against a person or to property; civil law that affects the practice of medicine include:
   a. Contract law: governs enforceable promises
   b. Tort law: governs intentional or accidental acts that bring harm to a person or that damage property
   c. Administrative law: governs regulations set forth by governmental agencies
2. Criminal law: a wrong committed against a person or to property in violation of a statute or ordinance; criminal laws that may affect the practice of medicine include:
   a. Infraction: a minor offense that usually results only in a fine
   b. Misdemeanor: violation of a law that includes as punishment a maximum imprisonment of no more than 1 year
   c. Felony: a major crime that includes as punishment imprisonment of more than 1 year

II. LICENSURE, REGISTRATION, CERTIFICATION

A. Licensure
1. Strongest form of administrative regulation
2. Mandatory credential to practice medicine
3. Granted by a state board; verifies that the person holding the license has met minimum standards; for physicians, defined by the Medical Practice Act; for licensed nurses, defined and governed by the Nurse Practice Act
   a. State statute that defines what is included in the practice of medicine within that state
   b. Governs the methods and requirements of licensure and establishes grounds for suspension and revocation of the license
4. Physicians can be licensed through:
   a. Examination: passing a written or oral examination
   b. Endorsement: acceptance of a national examination score
   c. Reciprocity: one state accepts another state's license
5. Licenses may be revoked or suspended for:
   a. Conviction of a misdemeanor or a felony
   b. Unprofessional conduct
   c. Personal or professional incapacity
6. License must be periodically renewed (if not renewed, will be suspended from practice)

B. Registration
1. Medical assistants can be registered
2. Voluntary process
3. Professional listed on a state or national registry
4. Process similar to certification
5. Usually accomplished by a written examination

C. Certification
1. Medical assistants can be certified
2. Voluntary process
3. Identifies a professional as meeting minimum standards to be able to practice
4. Usually accomplished by written examination
5. Governed by a professional organization

III. REGULATING ISSUES FOR THE MEDICAL OFFICE

A. CLIA '88
1. Clinical Laboratory Improvement Act (CLIA '88) of 1988
2. Identifies standards for laboratory testing
3. Any facility performing laboratory testing is subject to CLIA regulations

B. CON
1. Certificate of need
2. Process of acquiring approval, based on need to the community, to expand service

C. TJC
1. The Joint Commission (formerly the Joint Commission on Accreditation of Healthcare Organizations)
2. Accreditation of health care facilities

D. OSHA
1. Occupational Safety and Health Administration
2. Regulation of safety in the workplace

E. ADA
1. Americans with Disabilities Act
2. Sets up rules protecting people with physical or mental disability from being discriminated against

IV. CONSENT

A. Definition of Consent
1. Voluntary permission given by a capable person to receive medical care

B. Types
1. Express: oral or written expression of consent
2. Implied: actions or behavior that can be reasonably presumed to express consent

C. Informed Consent
1. Physician, or other caregiver, has an affirmative duty to explain to the patient information necessary to allow the patient to evaluate the medical care and make decisions on that information before having the medical care performed; implies an understanding of:
   a. What procedure is to be done
   b. Why the procedure should be done
   c. The risks involved in performing the procedure
   d. The expected benefits of having the procedure performed
   e. Any alternative treatments that can be performed
   f. The risks involved in performing the alternative treatment

D. Who May and May Not Give Consent
1. Persons who are mentally competent and of the age of majority can give consent
2. A parent, legal guardian, or someone legally charged with standing in place of the parent or guardian, can give consent for a minor (a minor is a person not yet of legal age, which is often 18); consent can legally be given by a minor under the following circumstances:
   a. Minor serving in the armed forces
   b. Emancipated minor
   c. Testing for sexually transmitted diseases
   d. Seeking contraception or abortion
3. Living will
   a. Also known as an *advanced directive*
   b. Authorizes in advance the withholding of artificial life-support methods in case of terminal illness or accident
   c. Encouraged by the Patient Self-Determination Act of 1990
4. Uniform Anatomical Gift Act of 1968: allows for competent adults to give their body or body parts in the event of their death for research, transplantation, or placement in a tissue bank
5. Persons who are *non compos mentis* ("not of sound mind") cannot give consent, and these persons require some form of guardianship to give consent
6. In emergencies, consent to treatment is implied only as long as the emergency exists; the Good Samaritan Act provides immunity from liability to non-negligent volunteers at the scene of an accident
7. Mentally competent persons have the right to refuse medical treatment (refused consent)
   a. Patient's refusal must be documented
   b. Patient must sign a document (*release*) absolving the caregiver of liability for not giving treatment
   c. Patient's *refused consent* can be overruled by a court of competent jurisdiction
8. Consent obtained by fraudulent means or misrepresentations is not binding
9. Without proper consent for treatment, a caregiver may be charged with:
   a. Assault: intentional, unlawful attempt of bodily injury to another by force
   b. Battery: willful and unlawful use of force or violence (or touching) on another person

V. CONTRACTS

A. General
1. An agreement creating an obligation
2. Can be oral or written, expressed or implied

B. Express Contract
1. Agreement between two or more parties
2. Contains the explicit terms of the agreement either orally or in writing

C. Implied Contract
1. Conclusion drawn from the actions of two or more parties
2. Patient-physician contract is implied

D. Necessary Elements of a Contract
1. Offer: one party makes an offer
2. Acceptance: another party agrees to the offer made
3. Consideration: mutual exchange of something of value between the parties
4. Capacity: all parties must be legally able to make the offer and to accept the terms
5. Legality: legal in nature and not against public policy

E. Patient and Physician Contract May Be Terminated by:
1. Patient: circumstances need to be fully documented in chart
2. Physician
   a. Must give patient notice (abandonment)
   b. Physician writes a certified letter with return receipt; copy in patient's record
   c. Letter should include:
      1) Reasons why care is being discontinued
      2) Assurance that physician will turn over patient records as directed
      3) Notice that patient should seek alternative care as soon as possible

VI. TORTS

A. Definition of a Tort
1. An act, intentional or accidental, that brings harm against another person or damage to another person's property

B. Negligence
1. Unintentional (accidental) tort
2. Characterized by commission of an act that an ordinary, reasonable, and prudent person would not have done or omission of an act that an ordinary, reasonable, and prudent person, would have done:
   a. Forms of negligence:
      1) Nonfeasance: failure to act when there was a duty to act causing or resulting in harm
      2) Misfeasance: improper performance of an act causing or resulting in harm
      3) Malfeasance: performance of an improper or unlawful act causing or resulting in harm
      4) Malpractice: negligence of a professional person, with the action or inaction compared with an ordinary, reasonable, and prudent professional

   b. *Four* Ds of negligence
      1) Duty: exists when a patient-physician relationship has been established
      2) Derelict: neglect of professional obligation
      3) Direct cause: injury was directly caused by the physician's poor actions or by the physician's failure to act
      4) Damages: harm resulting to the patient— three types:
         a) Nominal: the damage exists in name only; token compensation
         b) Compensatory: actual damages suffered by the patient because of the physician's negligence
         c) Punitive: damages above the actual damage suffered by the patient; to punish the physician for the negligent act

C. *Res Ipsa Loquitur*
1. Meaning: "the thing speaks for itself"
2. Describes a situation in which the nature of the injury implicates negligence

D. Intentional Torts
1. Assault: deliberate threat to make bodily contact
2. Battery: intentional physical contact
3. Abandonment: one-sided termination of the patient-physician relationship by the physician without proper notice to the patient
4. Invasion of privacy: giving out patient information without patient consent
5. Defamation: injury to a person's reputation caused by a false statement by another person
6. Libel: false or malicious writing against another person
7. Slander: false or malicious oral statement against another person
8. False imprisonment: unlawful restraint, or holding, of an individual against his or her will
9. Fraud: intentional misrepresentation that might cause harm

E. Product Liability
1. Liability of a manufacturer of products for injuries caused by defect of those products

F. Vicarious Liability
1. *Respondeat superior* (meaning: "let the master answer")
2. Employers are liable for the conduct of their employees while the employees are performing within the scope of their employment

VII. BUSINESS LAW

A. Employment Practices
1. National Labor Relations Act of 1935 (NLRA): defines unfair labor practices and provides hearing or mediation of complaints

2. Fair Labor Standards Act of 1938 (FLSA): defines minimum wage, equal pay for equal work, and child labor restrictions
3. Equal Pay Act of 1963 (EPA): amendment of FLSA that addresses wage disparities based on sex
4. Equal Employment Opportunity Act of 1972 (EEOA): prohibits employment discrimination based on age, race, color, religion, sex, or national origin
5. Age Discrimination in Employment Act of 1967 (ADEA): prohibits discrimination based on age
6. Americans with Disabilities Act of 1990 (ADA): prohibits discrimination against persons with physical or mental disabilities
7. Workers' compensation laws: state-mandated programs to provide wage continuation and medical treatment compensation for persons with work-related injuries or illnesses

B. Sexual Harassment
1. *Quid pro quo* ("something for something"); conditions of employment (raise, promotion) are based on a person's acceptance or rejection of unwelcome sexual conduct
2. Hostile work environment: creation of an intimidating, offensive, or hostile workplace resulting from unwelcome sexual conduct; interferes with a person's ability to perform job functions

C. Payroll
1. FLSA requires all employee records of hours worked to be continuously maintained
2. Federal Insurance Contributions Act (FICA): Social Security Tax; applied toward old-age benefits
3. Federal Unemployment Tax Act (FUTA): tax to provide income during unemployment
4. Payroll reports and forms
   a. Form 944: Employer's Quarterly Federal Tax Return; filed each 3 months, with payment of quarterly tax due
   b. Form 8109: Federal Tax Deposit Book; used to pay FICA and federal income tax
   c. Form W-2: Wage and Tax Statement; given to employees yearly, itemizing the wages earned and all taxes deducted from wages for that year
   d. Form W-3: Transmittal of Income and Tax Statement; submitted to Social Security Administration; compares W-2 forms with Form 941
   e. Form W-4: Employee's Withholding Allowance Certificate; employee decides the number of withholding allowances for the company to take out of wages earned, based on the number of dependents claimed

VIII. PUBLIC HEALTH DUTIES

A. General
1. States require physicians to report certain information
2. Reported information helps to provide for the health, safety, and welfare of the public

B. Births
1. Birth certificate completed by birth attendant

C. Deaths
1. Death certificate completed by physician in attendance
2. Medical examiner must be called in cases of:
   a. Violent or criminal activity death
   b. Death without a physician present
   c. Death from undetermined cause
   d. Death within 24 hours of admission to a hospital or health care facility
   e. Death without prior medical care

D. Communicable Diseases
1. Communicated to county health department
2. Includes smallpox, scarlet fever, rubella, measles, tuberculosis, plague, cholera, and sexually transmitted diseases

E. National Childhood Vaccine Injury Act
1. Requires providers who administer vaccines to report the following information to public health agencies:
   a. Date the vaccine was administered
   b. Lot number and manufacturer of vaccine
   c. Any adverse reactions to the vaccine
   d. Name, title, and address of the person administering the vaccine

F. Newborn Diseases
1. Inborn errors of metabolism (e.g., phenylketonuria [PKU])

G. Abuse
1. If suspected by the provider, the provider has the legal duty to report suspected abuse to the authorities
2. Medical assistants are also considered *mandatory reporters*
3. Types of abuse to be reported:
   a. Child abuse
   b. Spouse or domestic abuse
   c. Elder abuse
   d. Drug abuse
   e. Patient abuse in hospital and nursing homes

H. Criminal Acts
1. When identified by the provider, the provider has the legal duty to report suspected criminal acts to authorities

2. Types of criminal acts to be reported:
   a. Injuries by weapons
   b. Assault
   c. Attempted suicide
   d. Rape (may require a release by the victim because of confidentiality)

IX. INTRODUCTION TO ETHICS

A. General
1. A set of moral principles or values
2. Concerns the thoughts, judgments, and actions on issues that have greater implications of moral right and wrong

B. Duties
1. Obligations or commitments to act in certain ways
2. Includes:
   a. Non malfeasance: not doing any harm
   b. Beneficence: acting to create good
   c. Fidelity: meeting the patient's expectations through respect, competence, adherence to laws, and honoring agreements
   d. Veracity: telling the truth
   e. Justice: sharing of benefits and burdens

C. Rights
1. Claims made on a person or society
2. Correlated with duties

D. Virtues
1. Character traits that make a person act in a certain way
2. Principles are written in the form of a Code of Ethics

X. AMERICAN ASSOCIATION OF MEDICAL ASSISTANTS (AAMA) CODE OF ETHICS

A. General
1. As agent of physician, the medical assistant is governed by ethical standards
2. Decisions made in practice should be based on the professional nature of the professional and scope of practice
3. Code of Ethics is standard for all medical assistants to honor
4. Patterned after the American Medical Association (AMA) Code of Ethics
5. *Never* practice medicine; do not identify self as a "nurse"

XI. AMA CODE OF ETHICS

A. General
1. Written code of conduct for medical practice
2. Includes four components:
   a. Principles of medical ethics
   b. Fundamental elements of the patient-physician relationship
   c. Current opinions with annotation

   d. Reports of the Council of Ethical and Judicial Affairs; includes opinions on:
      1) Abortion: not prohibited by ethical standards
      2) Abuse: legal and ethical requirement to report
      3) Allocation of health resources: the physician must remain a patient advocate and allow institutional procedures to determine allocation
      4) Artificial insemination: requires informed consent; deals with who has parental rights
      5) Clinical investigation: the patient-physician relationship does not exist in clinical investigation
      6) Cost: quality of patient care should be the physician's first consideration, not cost
      7) Provision of adequate health care: an adequate level of health care for all persons
      8) Genetic counseling: concerns for the quality of life
      9) Organ donation: the donor should not receive payment for organ donation; involves protection of the right to privacy for both donor and recipient
      10) Quality of life: primary consideration of what is best for the patient
      11) Withholding or withdrawing life-prolonging treatment: the physician must be committed to saving life and relieving suffering; the patient may have his or her wishes known
      12) Euthanasia: incompatible with the physician's role

XII. PROFESSIONAL RELATIONSHIPS

A. Hospital Relations
1. Privileges granted based on competence and experience, not fees

B. Advertising
1. Only restrictions are those that protect the public from deceptive practices; physicians can advertise fees, identification of educational background, and specialty, but physicians cannot include any statements as to the quality of their services

C. Communication with the Media
1. Physician may not discuss a patient's condition with the press (unless a release has been granted); may release only authorized information that is in the public domain (births, deaths, accidents, and police cases)

D. Computers
1. The AMA has developed guidelines for the use and sharing of computerized information

E. Fees and Charges
1. Physician may not split patient fees with another physician for patient referral (fee splitting)
2. Physician's staff should assist in completing insurance forms without charge
3. Physician may request that the patient make payment at the time treatment is rendered
4. Insurance copayments may be waived or written off if access of care is threatened by inability to pay the copayment
5. Professional courtesy is a tradition

F. Physician's Records
1. Physician owns the notes prepared by him or her while treating a patient
2. Original medical records may not be released; records can be reproduced only on the physician's death, retirement, or sale of the physician's practice

XIII. PROFESSIONAL RIGHTS AND RESPONSIBILITIES

A. Discipline
1. Physician should expose dishonest, corrupt, incompetent, or unethical colleagues

B. Free Choice
1. Physician in private practice may decline to accept any individual as a patient

C. Patent
1. Physicians may patent any device that he or she discovers or invents

D. Patient–Physician Relationship
1. Both parties are free to enter into, or decline to enter into, the relationship

E. Infectious Disease
1. Physician who is infected with an infectious disease should not engage in any patient contact or activity that may create a risk for the patient

F. Substance Abuse
1. Physician should not practice under the influence of any controlled substance, of alcohol, or of chemical agents that impair the ability to render treatment

XIV. HIPAA

A. Health Insurance Portability and Accountability Act
1. Involved with privacy, security, and claims issues in the health care system
2. Standards for privacy of individually identifiable health information
3. Allows the flow of health information while protecting the privacy of patients
4. Issues identified by state and federal agencies
5. Failure to comply with mandates can lead to sanctions and fines
6. Enacted in 1996
7. Two provisions:
   a. Title I: Insurance Reform
   b. Title II: Administrative Simplification
8. Long-term benefits of HIPAA include:
   a. Lower administrative costs
   b. Increased accuracy of data
   c. Increased patient and customer satisfaction

B. Title I: Health Insurance Reform
1. General
   a. Provision of continuous insurance coverage for workers and their insured when the worker changes or loses a job
   b. Limits use of preexisting condition exclusions
   c. Prohibits discrimination for past or present poor health
   d. Guarantees individuals the right to purchase gap health insurance coverage after losing a job
   e. Allows renewal of health insurance coverage regardless of an individual's health condition

C. Title II: Administrative Simplification
1. General
   a. Focuses on the health care setting
   b. Intended to reduce administrative costs
   c. Accomplished by standardizing the exchange of health care data
   d. Includes provisions to ensure the privacy and security of an individual's health data
   e. Standardization of electronic transmissions will reduce the number of forms and methods used in claims processing
   f. Two parts to this provision include:
      1) Development and implementation of standardized electronic transactions using common sets of descriptors (code sets)
      2) Implementation of privacy and security procedures to prevent the misuse of health information and ensure confidentiality

D. Roles and Relationships
1. General
   a. Department of Health and Human Services (HHS): establishes and implements standards
   b. Centers for Medicare and Medicaid (CMS): enforces insurance portability and code set requirements of HIPAA
   c. Office of Civil Rights (OCR): enforces privacy standards
   d. Covered entity: may be a health plan (e.g., Blue Cross/Blue Shield), health care clearinghouse, or health care provider

e. Electronic media: mode of electronic transmission; may include the Internet, extranet, telephone lines, fax modems, or disks or magnetic tape

f. Transaction: transmission of information between two parties; can include:
1) Health care claims
2) Health care payments
3) Coordination of benefits
4) Claim status
5) Enrollment and disenrollment in a health plan
6) Eligibility for a health plan
7) Premium payments
8) Referral certification or authorization
9) First report of injury

E. Privacy Rule
1. General
   a. Privacy: condition of being secluded from the view or presence of others
   b. Confidentiality: use of discretion in keeping information private
   c. Disclosure: release, transfer, access to, or divulgence of information
   d. Individually identifiable health information (IIHI): any part of an individual's health information collected from an individual (e.g., demographic information, date of birth)
   e. Protected health information (PHI): IIHI that is transmitted by electronic media, maintained in electronic form, or transmitted or maintained in any other form or medium; all patient information is protected regardless of the way it is maintained; includes paper records, computerized practice management or billing systems, spoken words, and x-ray films
   f. Use: sharing, application, use, examination, or analysis of IIHI; PHI is protected both inside and outside of the organization unless the use is specifically required or permitted

F. Patient Rights under HIPAA
1. Right to notice of privacy practices
   a. Patients are entitled to receive written notice of privacy practices (Notice of Privacy Protection [NPP]) from the provider at the first appointment
   b. NPP outlines patient's rights
   c. Must be written in plain language; staff should obtain signature acknowledging receipt
   d. Can be done at front desk
2. Right to request restrictions on certain uses and disclosures of PHI
   a. Patient has right to ask for restrictions on how the office will use and disclose PHI
   b. Restrictions must be agreed on by the office; if agreed, restrictions must be documented and followed
   c. Practice may disclose confidential information without written authorization, such as communicable diseases, victims of abuse, and law enforcement purposes
   d. Patient may identify any other person whom information may be disclosed or not disclosed
3. Right to request confidential information
   a. Patient can request to receive confidential communication by alternative means or alternative location (call patient at work instead of home; test results sent in writing instead of over the telephone)
   b. Office must accommodate reasonable requests
   c. Requests may be required in writing
4. Right to access PHI
   a. Patient has the right to access, inspect, and obtain a copy of his or her PHI
   b. Request must be made in writing
   c. Request must be acted on within 30 days
   d. Reasonable fee for copies and postage may be applied
   e. Patients do not have the right to access psychotherapy notes, information compiled for use in legal proceedings, or information exempted under the Clinical Laboratory Improvement Acts of 1988 (CLIA)
   f. If health care provider has determined that the patient may be endangered by accessing information, access may be denied
   g. State law may take precedence
5. Right to request amendment of PHI
   a. Patient has the right to request that their PHI be changed
   b. Request should be made in writing
   c. Must be done in a timely manner
6. Right to receive an accounting of disclosures of PHI
   a. Providers should keep a log of disclosures
   b. Patients may request an accounting or tracking of their disclosures once a year without charge; additional accountings may be charged a fee
7. Organization and staff responsibilities
   a. General
   1) Organization must implement written policies and procedures
   2) Guidelines tailored to each practice
   3) Documentation must be maintained in written or electronic form and maintained for 6 years
   b. Verification of identity
   1) Office must verify identity of person requesting PHI
   2) Identification may be by date of birth, social security number, or password

c. Validation of patient permission
   1) Office must have appropriate permission
   2) Permission is maintained in practice management system or patient chart
d. Training
   1) Office must train all members
   2) Must include practice's policies and procedures that deal with PHI
   3) Each person's role should be addressed
e. Safeguards
   1) Ensure that information is secure
   2) Include administrative, technical, and physical measures that will safeguard PHI from any disclosure, intentional or accidental
f. Complaints
   1) Process must be in place for complaints
   2) Staff members are subject to appropriate sanctions for failure to comply (warning to termination)

8. Code set regulations
   a. General
      1) Transaction and code set (TCS): developed to streamline electronic data transactions
      2) Makes data processing transactions more efficient and reduces costs
      3) Single standard similar to a bank's automatic teller machine or grocery self-checkout
      4) Can be used by anyone to enter into a specific space on a form
      5) Electronic, not paper
      6) Documents why patients are seen (diagnosis, *International Classification of Diseases*, ninth edition, Clinical Modification [ICD-9-CM]) and what is done to them at the encounter (procedure, *Current Procedural Terminology*, fourth edition [CPT-4], Health Care Financing Administration Common Procedure Coding System [HCPCS])

9. Guidelines for HIPAA privacy compliance
   a. Reasonable and appropriate safeguards must be taken to ensure that all confidential information is protected
      1) Conversations can be overheard; consider privacy glass at the front desk and moving conversations away from populated settings; move dictation stations away from patient areas; telephone conversations in front of patients should be avoided
      2) Check medical record to see if any special instructions for contacting the patient are noted
      3) Limit the information (reason for visit) on patient sign-in sheets; change them throughout the day
      4) Patient must sign a form acknowledging the receipt of the NPP
      5) Formal policies for transferring and accepting PHI must be in place; these include couriers, billing services transcription services, and e-mail
      6) Computers should be turned so the screen is not visible to others; screensavers may be used; computer should automatically log off a user after a period of being idle
      7) Keep user names and passwords confidential, and change them often
      8) Safeguard the work area by keeping confidential information from patient view; keep PHI from cleaning services that may have access after business hours
      9) Medical records should be placed face down at reception area; when placing medical record on the door of the examination room, turn the chart so the identifying information faces the door
      10) Do not post the provider's daily schedule in areas accessible to patients
      11) Fax machines should not be placed in patient rooms or reception area where incoming documents may be viewed
      12) Direct mail and telephone calls to the appropriate persons
      13) For coding and billing purposes, recognize, learn, and use HIPAA TCS
      14) Send all privacy-related concerns and questions to the appropriate staff member
      15) Immediately report any suspected or known improper behavior to supervisor

Professionalism and Career Development   6

I. PROFESSIONALISM

A. Definition
1. Acting in a businesslike manner in the workplace
2. Conforming to the technical and ethical standards of a profession
3. Keeping calm in stressful situations
4. Not responding in anger when patients/coworkers are rude
5. Includes both appearance and attitude

B. Characteristics of Professional Behavior
1. Competence: ability to perform one's job to standards
2. Dependability: being punctual, efficient, reliable
3. Integrity: honest, straightforward
4. Compassion: using empathy to sense someone else's concerns/feelings
5. Respect for others: treating others with dignity
6. Responsibility: taking ownership of one's actions
7. Professional demeanor: acting in a thoughtful way; respect for self/others
8. Loyalty: devotion to another
9. Positive attitude: state of mind; way of carrying one's self; reflected in tone of voice, body language
10. Teamwork: working together
11. Ability to prioritize: determining which task must be completed before another
12. Flexibility: ability to adapt to a variety of situations
13. Courtesy: use of kind words, compassion and consideration

C. Professional Abilities
1. Competence: ability to get things done on time and correctly; understanding implications of actions; knowing when to ask for help
2. Dexterity: ability to move with skill or ease
3. Effective communication: ability to communicate on many levels with different types of people; includes English skills and facial expression

D. Professional Image
1. Personal appearance
   a. Bathe/shower daily; brush teeth
   b. Hair away from face, styled neatly; no extreme colors
   c. Clean nails; practical length; no artificial nails
   d. Minimal makeup; very little fragrance
   e. Minimal jewelry; no body piercings except earrings
   f. Uniform/scrubs clean and pressed; proper fit; worn with undergarments that should not be visible
   g. Socks/stockings should be worn
   h. Shoes should fit properly; no open-toes/sandals; no canvas shoes
   i. No gum, tobacco odor; cover visible tattoos

E. Barriers to Professionalism
1. Bringing personal problems into the workplace
2. Taking care of personal business while at work
3. Inappropriate discussions in front of patients
4. Procrastination of duties

F. Maintaining a Professional Image
1. Leave personal problems at home
2. Avoid office gossip
3. Do not conduct personal business during office hours
4. Stay out of office politics
5. Do not procrastinate

II. THE PROFESSIONAL MEDICAL ASSISTANT

A. Professional Duties
1. Administrative: having to do with the "front office"
2. Clinical: having to do with the "back office"; patient care
3. Transdisciplinary: general knowledge
4. Medical assistant works under the direct supervision of provider
5. Duties may vary from state to state

B. **Training Programs**
   1. Accredited programs: voluntary process to help programs set, achieve and maintain educational goals to meet guidelines and standards of the profession
   2. CAAHEP (Commission on Accreditation of Allied Health Education Programs)
   3. ABHES (Accrediting Bureau of Health Education Schools)

C. **Credentials**
   1. Promotes the profession
   2. AAMA (American Association of Medical Assistants): CMA
   3. AMT (American Medical Technologists): RMA
   4. Credentials awarded after passing exam
   5. Continuing education required to maintain credential, keep up with knowledge, and reinforce areas related to job responsibilities

D. **Continuing Education**
   1. Credits for courses, classes or seminars related to a person's profession
   2. Designed to promote education and keep individual up-to-date on current trends in his/her field
   3. Often required for licensing/certification

III. SCOPE OF PRACTICE

A. **Definition**
   1. Performance of delegated duties within the supervising provider's scope of practice consistent with the medical assistant's education, training and experience
   2. Duties performed by the medical assistant do not constitute the practice of medicine
   3. Medical assistant is not a nurse and should not refer to self as a nurse

B. **Provider Responsible for the Medical Assistant**
   1. Duties vary from state to state
   2. Medical assistant performs as an agent of the provider under supervision
   3. Medical assistant performs duties that he or she is told to perform; provider responsible for actions
   4. Duties can be related to the medical assistant verbally, through a supervisor, or by way of office policy/procedure manual
   5. *Respondeat superior*

C. **Medical assistant is not a nurse and should not refer to herself as a nurse.**

D. **AAMA Website: www.aama-ntl.org**

E. **AMT Website: www.amt1.com**

Computer Concepts, Written Communications, and Mail Processing

I. COMPUTER BASICS

A. General
1. Electronic device that accepts, processes, exports, and stores data
2. Classified according to size
   a. Mainframe: large computer that can handle many users at the same time
   b. Microcomputer: personal computer (PC)
   c. Laptop: portable PC

B. Hardware: Computer Equipment
1. Central processing unit (CPU)
   a. Control unit: supervises data processing operations
   b. Arithmetic logic unit (ALU): carries out arithmetic and logic operations
   c. Primary storage unit: stores data and program instructions
      1) Random access memory (RAM): computer's temporary memory
      2) Read-only memory (ROM): computer's permanent memory
2. Input devices
   a. Allows communication between the user and the computer hardware
   b. Allows data to be entered into the computer
   c. Keyboard: the *typewriter*; allows input of alphanumeric data
   d. Mouse: handheld pointing device; contains a ball that is moved when the mouse is rolled on a flat surface; movement of the mouse and thus the ball, moves the cursor on the computer screen
   e. Scanner: device that *reads,* or converts, printed matter directly into a computer-readable format
   f. Voice recognition: device that reads voices and creates a computer-readable format
3. Output devices
   a. Allows data to be displayed or recorded
   b. Monitor: device that resembles a television set; displays computer-generated information
   c. Printer: device that records computer-generated information onto paper (hard copy)
4. Storage
   a. Methods of saving the information input for future reference or for printing
   b. Hard drive: part of the computer hardware inside the computer box; contains the computer-operating information
   c. Compact disk (CD) ROM: allows the storage of data on a removable disk; holds more information than a diskette
   d. Disk drive: loads a program or data that is stored on a diskette into the computer; also can be used to transfer stored information from the computer onto a diskette for safekeeping; each microcomputer may have more than one drive
   e. Portable disk drives: ZIP drive, flash drive; jump drive; attached externally to the computer; contains a very high storage capacity; usually used as backup; can be stored somewhere other than the facility

C. Software
1. Typically referred to as a *program;* provides processing instructions to the computer
2. Systems software: manages the overall operations of the computer system; program instructions that control, interface with, and communicate between the applications software and the workstation
3. Applications software: mainly commercially prepared programs that perform specific data processing functions
4. Diskettes or CDs on which computer information may be stored

D. Data Processing
1. Transforms raw information (data) into useful information
2. The smallest piece of information processed is a *bit* (binary digit); an 8-bit unit is a *byte*
3. 1 byte is required to represent one character
4. 1 kilobyte (kb) equals 1024 bytes
5. 1 megabyte (MB) equals 1000 kilobytes
6. All data are processed in a cycle

7. Input: data are entered into the computer by an input device
8. Processing: data are manipulated
9. Output: processed information is accessed from an output device
10. Storage: information is stored for future use

II. WORD PROCESSING

A. General
1. Use of computer to produce documents
2. Software programs that allow the preparation of written documents

B. Keyboard Keys
1. Alphanumeric: keys that represent letters, numbers, and symbols
2. Backspace: allows the cursor to be moved to the left; erases character over which it is backspaced
3. Caps Lock: keeps the alphabet keys in uppercase
4. Ctrl and Alt (control and alternate keys): used in combination with other keys to increase the number of functions on the keyboard
5. Cursor control arrows: allows the cursor (the blinking arrow [or dash] on the screen that identifies where the data will be placed on the screen) to be moved up, down, to the left, or to the right
6. Del (delete): erases characters to the right of the cursor
7. End: moves the cursor to the end of a line of print
8. Enter (or Return): returns the cursor to the beginning of the next blank line
9. Esc (escape): allows the exit of a program or window
10. F1 through F12 (function keys): perform special program-directed moves
11. Home: moves the cursor to the upper, lower, left, or right margin
12. Page Up, Page Down: moves the cursor 1 page up or down
13. Print Screen: allows only the displayed screen to be printed (if allowed by the program)
14. Shift: places the alphabet key in uppercase when the Shift key is pressed simultaneously
15. Space bar: allows blank spaces to be placed between letters or words
16. Tab: moves the cursor a predetermined number of blank spaces; used to indent

C. Formatting
1. Determines the physical layout of the document
   a. Margins: the amount of blank space at the edges of the document
   b. Tab set: sets a specific number of blank spaces to be used in each tab
   c. Line spacing: sets a specific number of blank lines between each line of input text (usually set for single or double spacing)
   d. Pitch: number of characters per inch of type
   e. Justification: alignment of text to the left and/or right margin
   f. Header and footer: information to be included at the top (header) or bottom (footer) of each page
   g. Pagination: positions and prints the page numbers on each page
   h. Widows and orphans: eliminates a last paragraph line that appears alone at the top of the next page (widow), or eliminates a first paragraph line that appears at the bottom of the previous page (orphan)
   i. Font: style and size of the print used

D. Editing
1. Allows changes to be made within a document
   a. Highlight and Block: text can be highlighted for manipulation by using the cursor
   b. Delete: erases the highlighted text block
   c. Copy and paste: copies the highlighted text block for placement (paste) elsewhere in the document, at the new cursor location, without erasing
   d. Cut and paste: takes (cuts) the highlighted text block and places (pastes) it elsewhere in the document, at the new cursor location, without erasing
   e. Print: allows the document to be recorded (printed) on paper (hard copy)
   f. Save: allows data to be placed in storage on a diskette, on a CD, or on the hard drive
   g. Retrieve (open): allows stored data stored to be brought onto the screen

E. Word Processing Terminology
1. Default: predefined settings automatically loaded by the program used, unless changed by the user
2. Directory: index of files on a floppy or hard drive
3. Grammar check: application that identifies input grammar or punctuation errors
4. Help screen: provides explanations or instructions about a particular task within a particular program
5. Menu: display on the screen that gives a list of options for word processing
6. Page break: places the beginning of a new page where the cursor is positioned
7. Prompt: a message displayed on the screen that gives the user helpful information and/or instructions
8. Reveal codes: normally invisible word processing codes are made visible for quick editing

9. Sort: organizes a list in alphabetical or numerical order
10. Spell check: application that checks for misspelled words (medical spell check programs are available)
11. Thesaurus: identifies synonyms and antonyms for the word on which the cursor sits
12. Window: an application that allows more than one program to be in use at the same time
13. Word wrap: automatically moves the beginning of a line to the next line without having to press Enter (or Return)

III. COMPUTERS AND HIPAA

A. Information That May Be Used and Shared
1. Patient care and treatment coordination
2. To pay physicians/facilities for health care
3. With family whom the patient has identified as being involved in his or her care
4. To make certain good care is provided
5. To protect public health
6. To make required reports to law enforcement

B. Information That Cannot Be Shared or Used Without Patient Consent
1. Cannot give health information to an employer
2. Cannot use or share information for marketing
3. Cannot share mental health information obtained in counseling

C. Health Care Facility Must Train Anyone Using the System as to What Information Can and Cannot Be Shared
1. Individual log-ins and passwords
2. Patient information should not be accessed unless the user needs to know content for patient care
3. Care must be taken when releasing any kind of information

IV. WRITTEN COMMUNICATION SKILLS

A. Types of Written Communication within the Medical Office
1. Transcription from machine dictation; may be sent out to transcribe
2. Formal handwritten consultation and/or surgical reports
3. Composition of letters to patients, consulting physicians, and suppliers
4. Replies to inquiries
5. Responses to requests for information
6. Written collection letters
7. Supply orders
8. Documentation of treatment instructions for patients
9. Other types of office communication

B. Letters
1. Parts of a letter
   a. Heading
      1) Printed letterhead at the top of the page
      2) Dateline: three blank lines below the letterhead; name of the month written in full, followed by the day and year
   b. Opening
      1) Inside address
         a) Four blank lines below the dateline
         b) Title, name, and address of receiver
         c) Street, avenue, or boulevard; east, west, north, and south are all spelled out
         d) Street numbers 1 through 10 are spelled out
         e) Street numbers 11 and above are identified by numerals
         f) City is spelled out, followed by a comma
         g) State uses the standard two-letter abbreviation without any period
         h) Zip code uses the five, or nine if available, numerals one space after the state
      2) Attention line (optional)
         a) Placed two blank lines below the inside address
         b) Directs the letter to a particular department or person when the letter is addressed to an organization
      3) Salutation
         a) Opening greeting to the letter
         b) Two blank lines below the inside address
         c) Recipient's title and name followed by a colon (personal correspondence allows use of a comma)
         d) Use the courtesy title (Dr., Mr., Mrs., Ms.) when the letter is addressed to a specific individual
         e) Use the phrase *To Whom It May Concern:* or *Dear Sir or Madam:* when the letter is addressed to an unidentified individual within an organization
   c. Body
      1) Placed two blank lines below the salutation
      2) Contains the message of the letter
      3) Each line is single-spaced; a double space is placed between paragraphs
   d. Closing
      1) Complimentary closing
         a) Placed two blank lines below the body of the letter
         b) Only the first letter of the first word in the closing is capitalized
         c) Comma follows the complimentary closing
         d) May be formal (*Truly yours,* or *Very truly yours,*) or common (*Sincerely,* or *Sincerely yours,*)

2) Signature line
  a) Placed four or five blank lines below the complimentary closing
  b) Typed name of the person authoring the letter
  c) Author's title follows author's name, separated by a comma
  d) Author signs name above the signature line
3) Reference notation
  a) Placed two lines below the signature line
  b) Identifies the letter's author and the transcriber (DH:*lb* or DH/*lb*), with the author's initials in uppercase letters, the transcriber's initials in lowercase letters
  c) If the author types his or her own letter, then no reference notation is necessary
4) Enclosure notation
  a) Placed one or two blank lines below the reference notation (or signature line)
  b) Identifies any printed material accompanying the correspondence (*Enc:, Enclosure:, Enclosures:*)
5) Copy notation
  a) Placed one or two lines below enclosure notation
  b) Indicates that a copy of the correspondence, with any enclosures, was also forwarded to a third party (*cc: Rob David*)
  c) If more than one third-party recipient exists, then the recipients are listed alphabetically or in order of authority
  d) Blind carbon copy (*bcc: Rob David*) allows a short note to be typed on the copy to be sent to one third party; the short note is placed only on the one copy of the letter that is sent to the blind carbon copy recipient
6) Postscript
  a) An afterthought
  b) Placed two lines below the last typed line (*P.S.:*)

2. Letter styles
  a. Full block (see Figure 7-1)
    1) All lines begin flush at the left margin
    2) Most efficient style, although the least attractive on paper
  b. Modified block (see Figure 7-2): all lines begin flush at the left margin except for the dateline and the complimentary close (these two lines begin at the center of the page)
  c. Semiblock (see Figure 7-3): same as modified block, except the beginning of each new paragraph of the body of the letter is indented five blank spaces

---

Elizabeth Blackwell, M.D.
223 Orange Avenue, N.W.
Cottonwood, UT 84121

January 26, 20—

Mr. Richard Fluege
3678 North Willow Avenue
Palm Beach, FL 33480

Dear Mr. Fluege:

Please send me full particulars on the professional suites you expect to offer for sale or rent in the Medical Arts Professional Annex.

In about six months, I will be ready to open my practice, and I am interested in locating to Florida. My preference is a street-level suite of approximately 2,000 square feet.

After I have had an opportunity to study the information you send me, I will write or telephone you if I have further questions.

Very truly yours,

Elizabeth Blackwell, M.D.

EB:mek

FIGURE 7-1 Block letter style. (Young AP, Kennedy DB: *Kinn's the medical assistant: an applied learning approach*, ed 10, St Louis, 2007, Saunders.)

MEDICAL ARTS PROFESSIONAL ANNEX
3678 North Willow Avenue
Palm Beach FL 33480

January 29, 20—

Elizabeth Blackwell, M.D.
223 Orange Avenue, N.W.
Cottonwood, UT 84121

Dear Doctor Blackwell:

We have two remaining street-level suites available for occupancy about July 1. These are marked on pages 3 and 4 of the enclosed descriptive brochure. If one of these suites appeals to you, we will be pleased to customize it for your practice.

Please feel free to call me collect at the number on the brochure for further discussion of your needs.

Sincerely yours,

Richard Fluege
Business Manager

RF:ab
Enclosure

FIGURE 7-2 Modified block letter style. (Young AP, Kennedy DB: *Kinn's the medical assistant: an applied learning approach*, ed 10, St Louis, 2007, Saunders.)

WILLIAM OSLER, M.D.
1000 South West Street
Park Ridge, NJ 07656

January 26, 20—

Robert Koch, M.D.
398 Main Street
Park Ridge, NJ 07656

Dear Doctor Koch:

Mrs. Elaine Norris

Thank you for referring your patient, Mrs. Elaine Norris, for consultation and care. She was examined in my office today.

FINDINGS: The patient complained of pain in the left lower quadrant and some abdominal tenderness. She had a temperature of 100.2 degrees.

RECOMMENDATION: The patient was placed on a soft, low-residue, bland diet, antibiotics, and bed rest for a few days. Upper and lower gastrointestinal x-rays will be performed next week.

TENTATIVE DIAGNOSIS: Diverticulitis of large bowel.

Mrs. Norris has been asked to return here for reevaluation in about ten days.

Sincerely yours,

William Osler, M.D.

WO:gm

FIGURE 7-3 Modified block letter style with indented paragraphs. (Young AP, Kennedy DB: *Kinn's the medical assistant: an applied learning approach*, ed 10, St Louis, 2007, Saunders.)

d. Hanging indentation: same as the modified block, except that all lines of each new paragraph of the body of the letter are indented five blank spaces, except the first line of each paragraph

e. Simplified: same as the full block, except that no salutation and no complimentary close are inserted

3. Margins

a. Short letter (<100 words in the body): 2-inch margins

b. Medium letter (100 to 200 words): 1½-inch margins
c. Long letter (>200 words): 1-inch margins
4. Multiple pages
a. Use plain paper in same stock (weight) as letterhead
b. Type the recipient's name seven blank lines from the top of the page; type the page number one line below the recipient's name; type the current date one line below the page number
c. The body of the letter continues three blank lines below the page heading
d. The same page heading (with corresponding page number) on all subsequent pages

C. Envelopes
1. Sizes
a. #6¾: 6½ × 3⅝ inches
b. #10: 9½ × 4⅛ inches
2. Folding letters for insertion (see Figure 7-4)
a. #6¾ envelope
1) Fold the page in half, bottom up, and crease
2) Fold the right one third over the left, and crease
3) Fold the left one third over the right, and crease
4) Insert the last-creased edge into the envelope first
b. #10 envelope

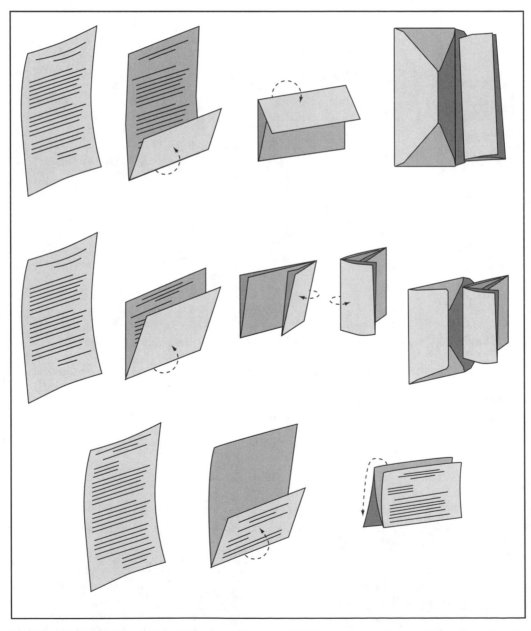

FIGURE 7-4 Correct methods of folding letters. (Young AP, Kennedy DB: *Kinn's the medical assistant: an applied learning approach*, ed 10, St Louis, 2007, Saunders.)

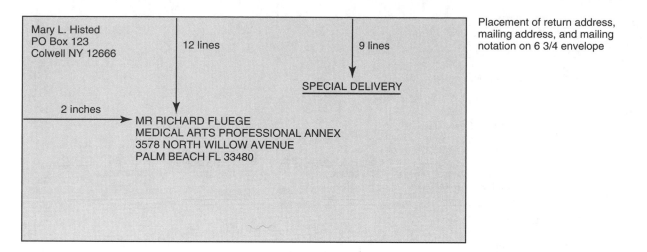

Placement of return address, mailing address, and mailing notation on 6 3/4 envelope

Mary L. Histed
PO Box 123
Colwell NY 12666

12 lines

9 lines

SPECIAL DELIVERY

2 inches

MR RICHARD FLUEGE
MEDICAL ARTS PROFESSIONAL ANNEX
3578 NORTH WILLOW AVENUE
PALM BEACH FL 33480

Placement of mailing address and Personal notation on No. 10 envelope

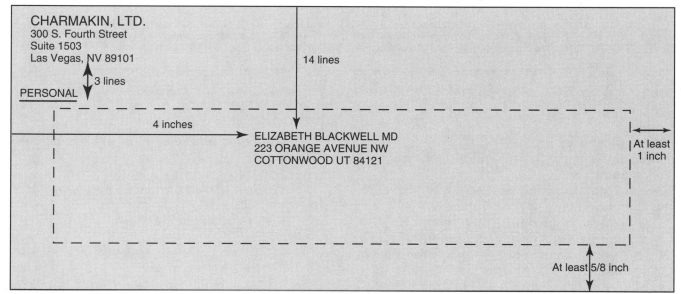

CHARMAKIN, LTD.
300 S. Fourth Street
Suite 1503
Las Vegas, NV 89101

14 lines

3 lines

PERSONAL

4 inches

ELIZABETH BLACKWELL MD
223 ORANGE AVENUE NW
COTTONWOOD UT 84121

At least 1 inch

At least 5/8 inch

FIGURE 7-5 Addressing envelopes. (Young AP, Kennedy DB: *Kinn's the medical assistant: an applied learning approach*, ed 10, St Louis, 2007, Saunders.)

1) Fold the bottom one third, bottom up, and crease
2) Fold the top one third, top down, and crease
3) Insert the last-creased edge into the envelope first

3. Return address

  a. Placed three blank lines from the top edge, five spaces from the left edge (if the return address is not preprinted on the envelope)

  b. Always place the complete return address on the envelope

4. Mailing address (see Figure 7-5)

  a. #6¾ envelope: placed 2 inches down from the top edge and 2 inches to the right of the left edge

  b. #10 envelope: placed 2 inches down from the top edge and 4 inches to the right of the left edge

  c. Type the address in block format; capitalize all letters; no punctuation used (copy the inside address from the letter to insert onto the envelope)

  d. Use standard two-letter state abbreviation

5. Notations

  a. Directed to the recipient (*Personal and Confidential*): placed two blank lines below the return address

  b. Directed to the post office (*Special Delivery* or *Certified Mail*): capitalize all letters in upper-right side, below the area of stamp placement

```
┌─────────────────────────────────────────────────────────────────────────┐
│  INTEROFFICE MEMORANDUM                                                   │
│                                                                           │
│     TO          All Staff                                                 │
│                                                                           │
│     FROM        Office Manager                                            │
│                                                                           │
│     DATE        December 1                                                │
│                                                                           │
│     SUBJECT     Holiday Schedule                                          │
│                                                                           │
│                 Our entire facility will be closed on December 24,        │
│                 December 25, December 31, and January 1. The office       │
│                 will be on reduced staff during the days of December 26,  │
│                 27, 28, 29, and 30. Assignments will be based on          │
│                 seniority of staff members. Please submit your            │
│  A              preferences as soon as possible.                          │
└───────────────────────────────────────────────────────────────────────┘
┌───────────────────────────────────────────────────────────────────────┐
│     MEMO TO:    George Walker                                             │
│                                                                           │
│     FROM:       Stanley Barr                                              │
│                                                                           │
│     DATE:       February 8                                                │
│                                                                           │
│     SUBJECT:    Office rental                                             │
│                                                                           │
│                 We are experiencing unexpectedly rapid growth in our      │
│                 business office and will soon need additional space for   │
│                 our increased number of employees. Do you have a larger   │
│                 facility available in this building? If so, I would like  │
│                 to hear from you regarding the location, square footage,  │
│  B              and anticipated rental costs.                             │
└───────────────────────────────────────────────────────────────────────┘
```

FIGURE 7-6 Examples of memoranda. (Young AP, Kennedy DB: *Kinn's the medical assistant: an applied learning approach*, ed 10, St Louis, 2007, Saunders.)

D. Memoranda (see Figure 7-6)

1. Written communication within an office or organization
2. Use headings, including Receiver, Sender, Date, and Subject of Memo; each office will have a template to be used in all memoranda
3. Information pertaining to the headings should be on the same line and two or three spaces after the heading, separated by a colon
4. Message should begin three blank lines below the last line of the headings
5. Can have a reference notation, and a copy notation (use the same format as for letters)

E. Manuscripts

1. Written document submitted for publication
2. Different professional organizations require different standard formats (template) for manuscript preparation and submission (each will forward its template on request)
3. Includes:
   a. Title page
      1) Identifies the title or theme of the manuscript
      2) Title, author, and author's credentials are normally centered horizontally and vertically on the title page (can vary depending on the organization's shell)
   b. Acknowledgments
      1) Identifies persons who have assisted the author in research or preparation
      2) Placed on a separate page following the title page
   c. Abstract
      1) Summary of the manuscript, normally in 100 to 200 words
      2) Placed on the third page
   d. Text
      1) Title is typed, in capital letters, 13 lines from the top of page
      2) Body of the manuscript begins three blank lines below the title
      3) Text of the manuscript is double-spaced
   e. References
      1) Identifies published works of others referenced within the text
      2) In the final version, each reference is indicated by numerical superscripts or numbers in parentheses after each citation (depending on the style of the journal to which the manuscript is being submitted); references are listed in numerical order at the end of the manuscript
   f. Footnote: cites references and their explanations near the bottom of the page on which the referenced material is written
   g. Bibliography: list of reference books, manuscripts, articles, or other sources that were used to prepare the manuscript; listed in alphabetical order by name of document or by last name of document author

h. Illustrations and tables: placed on separate sheets at the end of the manuscript and assigned consecutive numbers

F. E-mail
1. Electronic mail used for communication
2. Can be used to communicate with patients
3. Not the most secure form of communication

V. PROCESSING MAIL

A. Mail Classifications
1. Express mail, next-day service
   a. Available 7 days a week, 365 days a year
   b. Cost is normally one standard price per item
2. First class
   a. Sealed or unsealed material
   b. Includes letters, postcards, and business-reply mail
   c. Cost is based on weight (in 1-oz increments)
3. Priority mail
   a. First class mail weighing more than 11 oz (maximum weight is 70 lb)
   b. Postage calculated on the combined basis of weight and destination
4. Second class
   a. Regular rates
   b. Available to newspapers and periodicals preauthorized by the post office
5. Third class
   a. Includes catalogs, circulars, books, photographs, and other preprinted materials
   b. Must be marked *Third Class*
6. Fourth class: merchandise, books, and preprinted material (media mail) not included in first or second class and weigh 16 oz or more
7. Registered mail
   a. First class mail additionally protected by registration
   b. Post office receives an additional fee for this service
   c. Post office verifies delivery of the material
   d. Recipient may be required to sign a form to acknowledge receipt, if the sender requests

   e. Registered mail request form must be filled out before mailing
8. Certified mail
   a. Delivery of mail requiring the recipient's signature as proof of delivery
   b. Certified mail request form must be filled out before mailing

B. Equipment and Supplies
1. Postage scale: used to weigh mail to determine the correct postage
2. Postage meter
   a. Machine used to print prepaid postage directly on the envelope or on an adhesive label, depending on the weight of the material
   b. The date and the amount of postage are set by pressing the appropriate buttons
3. Stationery
   a. Standard size and weight, as determined by the office manager
   b. Normally light-colored paper with darker imprinting
4. Rubber stamps
   a. Can indicate the date of receipt of mail
   b. Can be used to endorse checks for deposit

C. Incoming Mail
1. Schedule a set time during which to sort and distribute received mail
2. Date-stamp the front (or the back) of each piece of paper within each envelope, and date-stamp the envelope, depending on the office method (except for checks)
3. *Personal* or *personal and confidential* noted mailings are delivered directly to the addressee without being opened
4. Any mail that is opened by mistake must be resealed with tape and noted on the envelope that it was opened by mistake
5. All checks received must be endorsed immediately and forwarded to the accounts receivable clerk

8 Records Management

I. THE MEDICAL RECORD

A. General
1. The "chart"
2. Chronological system used to annotate patient's medical care that the health care provider renders
3. Ensures competent and necessary (nonredundant) medical care
4. Legal document

B. Purpose
1. Establishes the patient database
2. Serves as a communication link between the health care provider and the staff
3. Helps with the planning of effective patient care
4. Provides evidence of care given to the patient
5. Can provide data for research or education

C. Content
1. Specific to the type of practice
2. Usually includes:
   a. Chief complaint (CC): main reason for the patient seeking care
   b. Past medical history (PH or PMH): gives information regarding usual childhood diseases (UCD), past illnesses, surgeries, and current health status; may be prepared by the patient, by the health care provider, or by the medical assistant
   c. Family history (FH): information regarding the patient's parents and siblings; may include health status, age, cause of death, and hereditary diseases
   d. Present illness (PI): expanded CC
   e. Social history (SH): information on patient's personal habits; may include exercise, sleep, diet, tobacco and/or alcohol use, drug use, sexual history, sexual preference, and hobbies
   f. Occupational history (OH): information regarding patient's employment
   g. Physical examination (PE): complete physical examination; gives information regarding each body system (review of systems [ROS]); may serve as a baseline against the future

   h. Test results: diagnostic and laboratory tests; arranged with most recent at top
   i. Consultations: reports on evaluations made by other health care providers
   j. Past medical records: records from other health care providers that have bearing on present treatment
   k. Correspondence: all correspondence related to patient care
   l. Progress notes: notes written in the chart by the health care provider regarding the patient's care, diagnosis, and treatment
   m. Medication/prescription record: record of all medications and prescriptions given or renewed in the office.
   n. Immunization record: record of all immunizations administered in the office

D. Organization
1. Source-oriented record
   a. Observations and data are categorized according to their source (health care provider, laboratory, radiography, nurse)
   b. Forms are filed in reverse chronological order (most recent on top)
   c. Information is filed in separate sections (e.g., laboratory reports section, x-ray reports section, progress notes section)
2. Problem-oriented medical record (POMR)
   a. Data are organized according to patient's disease or condition
   b. Divided into four parts:
      1) Database: includes CC, PI, PE findings, and laboratory results; each condition has its own page
      2) Problem list: numbered and titled list of every patient complaint; may include physical, psychological, and social problems related to the patient's condition
      3) Plan: diagnostic and treatment decisions for the condition; each plan is titled and numbered

4). Progress notes: structured notes that correspond to each problem number; uses the acronym SOAP
   a) S (subjective data): signs, symptoms, and feelings that the patient describes in the patient's own words
   b) O (objective data): clinical evidence that the health care provider determines
   c) A (assessment = S + O): describes the physical impression and finally diagnosis
   d) P (plan = S + O + A): action needed to solve the problem; may include treatment, medications, consultations, and surgery

E. Documentation
1. Chart in black ink
2. All entries must be dated and initialed, or signed, by the health care provider making the entry
3. All patient visits and telephone calls must be documented
4. No-shows must be recorded
5. Patient's name should appear on each page
6. Corrections are made by using the SLIDE rule:
   a. SL: single line through the error
   b. I: initials of the person correcting the error
   c. D: date and correct the error
   d. E: write the word *error*
7. Correspondence sent to the patient requires a note in the chart
8. *"If it was not charted, it was not done"*

F. Six "Cs" of Charting
1. Current
2. Complete
3. Concise
4. Correct
5. Confidential
6. Clean

G. Legalities and the Medical Record
1. The chart is a legal document
2. The chart belongs to the health care provider or the clinic, but the patient owns the information found on the chart
3. Records that patients or third parties request may be released only if the health care provider and the patient give consent, usually by a medical records release form
4. Records can be withheld from patients if the information can reasonably be expected to cause harm to the patient (doctrine of professional discretion)

5. Patient information is confidential and privileged (this patient confidentiality can be waived in writing by the patient or overruled in a courtroom)
6. Release of confidential patient information without the patient's written consent could lead to a charge of invasion of privacy by the patient
7. Medical records must be kept up to date, complete, and accurate
8. Records are retained according to the requirements of each state's statutes; medical records are usually retained permanently, until the patient's death
   a. Active records: belong to patients who have been seen within the past 2 to 5 years, depending on the practice; stored in the office
   b. Inactive records: records of patients who have not been seen within a time period specified by the practice; stored in a closed storage area onsite or offsite
   c. Inactive records are removed from active area at regular intervals
9. Medical records are destroyed by shredding or burning
10. Entries into medical records should be typewritten or written in black ink

H. Electronic Medical Record (EMR)
1. Entire patient record is stored in a database on the computer
2. Includes health history, progress reports, lab and diagnostic reports and hospital reports
3. Advantages:
   a. Speed and productivity: documents can be retrieved quickly; do not need to be filed; frees up space; saves paper costs
   b. Efficiency: facilitates entry of data; uses check boxes and drop-down lists; scan handouts and forms
   c. Accessibility: ready access to the record; available at any workstation
4. Diasadvantages:
   a. Initial cost
   b. Time investment for training
   c. Operational tasks
5. Information is entered during or immediately after each patient interaction
6. Paper reports are scanned into the record as soon as possible; originals are shredded
7. Password protected; access should be limited to the information a staff member needs to view
8. Signatures are taken electronically
9. EMRs should be backed up regularly and securely

II. RECORDS MANAGEMENT

A. Purpose
1. To classify, arrange, and store documents in an efficient, orderly, and accessible manner
   a. Records to be stored include:
      1) Medical records (charts)
      2) Financial records
      3) Patient correspondence
      4) Business records
      5) Research records
   b. Records can be stored as:
      1) Hard, printed, copies of the records
      2) Computer documents
      3) Microfiche and microfilm

B. Equipment and Supplies for Records Management
1. Storage cabinet
   a. Vertical: file cabinet style
   b. Lateral: chest of drawers style
   c. Shelf: open or closed storage
2. Guides
   a. Plastic or cardboard dividers; permit grouping of similar type files
   b. Outguide: guide used to replace a file taken from the cabinet; enables technician to replace the file in the proper place when ready
3. Folders
   a. Cardboard or plastic holders that contain the patients' medical records
   b. Have tabs within them for separating contents
4. Labels
   a. Small stickers placed onto folders to identify the contents or folder identity

C. Process
1. Condition
   a. Check for damage and, if found, repair it before refiling the record
   b. Date your work on the record, if required
2. Inspect and release
   a. Documents cannot be filed until the responsible parties have seen the document and have taken action on the record
   b. Release mark of some sort (office protocol) must be noted on the file
3. Index and code
   a. Determine where the document should be filed
   b. Identify the caption to be used in filing the document
4. Sort
   a. Arrange the documents according to the office protocol (system) used
5. Store
   a. Place the documents in the appropriate file folder and place in the filing cabinet

D. Filing Methods
1. Alphabetical
   a. Used with names of persons, businesses, or organizations; oldest, simplest, and most commonly used method
   b. Rules include:
      1) Names are divided into units and filed left to right
      2) Surname is unit 1, given name is unit 2, middle name (initial) is unit 3, and so on
      3) Names are alphabetized according to first unit letter; second unit considered if first units are the same; third unit considered if first two units are the same
      4) Initials filed before complete names starting with the same letter
      5) Units having no name filed before those that do (nothing before something)
      6) Hyphenated name is considered a single unit; if business name, each name is a separate unit
      7) Apostrophes are disregarded
      8) Abbreviations are indexed as if written in full
      9) Numbers as part of a name are indexed as if written out
      10) Titles and degrees are indexed last
      11) Married women are indexed by their own given name (first name)
      12) If two names are identical, patient's address is used as an index unit
      13) For names of organizations:
         a) Index in order as written, except when organization name includes a person's name (surname first, then given name)
         b) Numbers are indexed as if written out
         c) Disregard punctuation
         d) Directional terms are indexed as separate units
         e) Articles, conjunctions, and prepositions are disregarded unless *the* is the first word (if so, *the* is indexed as the last unit)
2. Numerical
   a. Used when each patient is assigned a number that is used on the patient's chart
   b. Patient number is cross-referenced with the patient's name and filed alphabetically
   c. Numerical filing is used in large clinics, group practices, and hospitals
   d. Types include:
      1) Consecutive numeric system
         a) Simplest system
         b) Patients are assigned consecutive numbers in the order of the date of their first visit to the facility

2) Terminal digit system
   a) Patients assigned consecutive numbers as they visit the facility
   b) Digits in the patient number are separated into groups of two or three
   c) Read in groups from right to left, instead of left to right, and filed backward in groups
3) Social security number
   a) Patient's social security number is patient's filing number
   b) Not every patient has a social security number

3. Subject
  a. Documents indexed by subject matter and then filed alphabetically, then filed numerically, or both
  b. Generally not used for medical records

4. Color coding
  a. Colored tabs are used to represent patient information at a glance
  b. Used on letters of the patient's surname
  c. Can help keep files from being misfiled
  d. Selection of colors and division of the alphabet are determined by the practice's needs
  e. Can be used as colored folders, adhesive labels, or a combination
  f. Can be filed alphabetically or numerically

5. Tickler file
  a. System that organizes items chronologically for follow-up
  b. Can be notations on the daily calendar, or a card file divided into months, with months divided into days
  c. To be effective, must be checked daily

9 *Patient Reception*

I. RECEPTION

A. General
1. Patient's first impression of the health care provider's office
2. Influences patient's perception of the office
3. Receptionist's attitude and appearance are important to set the tone of the office

II. RECEPTION AREA

A. General
1. Place to receive patients
2. Planned for patient comfort
3. Should be clean and uncluttered
4. Receptionist should be behind a counter that is high enough for health care provider privacy (of hard records, of patient information on computer screens, and of patient financial records)
5. Colors should be calming and restful
6. Lighting should be adequate for reading and safety
7. Adequate ventilation is essential
8. Temperature should be regulated for patients' comfort (average 72 °F)
9. Play area for children, if appropriate
10. Spacious coat rack to store patients' outerwear
11. Furniture arranged for patients' comfort, movement, and safety
12. Periodicals should be up to date and appropriate

III. RECEPTIONIST

A. General
1. First professional person with whom the patient comes in contact, either in person or by telephone
2. Medical assistant should display pride in him or herself and the job
3. Communication skills should demonstrate competence and a positive attitude
4. Clothing, hair, and makeup should be appropriate; follow office policies
5. Should have friendly, cheerful, caring, courteous, and respectful demeanor
6. Should be professional at all times
7. Greet every patient on arrival by name (using correct pronunciation)
8. A friendly farewell can show caring and courtesy
9. Duties may include:
    a. Answering telephones
    b. Scheduling appointments
    c. Registering patient and taking history
    d. Handling complaints
    e. Preparing charts
    f. Handling nonpatient visitors (vendors, sales representatives, pharmaceutical representatives)

IV. TELEPHONE TECHNIQUES

A. General
1. Majority of receptionist's communication occurs through the telephone
2. Telephone is the critical component of a successful health care provider's practice
3. Communication and listening skills are important
4. Incoming telephone calls may be from:
    a. Established patients calling for appointments or advice
    b. Patient emergencies
    c. Other physicians making patient referrals
    d. Laboratories reporting information regarding health care provider's patient
    e. New patients making a first contact
5. Telecommunication devices for the deaf (TDD)

B. Equipment
1. Six-button key set
    a. Several incoming lines
    b. Office intercom line
    c. Hold button
    d. Lights flash slowly for incoming calls, flash rapidly for reminder of call on hold

2. Two-line speakerphone
    a. Allows conversation without using the handset
    b. Last number redial
    c. Volume control
    d. Speed-dial and memory for frequent calls
    e. Intercom paging
    f. May have liquid crystal display (LCD) screen
3. Headset
    a. Lightweight plastic earphone and microphone combination
    b. Allows hands-free telephone use
4. Cellular telephone
    a. Mobile, transportable telephone
    b. Permits communication outside an office or within a vehicle
5. Pager
    a. Activated by calling the pager's number
    b. Can leave a voice message or digital message
6. Facsimile (fax) machine
    a. Transmits print material over telephone lines to other facilities that have fax capability
    b. Can send and receive copies of printed documents
    c. If sending sensitive patient information, call ahead to ensure that only the appropriate person receives the fax
7. Directories
    a. White pages: alphabetical listing by last name, includes last name, first name, sometimes middle initial, address, and telephone number
    b. Yellow pages: alphabetical listing by category of commercial business; in each category, alphabetical listing by company name (or businessperson's last name), includes company name (or businessperson's name), company address, and company telephone number or numbers
    c. Personal office directory: collection of frequently called telephone numbers within that office; can be stored in a Rolodex or in a 3 × 5 index card file
    d. Computerized directory: program that can hold names, information and phone numbers in order to access patients, providers, vendors, labs and referrals; many programs available

C. Incoming Calls

1. Answer promptly (ideally on the first ring, always by the third ring)
2. Hold the telephone instrument correctly (with the mouthpiece approximately 1 inch from your mouth)
3. Develop a pleasing telephone voice
4. Identify the health care provider's office; identify yourself
5. Gain the identity of the caller (ask to whom you are speaking if the caller does not first identify him or herself)
6. Offer assistance (using proper words and proper tone)
7. Screen incoming calls (follow any office policies about how incoming calls are to be handled and categorized)
8. Minimize caller waiting time (caller should experience no more than 1 minute without voice contact of some type)
9. When answering a second call, ask the first caller to please hold, transfer to the second incoming line, identify the second caller, ask the second caller to please hold, and return to the first caller
10. End each call pleasantly and graciously (say "thank you" and some form of "good-bye")

D. Telephone Messages

1. May be recorded on message sheet or in an office telephone log
2. Message should include the following information:
    a. Name of the person to whom the call is directed
    b. Name of the person calling
    c. Caller's daytime telephone number (include pager and/or cellular telephone numbers)
    d. Reason for the call
    e. Action to be taken by the recipient
    f. Date and time the call was received
    g. Initials of the person taking the call

E. Outgoing Telephone Calls

1. Know what needs to be said, how it is to be said, and have all pertinent information on hand before placing the call
2. Voice should convey warmth, friendliness, confidence, and intelligence
3. Address the person by name
4. Use "please" and "thank you"
5. Do not rush the call
6. Use discretion when conveying personal or confidential patient or medical information
7. Long distance (check with office manager to verify this procedure because different long-distance carriers have different calling requirements)
    a. Direct dial: 1 + area code + seven-digit telephone number
    b. Long-distance directory assistance: 1 + area code + 555-1212

    c. Operator assisted: 0 + area code + seven-digit telephone number
      1) Person-to-person (operator will not connect the line until the person to whom you requested answers the telephone)
      2) Station-to-station (operator will connect the line as soon as anyone at the receiving telephone number answers the telephone)
      3) Collect call (operator will not connect the line until a recipient agrees to be billed for the long-distance telephone call)
      4) Bill to third party (operator verifies that a third party [someone not a party to this long-distance telephone call] will accept the charges for the phone call)
      5) Request for time and charges (the operator, if asked before connecting the long-distance line, will call you back after the call is ended and will tell you the time of the long-distance call, as well as the cost of the long-distance call; you will then be able to verify the long-distance charge against the next telephone bill)
    d. Time zones
      1) Pacific Time: 1:00 (WA, OR, NV, CA)
      2) Mountain Time: 2:00 (MT, UT, ID, WY, CO, NM, AZ; parts of ND, SD, NE, KS)
      3) Central Time: 3:00 (MN, WI, IA, MO, AR, OK, TX, LA, MS, IL, AL; parts of TN, KY, ND, SD, NE, KS)
      4) Eastern Time: 4:00 (all other states, except for HI and AK)
    e. Wrong number dialed
      1) Verify the telephone number with the person answering
      2) Apologize
      3) If long distance, call the operator to credit the office account

F. Answering Services
1. Health care provider must be able to be contacted at all times in order to respond to emergencies (to prevent abandonment charges)
2. Answering services
    a. Provides coverage when the office is closed
    b. Answering services answer and screen incoming telephone calls
3. Electronic answering devices
    a. Recorded message that tells caller how to reach the health care provider (or health care provider's colleague) or invites the caller to leave a voice message
    b. Messages can be retrieved directly from the machine or can be remotely accessed
    c. Answering message may be changed as necessary

4. Voice mail: computerized system used to record, send, or retrieve voice message from the telephone system
5. Automatic routing
    a. Telephone calls answered by automated operator that announces a list of options from which the caller selects one
    b. This system is rather impersonal but may be good for the larger clinic

V. APPOINTMENT SCHEDULING

A. General
1. Process that determines which patients will be seen by the health care provider (*appointment*), the dates and times for the appointments, and the allotted time for each appointment
2. Allotted time for each appointment is based on the patient's complaint as compared with the health care provider's availability
3. Important factor in the success of health care provider's practice
4. Many approaches to scheduling

B. Guidelines
1. Understand the nature of the practice
2. Know the personalities and habits of the medical staff
3. Be aware of the time needed to assess each patient complaint type
4. Plan realistically

C. Materials Needed
1. Appointment book (see Figure 9-1)
    a. May be for one or several health care providers
    b. May show day, week, or month per page
    c. May be blank or preprinted
    d. May be loose-leaf or spiral bound
    e. Each block of time must have sufficient space to record the patient's name, the patient's telephone numbers, and the purpose of patient's visit to the health care provider
    f. Entire book must fit comfortably on the receptionist's desk and be easily accessible to all who are responsible for scheduling; the book must always be left in place
    g. Appointment book is a legal document and must be preserved as such
2. Pen or pencil
    a. Appointments should be written in black ink (because it is a legal document)
    b. Must be corrected in the same manner as correcting the patient chart (no erasing, no scribbling, no correction fluid)
    c. Use of pencil is more practical than a pen in anticipation of any appointment changes or cancellations
    d. Occasional use of colored ink (or pencil) may denote new or special patient

FIGURE 9-1 Sample appointment book. (Courtesy of Bibbero Systems, Inc., Petaluma, California 94954-1180, 800-242-2376; fax: 800-242-9330, *http://www.bibbero.com*.)

3. Appointment card
   a. Given to each patient after the follow-up appointment is made in the office
   b. Often preprinted with the clinic name, address, and telephone number, space on the card for date, day and time of appointment, and patient name

D. Methods of Scheduling
1. Open-office hours
   a. Clinic is open only for specified time period
   b. Patients are seen in the order of their arrival in the clinic (patients sign into a log-book on arrival), with provision that emergency treatment is given priority
   c. Least efficient method of scheduling
   d. Common among urgent care centers
   e. Triage: used to screen and classify sick or injured patients for priority
2. Flexible office hours
   a. Clinic is open at odd hours in addition to normal office hours (early morning or evening hours on certain days of the week)
   b. Accommodates various work schedules of patients
   c. Usually used in group practices
3. Time-specified hours
   a. Most common system
   b. Each patient is given a specific time on a specific day for the appointment
   c. Does not easily accommodate the unplanned illness or accident and does not allow any buffer time (unless one or two open appointments each day are kept for such use)
4. Wave
   a. Gives short-term flexibility within each hour
   b. Assumes that the average time needed for the appointments will average out over the course of the day
   c. Each hour is divided into the average time the health care provider should spend with each patient (hour divided into 10-minute, 15-minute, or 20-minute blocks)
   d. Patients are scheduled on the hour (6 per hour for 10-minute block, 4 per hour for 15-minute block, and so on) and are seen by the health care provider in the order in which they sign in with the receptionist
   e. This system allows for late arrivals, allows for the patient whose accident or illness needs more (or less) time than the average, allows for the failed appointment, and allows for unscheduled interruptions of the health care provider
   f. Variable waiting times may result from this method of scheduling

5. Modified wave: appointments are staggered throughout the health care provider hour
6. Double booking
   a. Scheduling two patients at the same time
   b. Not an efficient way to schedule
   c. Can be wavelike if two patients each needing 5 minutes are both scheduled in the same 15-minute block
7. Grouping
   a. Similar procedures (e.g., Pap smears, well-baby checks, complete physicals) are all scheduled at a specific time of a specific day of the week or at specific hours
   b. These like procedures can be color-coded for ease of view

E. Scheduling Procedures
1. Establish a matrix
   a. Block out times the health care provider is not available for appointments
   b. Establish a buffer time both in the morning and in the afternoon for catch-up
2. Chief complaint
   a. Identify the reason for patient visit
   b. Identify the level of urgency of the patient visit
   c. Identify the health care provider resources available
3. Referral: determine whether the patient has been referred by another health care provider
4. Locate the first available time to see the patient, as well as one alternative time; offer the dates and times to the patient
5. Enter the patient's name, telephone numbers, and complaint in the appointment book in the corresponding date and time block agreed to by the patient
6. Explain the pertinent office policies and instructions to the patient
7. Repeat the date and time to the patient for double-check before ending the call

F. Appointment Problems
1. Patient habitually late: schedule this patient near the end of the day
2. Consecutive appointments: schedule at the same time and day (different dates) for ease of remembering
3. Cancellations: offer the patient an alternative appointment
4. Missed appointment and no-show
   a. Prevent with a reminder telephone call the day before the appointment
   b. Patient may legally be charged for the missed appointment
   c. Patient may be discharged from health care provider's care for habitual no-shows
   d. Note all missed appointments in both the patient's chart and the appointment book

5. Emergencies
   a. Follow office protocol
   b. Emergencies take precedence over all other appointments
   c. Call 911 if the emergency is outside of the office protocol
6. Acute needs
   a. Provide the first available appointment to patient
   b. Double booking may be necessary
7. Referrals
   a. Process of sending patient to another health care provider (a specialist) for diagnosis and treatment
   b. Appointment may be made by the patient or by the referring health care provider
   c. Make sure all appropriate documents are provided to the referred health care provider (necessary patient records, x-rays, insurance referral letter)
8. Delays
   a. Attempt to call affected patients about health care provider delays, and request that they come later that day or reschedule for another date and time
   b. Explain courteously if the health care provider is called out of the office on an emergency
   c. Waiting patients should be given an explanation, an estimated time of the current delay, and the patients' option to wait on the health care provider or reschedule

G. Computerized Appointments
1. Software varies from simple to complex
2. Offer great flexibility
3. System searches for provider's schedule to locate available time
4. Schedule can be printed
5. More than one person can access the system at one time
6. Backup system should be in place (appointment book)

H. Self-Scheduling
1. Method by which a patient can log on to the Internet, view a facility's schedule, then select and make appointment
2. Confidentiality is provided by showing only times available, not names
3. Can reduce number of calls to office
4. Available 24 hours a day
5. Best used for uncomplicated appointments
6. Allowances must be made for patients who are computer illiterate or do not want their name on the Internet

I. Scheduling Other Types of Appointments
1. Inpatient surgery
   a. Call facility where procedure will be performed as soon as the operation is planned
   b. Provide all necessary information including special requests of the surgeon
   c. Provide patient's insurance information and phone number
2. Outpatient and inpatient procedures
   a. Can include laboratory, radiography, magnetic resonance imaging, computed tomography scans, and ultrasonography appointments
   b. Make sure all necessary information is available
   c. Inform patient of time, place, and any instructions; note this information in chart
   d. Must coordinate with the hospital instead of an outside facility

10 Office Management

I. INTRODUCTION

A. General
1. Process of developing, implementing, and achieving organizational goals
2. Administration (nonhuman resources) and leadership (human resources) work together to achieve goals
3. Chain of command is the line of authority in clinics

B. Process of Management
1. Planning: development of goals
2. Organizing: assembling resources needed to achieve the goals
3. Coordinating: bringing various resources together to achieve the goals
4. Directing: supervising the use of resources to achieve the goals
5. Controlling: making necessary adjustments to achieve the goals

C. Supervision
1. Begins with leadership
2. Leadership is the process of working with and through employees to achieve goals
3. Leadership requires two types of behavior:
   a. Task behavior: leader tells what, when, how, where, and who is to perform a specific task
   b. Relationship behavior: the way the leader communicates, listens, supports, and facilitates in assisting employees in performing a specific task
4. Leadership styles
   a. Telling: makes decisions and supervises employee performance
   b. Selling: makes and explains decisions to employees
   c. Participating: shares ideas and facilitates employee decision making
   d. Delegating: turns responsibility for making and implementing decisions over to the employees

D. Human Resources
1. Hiring process
   a. Recruiting: potential candidates are notified of an available position through advertisement
   b. Interviewing: face-to-face meeting and discussion with employee candidate
   c. Checking references: calling the references indicated by the employee candidate to verify the candidate's information
   d. Selection: choosing the best employee candidate based on the candidate's education, experience, references, and "fit"
   e. Offer: formally offering the position to the employee candidate, including wage and benefit information
   f. Negotiation: negotiating the specific terms of the employment offered
   g. Acceptance or rejection: employee candidate accepts the job offer and begins employment, or the candidate rejects the offer, and the employer again begins the process (or offers the position to the next-best candidate)
2. Job description should include:
   a. Job title
   b. Job summary
   c. Supervisor's title
   d. Job duties and employee responsibilities
   e. Job specifications
3. Orientation: transition from candidate to employee
4. Probation
   a. Time needed to determine whether the newly hired employee is a good "fit"
   b. Usually 60 to 90 days
5. Performance appraisal
   a. Objective employee performance assessment
   b. Should assess the employee's work, dependability, teamwork, appearance, and attitude
   c. Should be done regularly
   d. Result must be discussed with the employee

6. Discipline: all actions on employee performance should be recorded in the employee's personnel file
7. Professional development
   a. Encourage and subsidize professional development
   b. Encourage membership in professional organizations
   c. Promote the employee attendance at seminars, workshops, and conventions
   d. Enable the employee to obtain continuing education units (CEUs) or continuing medical education units (CMEs)

II. MEETINGS

A. General
1. Keep a calendar of all scheduled meetings (with date, time, place, and topic)
2. Meetings conducted in accordance with *Robert's Rules of Order*
3. Person chairing the meeting is responsible for all portions of the meeting process to ensure that objectives are met
4. Agenda should be typed and distributed to meeting members
5. Minutes are the record of the meeting; should include the date, time, place, and topic of the meeting; persons in attendance and those absent; issues discussed; and time of adjournment

III. EMPLOYER TRAVEL

A. General
1. Travel arrangements may be made by the medical assistant, a travel agent, or both
2. Itinerary should be typed; must include departure and arrival times and locations, contact telephone numbers, destination ground transportation, hotel accommodations, and a schedule of events and activities involved in the travel function; a copy of the travel itinerary must be kept in the office; a copy of the itinerary is given to the traveler
3. If the travel function is a speaking arrangement, then confirm the time, place, and topic; also confirm the honorarium (payment)
4. Check with the airlines before leaving for the airport in case of flight delays
5. Confirm ground transportation at the destination location (courtesy car, taxi service, hotel shuttle, rental car)
6. Confirm hotel accommodations; copy the reservation confirmation number onto the travel itinerary

IV. RESOURCE MANAGEMENT

A. Facility
1. Temperature: 68 °F to 74 °F, with proper ventilation
2. Lighting: fluorescent lighting in all examination and working areas
3. Floor covering: carpeting in waiting room, office, and hallways; sheet vinyl flooring in all examination, bathroom, and laboratory areas
4. Walls: soft or pastel colors, paint or wallpaper
5. Storage: locked space for supplies, equipment, and patient charts; locked and secure cabinets for drugs
6. Noise control: examination rooms and physician offices should be arranged to keep sounds at a minimum
7. Patient rooms: arranged so that the patient cannot be seen by others when the door is opened
8. Offices: separate from the patient examination areas
9. Clinical areas: checked between patients to maintain cleanliness and to keep neat and well stocked with supplies
10. Laboratory area: well ventilated; ensure that contamination is well controlled
11. Bathrooms: clean and well stocked; patient bathrooms should be separate from staff facilities
12. Janitorial services: staff should keep all areas neat, clean, and repaired; staff should schedule janitorial services for the remainder of cleaning duties
13. Safety: continually monitor the office for hazards; smoke alarms and fire extinguishers should be strategically placed and checked often to ensure that they are properly functioning; fire exits should be clearly marked and kept free of obstacles
14. Security: an adequate number of security personnel should be readily available
15. Regulated waste disposal: schedule regular regulated waste removal and sharps biohazard waste removal

B. Office Equipment
1. Keep warranties filed for future reference
2. Maintain a file for service agreements
3. Maintain a file with service technician telephone numbers
4. Keep inventories reports on file, with a physical inventory completed at least once a year; inventory should include:
   a. Name of item
   b. Model and serial number
   c. Date of purchase or lease (and price)

5. Inventory should be made of the following property:
   a. Laboratory equipment
   b. Clinical equipment
   c. Clinical instruments
   d. Office equipment
   e. Office furniture
   f. Anything of value that is not consumed in the treatment of patients

C. Supplies

1. Includes consumable items that are needed to operate the office, housekeeping supplies, and medical supplies
2. Ordered on an ongoing basis
3. One person within the office should be designated to order supplies and to maintain and inventory the supplies
4. Supply inventory (separate from office equipment inventory) should be kept up to date so that supplies never run out
5. Contents of supply deliveries should be checked in and verified against the purchase order and packing slip
6. Supplies must be stored in a neat and orderly fashion

V. RESOURCES FOR STAFF AND PATIENTS

A. Policy and Procedure Manuals

1. Information about the office for employees, which includes:
   a. Office or clinic mission statement
   b. Orientation information
   c. Dress code
   d. Job descriptions
   e. Holidays, leaves, vacations, and sick days
   f. Payroll and benefits
   g. Disciplinary actions
2. Procedure manual
   a. Description of steps taken to handle a situation or perform a certain task
   b. Regular review of procedures is necessary to be sure they are up-to-date and conform to legal regulations
   c. May be separate manuals for clinical and administrative procedures
   d. All personnel should be encouraged to use manuals as a reference

B. Emergency Preparedness and Evacuation Plan

1. Plan needs to be in place in order to respond to a fire, natural disaster, or emergency situation that affects the entire office
2. OSHA requires businesses to have a written plan to guide employees during an emergency

3. Written plan must include the following:
   a. Means of reporting emergencies
   b. Evacuation procedures and emergency escape routes
   c. Procedures to account for all employees
   d. Specific assignments for employees to follow
4. Map of the floor plan clearly showing marked escape routes should be posted

C. Community Resources

1. Help for patients who require community services to meet health needs
2. Office may keep a list of local organizations in the following areas:
   a. Support for alcoholism/addiction
   b. Support for caregivers of individuals with decreased mental or physical disability
   c. Visiting nurse and homemaker services
   d. Legal aid
   e. Local organizations to help children, families, older adults, and homeless
   f. Local health department
   g. Cardiopulmonary resuscitation and first aid training
   h. Immunization clinics
   i. Weight control and smoking cessation programs
3. Medical assistant may also assist patient in Internet search for resources

VI. RISK MANAGEMENT

A. Process of Assessing Risk and Putting Polices in Place to Minimize It

1. Office manager can be responsible
2. Policies are designed by provider working with an attorney and insurance company
3. When new policies are adopted, copy is given to each employee

B. Incident Reports

1. Report filed whenever anything happens in the office that could be considered liable
2. Initiated by staff member who is injured or closest to patient when injured
3. Reports vary, but usually ask for the following information:
   a. Date and time of incident
   b. Name of individual involved
   c. Address where incident happened
   d. Description of how the incident occurred and exactly what occurred
   e. Complete description of any injury
   f. Name of witness
   g. Name and contact information of person to whom the incident was reported
   h. Date of receipt/follow-up by supervisor

C. Liability Coverage
1. Adequate insurance protection against professional liability (malpractice) and accidents that may occur in the office
2. Medical assistant can purchase professional liability through a professional organization or may be covered by provider
3. Office should have adequate insurance to cover property damage to the office in case of fire, storm, or flooding
4. Office should have adequate coverage against personal injury sustained on the office's property
   a. If practice is in an office building, landlord is responsible for public areas
   b. If free-standing building, the practice is responsible for any occurrences on walkways, parking lot, or other outdoor areas

11 Finances

I. ACCOUNTING

A. General
1. Process of recording, classifying, summarizing, reporting, analyzing, and interpreting financial data
2. Provides financial information about the business operation

B. Accounting Elements
1. Asset
   a. Property owned or controlled by a business
   b. Includes:
      1) Land, buildings, fixtures, and furnishings
      2) Medical or office equipment
      3) Money
      4) Accounts receivable
      5) Stocks, bonds, and investments
2. Liability
   a. Debt obligation of the business
   b. Includes:
      1) Accounts payable
      2) Bank debts
3. Owner's equity
   a. Amount by which assets exceed liabilities; *net worth*
   b. Includes:
      1) Revenue (assets in)
      2) Expense (assets out)
      3) Drawing (personal use of assets)
4. Accounting equations
   a. Assets = Liabilities + Owner's Equity
   b. Liabilities = Assets − Owner's Equity
   c. Owner's Equity = Assets − Liabilities

II. BOOKKEEPING

A. Systems
1. Single-entry system
   a. Oldest and simplest method
   b. Simple to use, inexpensive, and requires little training
   c. Includes three basic records:
      1) Journal: also called the daily log, daybook, day sheet, or charge journal; records of charges and receipts are entered daily
      2) Cash payment journal: simple form of a checkbook
      3) Accounts receivable ledger: record of the amounts that patients owe the office; each patient has his or her own card; statements are prepared manually from these cards
   d. Lacks methods for cross-checking to prevent errors
2. Pegboard (write-it-once) system (see Figure 11-1)
   a. Most common manual method used in the physician's office
   b. All transactions are recorded at one time
   c. Uses the following materials:
      1) Pegboard
         a) Plastic board with pegs along the left edge
         b) Pegs hold perforated accounting entry pages
      2) Day sheet
         a) Page size of pegboard
         b) Keeps record of all daily charges and receipts
      3) Ledger card: record of all charges and payments for each patient
      4) Charge slip or charge receipt
         a) Form used to record a charge
         b) Serves as a bill or receipt if payment is made by the patient
         c) May be in the form of a *superbill* or *encounter form* (a multipage, carbonless charge slip; one copy of the form is given to the patient, and one copy is kept by the office; one copy of the form is forwarded to the patient's insurance company)
   d. Day sheet is affixed to the pegboard (perforations on the sheet are placed over the pegs on the pegboard)

FIGURE 11-1 Sample day sheet for pegboard bookkeeping system, with deposit list of checks and optional business analysis summaries. (Courtesy of Patterson Office Supplies, a division of Patterson Companies, Inc., 1-800-637-1140.)

e. Each patient ledger card is placed over the day sheet, hooked onto the pegs so that the columns and rows line up with the day sheet

f. Charge slip or charge receipt is placed over the patient ledger card

g. Bookkeeping entries are made and recorded simultaneously on all forms on the pegboard

3. Double-entry system
   a. Inexpensive method but requires some training
   b. Transactions may be recorded manually or by computer
   c. Each transaction is recorded in a way that keeps a balance of accounting equation
   d. Each transaction affects two accounts: one is debited, the other is credited

B. Accounts Receivable
1. Fees that patients owe for services performed
2. Most receipts come from third-party payments (e.g., insurance carrier); payments might not be received for 30 to 90 days after service
3. Accounts are classified according to the amount of time that the balance remains unpaid (current, 30 days, 60 days, over 90 days, past due)

C. Accounts Payable
1. Money owed to vendors
2. Payments to vendors for purchases and services
3. Invoice normally accompanies the purchase
4. Record of payments kept by making an entry into the appropriate accounts payable record

D. Petty Cash
1. Cash kept within the office to cover minor purchases
2. Usual amount is $50.00
3. Eliminates the need to write a check for minor purchases
4. Fund is established by writing a check on the office account; this check is cashed by the bank, and the cash is placed in a safe place within the office
5. One person is designated to make disbursements from the petty cash fund
6. A voucher is normally required to draw cash out of the fund; the voucher should show the name of the person taking the cash, the amount of cash taken, and the purpose of the petty cash draw; this voucher is used to balance the account
7. A register should be maintained to track the vouchers
8. The petty cash fund is replenished by again writing and cashing a check

III. BILLING

A. Fees
1. Should reflect the revenue necessary to maintain the financial stability of the practice
2. Influenced by the time to be spent and the degree of difficulty in providing the service

3. Set up by a schedule that includes code numbers, detailed description, and cost of each particular service rendered within the practice
4. The schedule must be available to all patients
   a. Usual fee: fee most frequently charged for a particular service
   b. Customary fee: range of usual fees charged for the particular service by practitioners of similar training and experience
   c. Reasonable fee: fee assigned to an unusual service or a service that has complex features; meets the criteria of usual and customary fees

B. Forms
1. Patient information form
   a. Used to collect and maintain general information about the patient for billing purposes
   b. Includes the patient's name, home address, home telephone number, occupation, business address, business telephone number, social security number; name of the insured, insurance carrier, and policy number; the spouse's name, occupation, business address, and business telephone number; and an emergency contact telephone number
2. Release of information form
   a. Used to request information gathered by other medical providers
   b. Patient's signature authorizes a third party (e.g., insurance company) to be given information about the patient's treatment
3. Assignment of benefits form: patient's signature requests the insurance company to send insurance proceeds directly to the provider

C. Billing Methods
1. Time-of-service
   a. Fee collected when the service is provided
   b. Reduces collection costs
   c. Increases cash flow
2. Monthly billing: a bill is sent to each patient on a monthly basis
3. Cycle billing: a bill is sent to certain segments of the patient population at a consistent time each month, with each segment being sent at a different time during the month
4. Billing service: the office may contract with an outside agency to prepare and send the bills to the patients

D. Statements
1. Typed: each patient bill is individually typed
2. Ledger cards: copies are made of the patient's ledger card entries and mailed to the patient
3. Superbill (encounter form, routing slip) (see Figure 11-2)

STATE LIC. # 123456789
SOC. SEC. # 000-11-0000
PIN # _____

JOHN R. JOHNSON, M.D.
Family Practice
1000 MAIN STREET, SOME PLACE, USA 70000

TELEPHONE: (123) 234-5678

☐ PRIVATE   ☐ BLUECROSS   ☐ IND.   ☐ MEDICARE   ☐ MEDI-CAL   ☐ HMO   ☐ PPO

PATIENT'S LAST NAME	FIRST	ACCOUNT #	BIRTHDATE / /	SEX ☐ MALE ☐ FEMALE	TODAY'S DATE / /
INSURANCE COMPANY	SUBSCRIBER		PLAN #	SUB. #	GROUP

ASSIGNMENT: I hereby assign my insurance benefits to be paid directly to the undersigned physician. I am financially responsible for non-covered services.
SIGNED: (Patient, or Parent, if Minor)   DATE: /   /

RELEASE: I hereby authorize the physician to release to my insurance carrers any information required to process this claim.
SIGNED: (Patient, or Parent, if Minor)   DATE: /   /

✔	DESCRIPTION	M/Care	CPT/Mod	DxRe	FEE	✔	DESCRIPTION	M/Care	CPT/Mod	DxRe	FEE	✔	DESCRIPTION	M/Care	CPT/Mod	DxRe	FEE
	OFFICE CARE						PROCEDURES						INJECTIONS/IMMUNIZATIONS				
	NEW PATIENT						Treadmill (In Office)		93015				Tetanus Toxoid		90703		
	Focused		99201				24 Hr. Holter Monitor		93224				Hypertet	J1670	90782		
	Expanded		99202				Recording Only		93225				Pneumococcal		90732		
	Detailed		99203				Interp. & Report		93227				Influenza		90724		
	Comprehensive-Mod.		99204				EKG w/Interpretation		93000				TB Skin Test (PPD)		86585		
	Comprehensive-High		99205				EKG (Medicare)		93005				Antigen Injection-Single		95115		
							Sigmoidoscopy		45300				Multiple		95117		
	ESTABLISHED PATIENT						Sigmoidoscopy, Flexible		45330				B12 Injection	J3420	90782		
	Minimal		99211				Sigmoidos. . Flex. w/Bx.		45331				Injection, IM		90788		
	Focused		99212				Spirometry, FEV/FVC		94010				Compazine	J0780	90782		
	Expanded		99213				Spirometry, Post-Dilator		94060				Demerol	J2175	90782		
	Detailed		99214										Vistaril	J3410	90782		
	Comprehensive-Mod.		99215										Susphrine	J0170	90782		
	Comprehensive-High		99215				LABORATORY						Decadron	J0890	90782		
							Routine Venipuncture		36415				Estradiol	J1000	90782		
	CONSULTATION-OFFICE						Urinalysis, Chemical		81005				Testosterone	J1080	90782		
	Focused		99241				Throat Culture		87081				Lidocaine	J2000	90782		
	Expanded		99242				Occult Blood		82270				Solumedrol	J2920	90782		
	Detailed		99243				Pap Handling Charge		99000				Solucortef	J1720	90782		
	Comprehensive-Mod.		99244				Pap Life Guard		88150-90				Hydeltra	J1690	90782		
	Comprehensive-High		99245				Gram Stain		87205				Pen Procaine	J2510	90788		
	Dr.						Wet Mount		87210								
	Post-op Exam		99024				Urine Drug Screen		99000				INJECTIONS - JOINT/BURSA				
	EVALUATION/CASE MANAGEMENT												Arthrocentesis-Small Jt.		20600		
	Brief Eval.-30 Mins.		99361										Arthrocent.-Interm. Jts.		20605		
	Intermed. Eval.-60 Mins.		99362				SUPPLIES						Arthrocent.-Major Jts.		20610		
	Telephone-Brief		99371										Trigger Point Injection		20550		
	Telephone-Intermed.		99372										MISCELLANEOUS				
	Telephone-Complex		99272														

DIAGNOSIS:	ICD-9												
Abdominal Pain	789.0_	Gout	274.0	C.V.A. - Acute	436.	Electrolyte Dis.	276.9	Herpes Simplex	054.9
Abscess (Site)	682.9	Asthma	493.90	Cere. Vas. Accid. (Old)	438	Fatigue	780.7	Herpes Zoster	053.9
Adverse Drug Rx	995.2	Asthmatic Bronchitis	491.20	Cerumen	380.4	Fibrocys. Br. Dis	610.1	Hydrocele	603.9
Alcohol Detox	291.8	Atrial Fib.	427.31	Chestwall Pain	786.59	Fracture (Site)	829.0	Hyperlipidemia	272.4
Alcoholism	303.90	Atrial Tachycardia	427.89	Cholecystitis	575.0	Open/Close		Hypertension	401.9
Allergic Rhinitis	477.9	Bowel Obstruct.	560.9	Cholelithiasis	574.00	Fungal Infect. (Site)	117.9	Hyperthyroidism	242.9
Allergy	995.3	Breast Mass	611.72	COPD	496	Gastric Ulcer	531.90	Hypothyroidism	244.9
Alzheimer's Dis.	290.1_	Bronchitis, Acute	466.0	Cirrhosis	571.5	Gastritis	535.0	Labyrinthitis	386.30
Anemia	285.9	Bursitis	727.3	Cong. Heart Fail.	428.9	Gastroenteritis	558.9	Lipoma (Site)	214.9
Anemia - Pernicious	281.0	Cancer, Breast (Site)	174.9	Conjunctivitis	372.30	G.I. Bleeding	578.9	Lymphoma	202.8
Angina	413.9	Metastatic (Sito)	108.2	Contusion (Site)	924.9	Glomerulonephritis	583.89	Mit. Valve Prolapse	424.0
Anxiety Synd.	300.00	Colon	153.9	Costochondritis	733.99	Headache	784.0	Myocard. Infarction (Area)	410.9
Appendicitis	541	Cancer, Rectal	154.1	Depression	311.	Headache, Tension	307.81	M.I., Old	412
Arterioscl. H.D.	414.0_	Lung (Sito)	162.0	Dermatitis	692.9	Migraine (Type)	346.9	Myositis	729.1
Arthritis, Osteo.	715.90	Skin (Site)	173.9	Diabetes Mellitus	250.00	Hemorrhoids	455.6	Nausea/Vomiting	787.01
Rheumatoid	714.0	Card. Arrhythmia (Type)	427.9	Diabetic Ketosis	250.10	Hernia, Hiatal	553.3	Neuralgia	729.2
Lupus	710.0	Cardiomyopathy	425.4	Diverticulitis	562.11	Inguinal	550.9	Nevus (Site)	216.9
		Cellulitis (Site)	682.9	Diverticulosis	562.10	Hepatitis	573.3	Obesity	278.00

DIAGNOSIS: (IF NOT CHECKED ABOVE)

SERVICES PERFORMED AT: ☐ Office   ☐ E.R.
☐   ☐   ☐ CLAIM CONTAINS NO
                                            ORDERED REFERRING SERVICE

REFERRING PHYSICIAN & I.D. NUMBER

RETURN APPOINTMENT INFORMATION:
5 - 10 - 15 - 20 - 30 - 40 - 60

[DAYS] [WKS.] [MOS.] [PRN]

NEXT APPOINTMENT
M - T - W - TH - F - S
DATE   /   /   TIME:

AM
PM

ACCEPT ASSIGNMENT?
☐ YES
☐ NO

DOCTOR'S SIGNATURE

INSTRUCTIONS TO PATIENT FOR FILING INSURANCE CLAIMS:

1. Complete upper portion of this form, sign and date.
2. Attach this form to your own insurance company's form for direct reimbursement.

**MEDICARE PATIENTS - DO NOT SEND THIS TO MEDICARE.
WE WILL SUBMIT THE CLAIM FOR YOU.**

☐ CASH
☐ CHECK
   # _____
☐ VISA
☐ MC
☐ CO-PAY

TOTAL TODAY'S FEE	
OLD BALANCE	
TOTAL DUE	
AMOUNT REC'D. TODAY	

FIGURE 11-2 Superbill. (Courtesy of Bibbero Systems, Inc., Petaluma, California 94954-1180, 800-242-2376, fax 800-242-8330, http://www.bibbero.com.)

a. Presented to the patient at each visit
b. Payment is made at the time of the office visit or mailed in at a later date

4. Computerized: data are keyed into an accounting computer program; statements are automatically generated by the accounting software

IV. COLLECTIONS

A. General
1. Revenue from services rendered must be collected to cover expenses
2. Harassing debtors is illegal

B. Telephone Collections
1. Making threatening or abusive calls when attempting to collect a debt is illegal
2. Call between 8:00 AM and 8:00 PM and only to the patient's home telephone when attempting to collect a debt
3. Determine the identity of the person with whom you are discussing debt collection by using the debtor's full name
4. Be positive and assertive
5. State the purpose of your call
6. Attempt to obtain a commitment by the debtor before ending the debt collection call; attempt to get the debtor to promise to deliver a certain sum by a certain date
7. After this initial debt collection contact, follow up with another confirmation call

C. Mailings
1. Use letters within opaque envelopes for debt collection, never postcards
2. Prepare correspondence to meet the situation (begin debt collection process with a friendly tone, progressing to a more assertive tone as debt collection lags)
3. Debt collection letters should be signed by the office manager
4. Inform the patient by Certified Mail or Return Receipt Requested of possible collection agency action or legal action to collect the debt

D. Progressive Collection Process
1. Office should have developed a color-coded or written stage-by-stage process by which the office can keep track of debt collection efforts (with the process identified first by friendly tones, progressing to more assertive tones as debt collection lags)

E. Collection Agency
1. Forward the past due account to the collection agency once the account has been determined uncollectible by office personnel

2. Once the account is given to a collection agency, the clinic may not continue collection efforts on the debt
3. Patients should make payments on their debt only to the collection agency once the account has been turned over to the agency
4. The collection agency will keep a percentage of the amount collected as their fee

V. PAYROLL

A. General
1. Affected by federal and state laws and regulations
2. Income tax, Federal Insurance Contributions Act (FICA), and Federal Unemployment Tax Act (FUTA) amounts withheld from employee checks must be paid to the Internal Revenue Service (IRS) and to the state tax commissioner at regular intervals
3. Payroll procedures must be explained to all new employees

B. Laws and Regulations
1. Detailed records must be kept in the office for each employee, including:
   a. Name, address, social security number
   b. Amount and date of each wage payment and period covered by the payment
   c. Amount of wages subject to taxes
   d. Amount and type of taxes withheld from employee's pay
   e. Date when employee begins work; date when employee leaves the employment
2. Fair Labor Standards Act
   a. Sets minimum wage
   b. Requires employers to pay 1½ times employee's regular wage for time worked over 40 regular hours
3. Title VII, Civil Rights Act of 1964: prohibits discrimination based on employee's race, color, religion, or gender in hiring, firing, or promoting employees
4. Age Discrimination in Employment Act: prohibits unfair practices in employment decisions regarding people over 40 years of age
5. Americans with Disabilities Act: prohibits unfair practices in employment decisions (and in many other areas) regarding people with physical, mental, or medical disabilities
6. Family Medical Leave Act of 1993
   a. In the case of birth, adoption, sick or injured family member, an employee is entitled to unpaid leave to care for the child, spouse, parent, or for him or herself
   b. The employee is entitled to benefits and job protection while on leave

C. Taxes

1. Income tax
   a. Employers are required by law to withhold employee income tax
   b. Amount withheld from the employee's paycheck is based on a graduated rate table
2. FICA
   a. Social Security and Medicare tax
   b. Employers are required to withhold (collect) these taxes from employee wages
   c. Employer submits amounts withheld to the IRS when the employer pays the employer's taxes
   d. Taxes are deducted from the employee's earnings each pay period
   e. Every dollar paid by the employee is matched, dollar for dollar, by the employer
3. FUTA
   a. Federal law requires employers to withhold tax to support the unemployment insurance programs
   b. Amount of tax withheld is computed on a graduated rate table based on employee earnings

D. Forms and Reports

1. Form SS-4
   a. Federal Tax Identification Number application form
   b. Required for employers who hire employees and who withhold taxes from employee pay
2. Form SS-5
   a. Social security number application form
   b. All employees are required to have a social security number
3. Form W-2
   a. Wages and Tax Statement
   b. Given to all employees
   c. Lists the wages earned (by one employee) and taxes withheld on wages for the preceding year
   d. Used to prepare personal income tax return
   e. Must be provided to employees by January 31 of the following year
   f. Consists of six parts:
      1) Copy A: sent to the Social Security Administration
      2) Copy 1: sent to the state tax department
      3) Copy B: filed with the employee's federal tax return
      4) Copy C: kept by the employee
      5) Copy 2: filed with employee's state tax return
      6) Copy D: retained by the employer
4. Form W-3
   a. Transmittal of Income and Tax Statement
   b. Used to report the total amount of income and FICA tax withheld during the year

   c. Filed by the employer with the Social Security Administration
5. Form W-4
   a. Employee's Withholding Allowance Certificate
   b. Identifies the total number of withholding allowances claimed by the employee
6. Form 940: employer's annual federal unemployment tax return
7. Form 941
   a. Employer's quarterly federal tax return
   b. Filed quarterly to report FUTA and income tax amounts to the federal government
8. Form 8109
   a. Federal Tax Deposit Coupon Book
   b. Used to make quarterly federal income tax and FUTA payments
9. Form 1099
   a. IRS form to report income other than wages
   b. A physician-employer's honoraria from speaking engagements would be claimed on this form
10. Form I-9: confirms U.S. citizenship or legality of working papers if a foreign national

E. Payroll Systems

1. Manual
   a. Most common for smaller organizations
   b. Payroll is computed and processed by hand
2. Computerized
   a. Data are entered into accounting management computer program
   b. Payroll calculations automatically prepared by the software
   c. Detailed records and reports are automatically prepared by the software
3. Payroll services
   a. Payroll data are sent to the payroll service
   b. Service prepares the payroll and delivers detailed records, reports, and the payroll checks to the office

VI. CHECKING ACCOUNTS

A. General (see Figure 11-3)

1. The majority of money transactions out of the office are conducted by check
2. A check is a commercial paper drawn on funds deposited in a bank account
3. A check is a written order for the bank to pay a person a specific amount of money
4. A check is negotiable; anyone who properly endorses the check is entitled to receive the money
5. Parties involved in a check:
   a. Drawer: the person writing the check
   b. Drawee: the bank
   c. Payee: the person who is to receive the money from the check

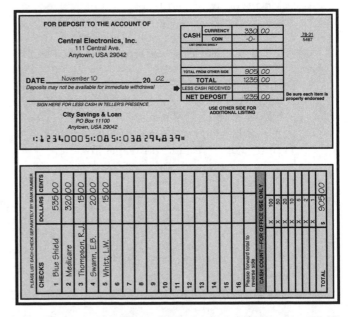

FIGURE 11-3 The first four examples illustrate the correct method of writing a check. The last example (bottom right) shows the incorrect method of writing a check, with incomplete name and space for altering (e.g., 6.00 might be made into 26.00 or more, and 00 could be made into 88). (Young AP, Kennedy DB: *Kinn's the medical assistant: an applied learning approach,* ed 10, St Louis, 2007, Saunders.)

B. Opening a Checking Account

1. Requires approval from a bank official
2. Requires an initial deposit, in accordance with the bank's rules
3. Requires a signature card: the signature card contains the names and signatures of all persons who are authorized to access the checking account

C. Deposits

1. Can be made by using:
   a. Paper money
      1) Arranged in order of denomination (smallest value bill on top)
      2) All bills should be arranged face up and top up
   b. Coins: a large quantity of coins should be wrapped in coin wrappers before deposit
   c. Checks
      1) Office personnel should verify each check for completeness
      2) Each check must be endorsed (in writing or by stamp) directing how the check is to be applied
   d. Deposit slip: a preprinted form with account information; identifies all items being deposited (see Figure 11-4)

FIGURE 11-4 Front and back of a deposit slip. (Young AP, Kennedy DB: *Kinn's the medical assistant: an applied learning approach,* ed 10, St Louis, 2007, Saunders.)

1) Enter the date of the deposit
2) Enter the total amount of coins and currency being deposited
3) Enter and note separately each check to be deposited

4) Record the total amount of the deposit
5) Withdraw cash by entering the amount to be withdrawn on the designated space on the deposit slip and subtracting this amount from the deposit total; if a withdrawal of cash is needed, the deposit slip must be signed

D. Dishonored Checks

1. A check that the bank refuses to pay
2. Usually the result of insufficient funds in the account (NSF: not sufficient funds)
3. If a check is deposited and not accepted by the bank it is written on, the payee's bank will return the dishonored check back to the payee, will deduct the amount of that check from payee's account, and will normally assess the payee a fee for the work caused
   a. Overdraft
      1) Issuing a check without sufficient funds in the writer's account
      2) Knowingly issuing an NSF check is illegal
   b. Postdated check: issuing a check but putting a date in the future on the check; a bank may not honor a check until the date on the check

E. Bank Statements

1. Statement of account sent to each depositor once a month by the bank
2. Gives the account holder the following information:
   a. Account balance at the beginning of the period
   b. Amount of deposits made during the period
   c. Amount of checks paid during the period
   d. Other items paid or credited during the period
   e. Account balance at the end of the period
3. Canceled checks may be enclosed with the statement
4. Statement needs to be reconciled (to ensure that the bank's balance agrees with the office's balance)
   a. Compare the deposited amounts recorded in the office files with the amounts recorded on the statement
   b. Compare the canceled check amounts with those on the statement and on the office check register
   c. Identify all debits and credits to the account between the bank's and the office's records
   d. Identify any errors found on the bank statement or on the office register
   e. Add and subtract all adjustments made to the bank statement and to the office register; both balances should be equal

12 Coding

I. INTRODUCTION TO CODING

A. Purpose

1. Coding system translates descriptions of diseases, illnesses, injuries, and procedures into numeric codes
2. Helps insurance company quickly and accurately review what services the patient received and how they are related to the illness or injury
3. Facilitates the use of computers in insurance claim processing
4. Developed for:
   a. Tracking disease processes
   b. Classification of medical procedures
   c. Medical research
   d. Evaluation of hospital utilization
   e. Reimbursement

B. Types of Coding Systems

1. ICD-9-CM
   a. *International Classification of Diseases,* ninth edition, Clinical Modification
   b. Used to code disease conditions or diagnosis
2. CPT-4
   a. *Current Procedural Terminology,* fourth edition
   b. Used to code procedures and medical services provided by practitioner
3. HCPCS
   a. Health Care Financing Administration (HCFA) Common Procedural Coding System
   b. Used to report services performed to Medicare program
4. RVS
   a. Relative value scale
   b. Assigned unit value given to commonly performed medical procedures
   c. Based on time, knowledge, and skill required by the practitioner
   d. Point value is multiplied by a dollar factor to find a final fee amount

5. RBRVS
   a. Resource-based relative value scale
   b. Fee schedule for Medicare for services based on level of resources needed to provide the service
6. DRG
   a. Diagnosis-related groups
   b. Medicare-fixed fee structure for hospital billing of inpatient services
   c. Based on principal diagnosis

II. ICD-9-CM

A. General

1. Assigns numeric codes to illnesses, diseases, injuries, and health-related condition

B. ICD-9-CM System

1. Volume I (Tabular List of Diseases): numeric arrangement of conditions
   a. 110 to 799: codes that refer to specific conditions by body systems
   b. 800 to 959, 990 to 999: codes that refer to injury
   c. 960 to 989: codes that refer to poisoning
   d. V-codes (V01 to V82): codes that refer to factors that influence health status (e.g., well-baby checks, annual physicals)
   e. E-codes: external causes of injury (poisonings, adverse effects of drugs, accidents/falls, suicide/self-inflicted injuries)
   f. M-codes: morphology of neoplasms
2. Volume II (Disease: Alphabetical List): three-part index for volume I
   a. Section I: alphabetical index of disease and injury
   b. Section II: table of adverse reactions to drugs and chemicals
   c. Section III: index of external causes (E-Codes)
3. Volume III (Tabular List and Alphabetical Index of Procedures)
   a. Used primarily in hospitals
   b. Procedures are arranged both alphabetically and numerically

C. **Organization of Volumes**
1. Volume I
   a. Codes 001 through 999 use a three-digit main number, with a specificity to cause identified with a fourth digit; a fifth digit may be required
   b. Chapter headings in bold uppercase letters
   c. Notes following the chapter headings give guidelines for coding within the chapter
   d. Major topic headings are in uppercase letters followed by inclusive codes in parentheses
   e. Exclusion statements tell what is *not* included in the specific code number
   f. Category headings further divide major topic headings
   g. Subcategory headings are indented and include a fourth-digit modifier
   h. Fifth-digit modifiers further subdivide the subcategory heading; generally flagged in some way (a section mark)
2. Volume II
   a. Alphabetical listing of conditions
   b. May be expressed as nouns, adjectives, or eponyms
   c. Main terms are highlighted in bold type followed by the code number
   d. Modifiers in parentheses may be present between the main term and the code number
   e. Subterms are indented, giving further subclassifications

D. **Conventions**
1. Volume I
   a. Colon (:): modifiers after the colon complete the statement before the colon
   b. Brace (}): term after the brace is a required modifier
   c. Section mark (§): identifies a code that needs a fifth-digit modifier
   d. Excludes (/): enclosed within a rectangle; conditions following this mark do not qualify for code assignment
   e. Includes: clarifies a description
2. Volume II
   a. Diagnoses are organized by main terms printed in boldface type
   1) Modifiers: specific factors that influence a diagnostic code
      a) Nonessential: main term followed by terms in parentheses; may be included with the main term
      b) Subterm: specific manifestations of a condition; these have a specific code number; indented below the main term
      c) Adjectives: appear as main terms with no code numbers; reference to *see condition*

   2) *See also:* directs researcher to another code number
   3) *See category:* directs the researcher to look into a synonym for the condition
   4) *See condition:* directs the researcher that the wrong word is being looked up
3. Volumes I and II
   a. Brackets ([ ]): enclosed terms are synonyms, explanatory phrases, or alternative words
   b. Slanted (italicized) brackets (*[]*): indicate a need for another code
   c. Parentheses (( )): enclosed terms may or may not affect a main term
   d. NEC (not elsewhere classified): used for ill-defined terms for which more precise information is not available
   e. NOS (not otherwise specified): general diagnosis term that may require more specific information
   f. Note: defines terms, or provides directions (fifth-digit modifier)
   g. *See:* directs researcher to look at another code

E. **Coding Steps (see Figure 12-1)**
1. Locate the term in the alphabetical index of volume II
2. Read and act on the notes printed after the term
3. Consider modifiers of the term
4. Follow cross-references
5. Verify the code number in volume I and make modifications as instructed
6. Record the code assignment

F. **Table Guidelines**
1. Two coding tables in volume II:
   a. Hypertension table: three main column headings:
   1) Malignant: severe; vascular damage; diastolic blood pressure > 130 mm Hg
   2) Benign: mild; in control
   3) Unspecified: no note of malignant or benign
   b. Neoplasm table
   1) Arranged by site
   2) Six classifications:
      a) Primary malignancy: original tumor site
      b) Secondary malignancy: tumor metastasized
      c) Carcinoma in situ: localized: noninvasive malignant tumor
      d) Benign: nonspreading, noninvasive tumor
      e) Uncertain behavior: impossible to predict behavior or morphology
      f) Unspecified: tumor with no indication of histology

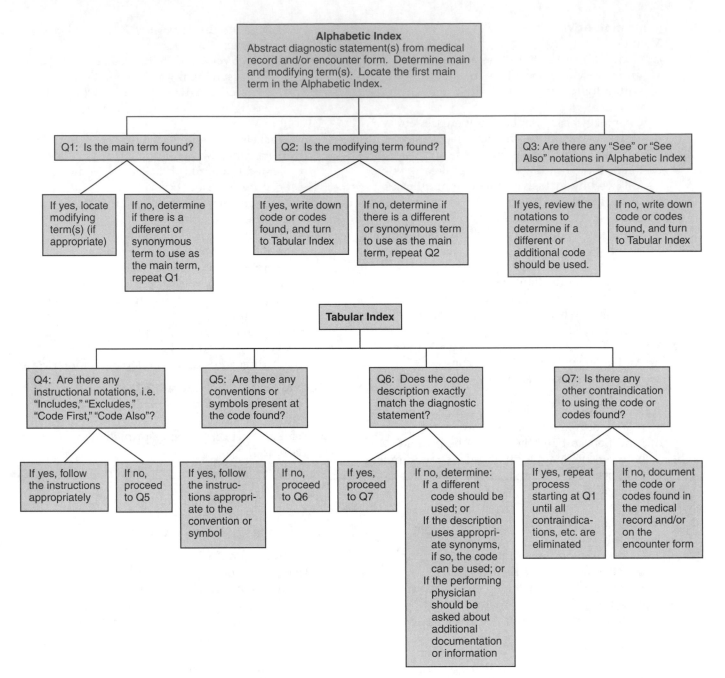

Alphabetic Index
Abstract diagnostic statement(s) from medical record and/or encounter form. Determine main and modifying term(s). Locate the first main term in the Alphabetic Index.

Q1: Is the main term found?

If yes, locate modifying term(s) (if appropriate)

If no, determine if there is a different or synonymous term to use as the main term, repeat Q1

Q2: Is the modifying term found?

If yes, write down code or codes found, and turn to Tabular Index

If no, determine if there is a different or synonymous term to use as the main term, repeat Q2

Q3: Are there any "See" or "See Also" notations in Alphabetic Index

If yes, review the notations to determine if a different or additional code should be used.

If no, write down code or codes found, and turn to Tabular Index

Tabular Index

Q4: Are there any instructional notations, i.e. "Includes," "Excludes," "Code First," "Code Also"?

If yes, follow the instructions appropriately

If no, proceed to Q5

Q5: Are there any conventions or symbols present at the code found?

If yes, follow the instructions appropriate to the convention or symbol

If no, proceed to Q6

Q6: Does the code description exactly match the diagnostic statement?

If yes, proceed to Q7

If no, determine:
If a different code should be used; or
If the description uses appropriate synonyms, if so, the code can be used; or
If the performing physician should be asked about additional documentation or information

Q7: Is there any other contraindication to using the code or codes found?

If yes, repeat process starting at Q1 until all contraindications, etc. are eliminated

If no, document the code or codes found in the medical record and/or on the encounter form

FIGURE 12-1 Decision tree for ICD-9-CM diagnostic coding. (Young AP, Proctor DB: *Kinn's the medical assistant: an applied learning approach*, ed 10, St. Louis, 2007, Saunders.)

III. CPT-4

A. General

1. Lists and codes procedures and services performed by practitioners
2. Each procedure is identified by a five-digit code
3. Simplifies reporting to insurance carriers
4. CPT book is divided into six sections; subsections include anatomic, procedural, conditions, and descriptors:
   a. Evaluation and Management (E&M): 99200 to 99499
   b. Anesthesia: 00100 to 01999
   c. Surgery: 10000 to 69999
   d. Radiology, Nuclear Medicine, and Diagnostic Ultrasound: 70000 to 79999
   e. Pathology and Lab: 80000 to 89999
   f. Medicine: 90701 to 99199

B. Format and Conventions

1. Main statement followed by semicolon; subordinate statement describes procedure or extent of services
2. Terms: indented below main statement giving additional statements

3. Guidelines: specific directions at the beginning of each section; necessary to code correctly
4. Modifiers: two-digit, terminal code; represents an alteration of the procedure or circumstances
5. Major headings are boldface
6. Notes: provide coding instructions
7. Descriptive qualifiers: descriptions surrounding a code provide more detailed information; sometimes in parentheses

C. Coding Steps (see Figure 12-2)
1. Review the guidelines beginning each section
2. Turn to the index and locate the main term
3. Locate the subterm and follow the cross-references

4. Read the code descriptors of all code numbers
5. Record the proper code

D. E&M
1. Includes basic diagnostic and treatment services
2. E&M section divided into broad categories with two or more subdivisions
   a. New patient: patient who is new to the practice or who has not received any professional services by the practitioner for 3 or more years
   b. Established patient: patient who has received professional services from the practitioner within the last 3 years

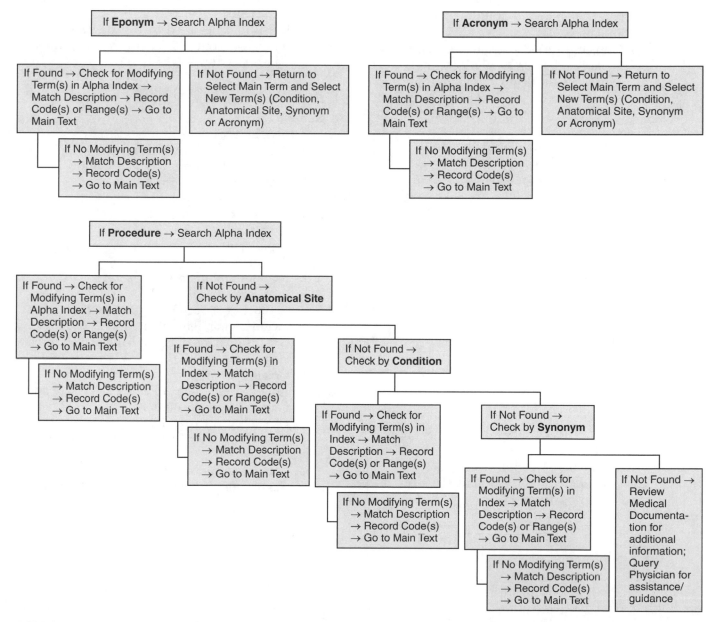

FIGURE 12-2 Decision tree for CPT-4 main text. (Young AP, Proctor DB: *Kinn's the medical assistant: an applied learning approach,* ed 10, St. Louis, 2007, Saunders.)

c. Concurrent care: rendering of similar services to the same patient by more than one practitioner on the same day

d. Counseling: discussion with the patient and/or family regarding diagnosis, treatment, and patient education

3. The following *must* be determined within each category to select the correct E&M code:

   a. History

      1) Problem-focused: chief complaint and brief history of problem

      2) Expanded problem-focused: chief complaint, brief history, and review of system affected by the problem

      3) Detailed: chief complaint, expanded history of the problem, expanded review of system affected and pertinent past, family, and/or social history

   b. Examination

      1) Problem-focused: examination is limited to the affected body area or system

      2) Expanded problem-focused: examination is limited to the affected body area or system and other closely related systems

      3) Detailed: extended examination of the affected body area or system and other closely related systems

      4) Comprehensive: complete single-system specialty examination or a complete multisystem examination

   c. Complexity of medical decision-making (diagnosis and/or management)

      1) Straightforward: all three criteria are minimal

      2) Low complexity: low degree in each criterion

      3) Moderate complexity: moderate degree in each criterion

      4) High complexity: high degree of complexity in each criterion

4. Criteria to be considered at each complexity level:

   a. Number of diagnoses or management options available

   b. Amount and/or complexity of data

   c. Risk of complication, morbidity, and/or mortality

IV. HCPCS

A. General

1. HCFA: Health Care Financing Administration; government agency that regulates Medicaid and Medicare

2. Coding system that expands the CPT system

3. Provides a temporary list of new codes prior to inclusion in the CPT system

4. Three levels:

   a. Level I: existing CPT codes

   b. Level II: additional codes that provide greater precision in CPT categories; five-character alphanumeric system (A0000 to V5999); includes:

      1) Nonphysician services

      2) Codes not found within the existing CPT system

   c. Level III: codes used by private insurance companies contracted to process government claims (Medicare)

V. ICD-10-CM AND ICD-10-PCS

A. General

1. Two separate systems:

   a. ICD-10-CM: diagnostic coding

      1) Replacement for Volumes I and II

   b. ICD-10-PCS: procedural coding

      1) Replaces Volume III

2. WHO (World Health Organization) published tenth edition in 1992

   a. Expands the content, purpose, and scope of system

   b. Includes ambulatory care services

   c. Increases clinical details

   d. Captures risk factors in primary care

   e. Includes emergent diseases

   f. Groups diagnoses for epidemiologic purposes

3. Benefits

   a. Greater specificity

   b. Added descriptions to ambulatory care and managed care encounters

   c. Possibility of expansion

   d. Extends beyond classification of diseases and injuries

   e. General terminology and disease classification updated to current standards

I. DEFINITION

A. Protection Against Financial Loss by Unplanned Events

B. Types of Health Insurance Programs
1. Commercial: policies created and sold by private companies
   a. Fee-for-service
   b. Usually have a deductible
   c. Commonly pay for percentage of allowed charges (commonly 80%)
   d. Patient can make appointment with any doctor in any specialty; insurance will pay designated amount for services
2. Managed care plans: movement to control healthcare costs while improving preventive care
   a. Each patient chooses one provider as a primary care provider
   b. Care may be restricted to providers, labs, and hospitals unless they accept payment
   c. Patient may not have access to providers or services outside the plan
   d. Plan may require referrals from primary care provider (gatekeeper) for consults, therapy, and testing
   e. Plan usually requires preauthorization for surgery or other procedures
   f. Types of plans include:
      1) Health Maintenance Organization (HMO): organization that provides a comprehensive range of services for a prepaid fee
      2) Preferred Provider Organization (PPO): agreement between employers and physician to provide services to employee subscribers at a discount
      3) Exclusive Provider Organization (EPO): members must receive services within the network only
      4) Point-of-Service Plans: in-network combined with out-of-network
3. Government plans
   a. Medicare
      1) Federal program administered by Health Care Financing Administration (HCFA)
      2) Established in 1965 as Title 18 of the Social Security Act
      3) Eligibility
         a) Age 65 or older
         b) Disabled under Medicare rules
      4) Benefits
         a) Part A: covers inpatient care after applicable deductible is satisfied
         b) Part B: voluntary program; covers certain outpatient services
         c) Part C: Medicare + Choice, Medicare Advantage; expanded benefits for a fee through private health insurance programs
         d) Part D: drug and prescription benefits
      5) Medigap: commercial insurance policies available to cover the Medicare deductible, the co-insurance, and some specific treatments not covered by Medicare
   b. Medicaid
      1) Federal program administered by each state
      2) Established in 1965 as Title 19 of the Social Security Act
      3) Eligibility
         a) Determined by the state
         b) Available to persons with income levels below the federal poverty level
         c) Eligible patients receive an official identification card for their periods of eligibility
         d) Persons may be covered by both Medicare and Medicaid (Medi/Medi); Medicare is the primary carrier and is always billed first

    c. State Children's Health Insurance Plan
      1) Federal government funding for states to further assist children whose parents cannot afford insurance for them
      2) Administered by the state
    d. Workers' compensation
      1) State-administered program
      2) Established to help pay the cost of medical care and lost wages associated with work-related injuries or illnesses
      3) Patients are compensated in full for their related medical expenses and for a portion of their lost wages
      4) Eligibility: patients must sustain an injury or illness while carrying out their job duties
      5) Classification of cases
        a) Claim with no disability: filed for minor injuries or illnesses; patient returns to work in a few days
        b) Temporary disability: filed for injuries and illnesses requiring more than a few days of recuperation before returning to work
        c) Permanent disability: filed for injuries and illnesses resulting in diminished capacity of the patient; ranges from 10% to 100% disability
        d) Vocational rehabilitation: filed for permanently or temporarily disabled persons who require training or education to return to work
    e. Armed Services and Veteran Insurance Plans
      1) TRICARE
        a) Comprehensive health benefits program offering three types of plans for the dependents of men and women in the uniformed services
          (1) TRICARE Standard: fee for service
          (2) TRICARE Extra: PPO plan
          (3) TRICARE Prime: HMO plan with a point-of-service option
      2) CHAMPVA
        a) Provides inpatient and outpatient benefits for dependent spouses and children of veterans who have suffered total, permanent service-connected disabilities

C. Insurance Terms

1. Beneficiary: person designated to receive the benefits of the insurance policy
2. Birthday rule: rule stating that when an individual is covered under two insurance policies, the insurance plan of the policyholder whose birthday comes first in the calendar years (month and day) becomes the primary insurance.
3. Carrier: insurance company; insurer
4. Co-insurance: percentage of the allowed amount that is the patient's responsibility; policyholder and insurance company share the cost of covered losses in a specified ratio
5. Copayment: portion of the cost of service to be paid by the insured
6. Deductible: annual amount to be paid by the insured toward the cost of service before insurance policy benefits are paid
7. Exclusion: treatment or conditions not covered by the insurance policy
8. Explanation of benefits: document prepared by the carrier that identifies the services covered by the policy, the amount billed by the provider, and the amount paid by the carrier
9. Fee-for-service: provider bills for each service rendered
10. Group policy: policy purchased by an organization for the benefit of its members
11. Insured: policyholder; subscriber
12. Managed care: health care program that designates a primary care physician
13. Preauthorization: process required by some insurance carriers where the provider obtains permission to perform certain procedures/services or refer a patient to a specialist
14. Preexisting condition: medical conditions present or being treated at the time a health insurance application is made
15. Premium: the fees paid for the health insurance coverage
16. Provider: health professional who provides services
17. Rider: clauses to the health insurance policy designating coverage items in addition to those included within the standard contract

D. Plan Options

1. Basic benefits include the following:
    a. Diagnostic studies
    b. Hospitalization
    c. Surgical treatments
    d. Obstetrical care
    e. Intensive care
    f. Chemotherapy
2. Major medical services not normally covered by a basic plan may include the following:
    a. Outpatient visits
    b. Minor surgery
    c. Physical and occupational therapies
    d. Cost of medical equipment
    e. Mental health care
    f. Dental care
    g. Prescriptions

3. Companion plan: policy that pays in addition to health insurance policies carried; pays the fees not covered by conventional plans

E. Methods of Payment

1. Physician fee profile: usual, customary, and reasonable charges
2. Assignment of benefits
   a. Gives the carrier instructions to send insurance payments directly to the provider
   b. Most commercial carriers will reimburse the patient unless instructed not to do so
   c. Assignment of benefits is accomplished by the patient (insured) signing the appropriate box on insurance claim form or completing a separate assignment of benefits form
   d. Patient is responsible for paying the difference between the provider charge and the insurance benefits paid
   e. If the provider accepts the assignment, the carrier then makes payment to the provider (in accordance with the policy language); if the claim is a government plan claim, the provider must then indicate on the claim form whether the assignment is accepted or rejected
   f. If the provider rejects the assignment of benefits, then the provider may bill the patient the difference between the fee charged and the fee reimbursed
3. Medicaid and workers' compensation: provider must accept government reimbursement as payment in full if the provider agrees to treat Medicaid and/or workers' compensation patients
4. Deductibles and copayments: patients are responsible to pay any deductible or copayment according to the terms of the insurance policy

F. Coordination of Benefits

1. Term for the rules insurance companies use to coordinate payments so no provider is paid more than 100% for services
2. If patient has more than one insurance policy, claim is first sent to primary insurance
   a. Private insurance must be billed before government insurance; Medicaid is always last insurance billed
3. If both members of a couple have insurance
   a. Patient's insurance is primary and spouse's is secondary
   b. If a child is the patient, "birthday rule" applies: parent whose birthday comes first becomes the primary insurance
4. Medicare recipients may also have private insurance: private insurance is primary

II. INSURANCE CLAIMS

A. CMS-1500 Claim Form (see Figure 13-1)

1. Universal health claim form developed by HCFA
2. Standardizes data required by most carriers so that claims can be processed
3. Before submitting a claim for payment, make sure patient information release forms are current
4. Type information onto the form using uppercase letters
5. Do not use periods, hyphens, commas, dollar signs, or slashes
6. Use two zeros (00) in the cents column for whole dollar amounts
7. Dates should be filled in using the eight (8)-digit year (mmddyyyy)
8. Boxes that should be checked are filled in with an X
9. Type corrections are made by permanent correction methods (correction fluid)
10. Completed forms should be maintained in provider files for 6 years

B. Medicare

1. Requires the provider to report to the primary carrier on HCFA form
2. Filing deadline is December 31 of the year following service

C. Medicaid

1. File this claim as soon as possible after service
2. Providers treating Medicaid patients must accept the assignment and accept Medicaid reimbursements as payment in full for the service
3. Patients cannot be billed for qualified services, regardless of the Medicaid amount reimbursed to the provider
4. Services not covered by Medicaid may be billed directly to the patient
5. Keep a copy of the patient's Medicaid identification card within his or her chart

D. Workers' Compensation

1. Form completed in quadruplicate at patient's first visit to report the injury; copies are sent to the state workers' compensation board, compensation carrier, and employer; a copy is also inserted in the patient's chart
2. Filing deadlines may vary by state
3. Progress reports should be a narrative and should indicate any significant changes on the patient's current status
4. If an established patient seeks treatment for a work-related condition, create a separate chart and separate ledger card for the work-related condition
5. Provider must accept assignment and reimbursement as payment in full

1500

HEALTH INSURANCE CLAIM FORM

APPROVED BY NATIONAL UNIFORM CLAIM COMMITTEE 08/05

CARRIER

PICA ☐☐ | PICA ☐☐

1. MEDICARE MEDICAID TRICARE CHAMPUS CHAMPVA GROUP HEALTH PLAN FECA BLK LUNG OTHER
☐ (Medicare #) ☐ (Medicaid #) ☐ (Sponsor's SSN) ☐ (Member ID#) ☐ (SSN or ID) ☐ (SSN) ☐ (ID)

1a. INSURED'S I.D. NUMBER (For Program in Item 1)

2. PATIENT'S NAME (Last Name, First Name, Middle Initial)

3. PATIENT'S BIRTH DATE MM ∣ DD ∣ YY SEX M ☐ F ☐

4. INSURED'S NAME (Last Name, First Name, Middle Initial)

5. PATIENT'S ADDRESS (No., Street)

6. PATIENT RELATIONSHIP TO INSURED
Self ☐ Spouse ☐ Child ☐ Other ☐

7. INSURED'S ADDRESS (No., Street)

CITY STATE

8. PATIENT STATUS
Single ☐ Married ☐ Other ☐
Employed ☐ Full-Time Student ☐ Part-Time Student ☐

CITY STATE

ZIP CODE TELEPHONE (Include Area Code) ( )

ZIP CODE TELEPHONE (Include Area Code) ( )

9. OTHER INSURED'S NAME (Last Name, First Name, Middle Initial)

10. IS PATIENT'S CONDITION RELATED TO:

11. INSURED'S POLICY GROUP OR FECA NUMBER

a. OTHER INSURED'S POLICY OR GROUP NUMBER

a. EMPLOYMENT? (Current or Previous) ☐ YES ☐ NO

a. INSURED'S DATE OF BIRTH MM ∣ DD ∣ YY SEX M ☐ F ☐

b. OTHER INSURED'S DATE OF BIRTH MM ∣ DD ∣ YY SEX M ☐ F ☐

b. AUTO ACCIDENT? PLACE (State) ☐ YES ☐ NO

b. EMPLOYER'S NAME OR SCHOOL NAME

c. EMPLOYER'S NAME OR SCHOOL NAME

c. OTHER ACCIDENT? ☐ YES ☐ NO

c. INSURANCE PLAN NAME OR PROGRAM NAME

d. INSURANCE PLAN NAME OR PROGRAM NAME

10d. RESERVED FOR LOCAL USE

d. IS THERE ANOTHER HEALTH BENEFIT PLAN?
☐ YES ☐ NO If yes, return to and complete item 9 a-d.

READ BACK OF FORM BEFORE COMPLETING & SIGNING THIS FORM.

12. PATIENT'S OR AUTHORIZED PERSON'S SIGNATURE I authorize the release of any medical or other information necessary to process this claim. I also request payment of government benefits either to myself or to the party who accepts assignment below.

SIGNED _____ DATE _____

13. INSURED'S OR AUTHORIZED PERSON'S SIGNATURE I authorize payment of medical benefits to the undersigned physician or supplier for services described below.

SIGNED _____

PATIENT AND INSURED INFORMATION

14. DATE OF CURRENT: MM ∣ DD ∣ YY ◄ ILLNESS (First symptom) OR INJURY (Accident) OR PREGNANCY(LMP)

15. IF PATIENT HAS HAD SAME OR SIMILAR ILLNESS. GIVE FIRST DATE MM ∣ DD ∣ YY

16. DATES PATIENT UNABLE TO WORK IN CURRENT OCCUPATION MM ∣ DD ∣ YY FROM TO MM ∣ DD ∣ YY

17. NAME OF REFERRING PROVIDER OR OTHER SOURCE

17a.
17b. NPI

18. HOSPITALIZATION DATES RELATED TO CURRENT SERVICES MM ∣ DD ∣ YY FROM TO MM ∣ DD ∣ YY

19. RESERVED FOR LOCAL USE

20. OUTSIDE LAB? ☐ YES ☐ NO $ CHARGES

21. DIAGNOSIS OR NATURE OF ILLNESS OR INJURY (Relate Items 1, 2, 3 or 4 to Item 24E by Line)

1. |____.____
2. |____.____
3. |____.____
4. |____.____

22. MEDICAID RESUBMISSION CODE ORIGINAL REF. NO.

23. PRIOR AUTHORIZATION NUMBER

24. A. DATE(S) OF SERVICE			B. PLACE OF SERVICE	C. EMG	D. PROCEDURES, SERVICES, OR SUPPLIES (Explain Unusual Circumstances)		E. DIAGNOSIS POINTER	F. $ CHARGES	G. DAYS OR UNITS	H. EPSDT Family Plan	I. ID. QUAL.	J. RENDERING PROVIDER ID. #
From MM DD YY	To MM DD YY				CPT/HCPCS	MODIFIER						
1											NPI	
2											NPI	
3											NPI	
4											NPI	
5											NPI	
6											NPI	

25. FEDERAL TAX I.D. NUMBER SSN ☐ EIN ☐

26. PATIENT'S ACCOUNT NO.

27. ACCEPT ASSIGNMENT? (For govt. claims, see back) ☐ YES ☐ NO

28. TOTAL CHARGE $

29. AMOUNT PAID $

30. BALANCE DUE $

31. SIGNATURE OF PHYSICIAN OR SUPPLIER INCLUDING DEGREES OR CREDENTIALS (I certify that the statements on the reverse apply to this bill and are made a part thereof.)

SIGNED _____ DATE _____

32. SERVICE FACILITY LOCATION INFORMATION

a. b.

33. BILLING PROVIDER INFO & PH # ( )

a. b.

PHYSICIAN OR SUPPLIER INFORMATION

NUCC Instruction Manual available at: www.nucc.org

OMB APPROVAL PENDING

FIGURE 13-1 CMS-1500 insurance claim form. (Courtesy U.S. Department of Health and Human Services, Centers for Medicare and Medicaid Services.)

E. Reasons Claims Can Be Delayed or Rejected
   1. Coding errors
   2. Typographical errors
   3. Missing dates
   4. Incorrect identification or policy numbers
   5. Diagnosis does not support treatment rendered
   6. Patient names do not match the policyholder's names
   7. Dates of treatments do not correspond with the dates on the documents
   8. Missing attachments
   9. Defacement of bar code area of the claim form
   10. Submission of claim to the wrong carrier
   11. Patient ineligible for benefits
   12. Fee total calculated incorrectly

I. CHAIN OF INFECTION (See Figure 14-1)

A. General
1. Growth of microorganisms in cycle
2. Break the cycle, break the process

B. Reservoir Host
1. Start of the chain
2. May be an insect, animal, or human
3. Supplies nutrition to the microorganism
4. May not cause disease in the reservoir

C. Means of Exit
1. How the organism escapes the reservoir host
2. Exits include the mouth, nose, eyes, ears, intestines, urinary tract, reproductive tract, and open wounds

D. Means of Transmission
1. Way organisms are spread
   a. Direct transmission: occurs from contact with an infected person or discharges of an infected person
   b. Indirect transmission: occurs from droplets in the air, vectors (insects) that harbor pathogens, contaminated food or drink, and fomites (contaminated objects)

E. Means of Entry
1. How the organism gains entry into a new host
2. Entries include the mouth, nose, eyes, intestines, urinary tract, reproductive tract, and open wounds

F. Susceptible Host
1. One that is capable of supporting the growth of a microorganism
2. Factors that affect susceptibility include:
   a. Location of entry
   b. Dose of organisms
   c. Physical condition of individual
3. If conditions are right, susceptible host becomes reservoir host; the chain or cycle begins again

G. Inflammation
1. Trauma to the body alerts the protective mechanisms

2. The body responds
   a. Blood vessels at the site dilate; the number of white blood cells in the area increases, which causes redness
   b. White blood cells overpower and consume microorganisms (phagocytosis), which causes swelling
   c. Fluids in tissues increase and put pressure on nerves, which causes pain
   d. Blood supply to area increases and causes heat
3. The process creates four classic signs of inflammation: redness, swelling, pain, and heat

II. OSHA STANDARDS

A. General
1. Occupational Safety and Health Administration (OSHA)
2. Sets standards and protocols for health and safety

B. Blood-borne Pathogens
1. Disease-causing microorganisms that may be present in the blood or bodily fluids
2. Concerned mainly with hepatitis B virus (HBV), hepatitis C virus (HCV), and human immunodeficiency virus (HIV)
3. Blood-borne pathogens are transmitted when infected blood comes into contact with nonintact skin or mucous membranes

C. Standard Precautions
1. Concept of treating all blood and body fluids as if they are infected
2. Includes blood, body fluids, excretions, and secretions

D. Prevention of Exposure
1. Immunization: all persons who come in contact with blood or body fluids should receive hepatitis B series
2. Engineering controls: mechanical devices designed to minimize exposure; include:
   a. Eyewash stations
   b. Sharps containers
   c. Biohazard waste containers and labels
   d. Hand-washing stations

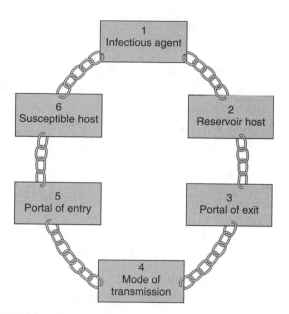

FIGURE 14-1 The chain of infection. (Young AP, Kennedy DB: *Kinn's the medical assistant: an applied learning approach*, ed 10, St Louis, 2007, Saunders.)

3. Personal protection equipment: equipment that minimizes exposure beyond engineering controls; includes:
   a. Gloves
   b. Laboratory coats
   c. Eye and/or face shields

E. Exposure Control
1. Contaminated sharps placed in sharps container (puncture-resistant, leak-proof container) immediately after use
2. Do not bend, break, or recap used needles
3. Work surfaces and equipment should be cleaned and decontaminated with disinfectant after each use
4. Contaminated waste (except sharps) should be discarded in a clearly labeled biohazard waste container (*"red bag trash"*)
5. Employee exposure incidents should be reported as directed and properly followed up to ensure that they do not again occur

F. Postexposure Follow-up
1. If exposed through accidental needlestick, human bite, exposure to broken skin or a splash/ splatter onto mucous membranes
   a. Immediately flush/wash exposed area
   b. Report to supervisor
   c. Receive confidential medical evaluation; all documentation kept confidential
   d. Incident report filled out
   e. Source, if known, screened for HIV and HBV; consent may or may not be required depending on state law
   f. Exposed worker tested for HIV and HBV
   g. Exposed worker must receive health counseling

2. Follow Material Safety Data Sheets (MSDS) guidelines

III. HAND WASHING

A. General
1. Single most important defense against transmission of microorganisms
2. Proper hand washing depends on friction and running water
3. Hands should be washed:
   a. Between patients
   b. After handling specimens
   c. Before and after using the restroom
   d. After handling contaminated materials
   e. Before leaving the clinic at the end of the day
4. Hand-washing procedure
   a. Remove all jewelry except plain wedding band
   b. Using warm water, thoroughly wet the hands
   c. Apply soap; lather while keeping the fingers pointed downward
   d. Rub, using friction for 30 seconds; wash between the fingers
   e. Rinse; allow water to flow from the wrist to the fingertips
   f. Thoroughly dry the hands with paper towels, and turn off the faucet or faucets with the paper towels
   g. Apply lotion if desired

IV. SANITIZATION

A. General
1. Process of cleaning or removing materials from objects
2. Requires scrubbing objects with detergents and brushes
3. First step in the sterilization process
4. Methods include:
   a. Detergents: agents that remove bacteria, fats, oils, and protein substances (blood)
   b. Ultrasound: machine that uses sound waves through a liquid to cause a vibration
   c. Antiseptic: agent that sanitizes skin

V. DISINFECTION

A. General
1. Process of removing infectious material from objects
2. Processes include:
   a. Chemical
      1) Surface germicide
      2) Used on inanimate objects sensitive to heat
         a) Soap: mechanically removes bacteria but does not destroy them unless the soap is germicidal
         b) Alcohol: commonly used on skin
         c) Acids: solutions containing phenol

d) Alkalis: bleach; used in the laboratory on flat surfaces

e) Formalin: solution requires rinsing

b. Ultraviolet radiation: ultraviolet light can have an effect on surfaces but does not penetrate surfaces

c. Desiccation: drying; does not kill spores

d. Boiling: kills most bacteria; does not kill some spores and viruses

VI. STERILIZATION

A. General

1. Complete destruction of microorganisms
2. Processes include:
   a. Chemical
      1) May be used for heat-sensitive materials
      2) Objects must be completely submerged for long periods
      3) Glutaraldehyde solutions commonly used
   b. Steam under pressure
      1) Autoclave
      2) Most common and effective sterilization method
   c. Gas: special chamber that uses a gas
   d. Oven: dry heat

VII. USE OF THE AUTOCLAVE

A. Preparing Instruments and Supplies

1. Instruments are sanitized and dried before wrapping
2. Wrapping materials include:
   a. Muslin
   b. Disposable paper
   c. Peel-back pouches
3. Open any hinged instruments to allow steam to reach all surfaces
4. Items to be wrapped are placed in the center of the wrapping material, with corners of the wrap at the top, bottom, and sides; bring the bottom of the wrapper up over the instrument, folding back a small corner for a handle; bring in the sides, one at a time, also folding back the small corners; the top of the wrapper is brought

around the object and secured with sterilizer tape

5. Label the tape with the identity of the contents, date, and operator's initials
6. Packs should be no larger than $12 \times 12 \times 20$ inches
7. Sterilization indicator should be included in the pack to show that the proper time and temperature were achieved

B. Loading the Autoclave

1. Packs should be placed vertically, 1 to 3 inches apart, away from the sides of the chamber
2. Place hard goods underneath soft goods
3. Open glassware should be placed on its side

C. Autoclave Procedure

1. Autoclave is a piece of equipment that provides steam under pressure
2. Autoclave is normally run at 250 °F, 20 to 30 lb pressure, for 15 to 30 minutes
3. Moist heat in the form of steam circulates in a pattern throughout the autoclave chamber
4. Check the autoclave water level; add distilled water if necessary
5. Properly load the autoclave
6. Close the autoclave door securely; turn the unit on
7. Begin timing when the proper temperature and pressure are achieved
8. After the autoclave cycle is completed, vent the autoclave chamber
9. Open the autoclave door just slightly to allow the contents to dry
10. Remove the items and check the indicator on the sterilizer tape; wrapped items may be handled with clean hands
11. Store sterilized items in a clean, dust-proof area; the shelf life of sterilized items is approximately 28 days (resterilize the items after 28 days)

Vital Signs and Anthropometric Measurement

I. VITAL SIGNS

A. General

1. Measurements that indicate the patient's general state of health and homeostasis
2. Can indicate a change in health and/or the presence or disappearance of a disease
3. Accuracy is essential
4. Includes temperature, pulse, respiration (TPR) and blood pressure (BP)
5. Can also include pain assessment

B. Temperature

1. Balance between heat lost by the body and heat that the body produces
2. Heat is produced by metabolism
3. In illness, metabolism increases, increasing internal heat production and increasing the body temperature
4. Variation in patient's baseline temperature may be the first warning of an illness or change in condition
5. Body temperature is regulated by hypothalamus
6. Factors affecting body temperature
   a. Age: body heat decreases with age
   b. Environment: exposure, wind chill, and temperature
   c. Activity: physical activity increases body temperature
   d. Diurnal variation: body temperature is lowest in the morning, highest in the evening
   e. Emotions: agitation increases body temperature; depression lowers body temperature
   f. Physiologic processes: body temperature increases with digestion, ovulation, and pregnancy
7. Normal ranges
   a. Oral: 97 °F to 99 °F; 36 °C to 37.8 °C
   b. Rectal: 1 °F higher than oral (most accurate measurement)
   c. Axillary: 1 °F lower than oral (least accurate measurement)
   d. Tympanic (aural): same as oral
   e. Temporal artery: 1 °F higher than oral
8. Characteristics
   a. Fever: temperature >100 °F; pyrexia; temperature ≥105 °F can cause brain damage or death if untreated
   b. Febrile: having fever
   c. Afebrile: without fever
   d. Intermittent: fluctuation among normal, abnormal, and fever
   e. Remittent: elevated fluctuations that do not return to normal
   f. Lysis: gradual return to normal
   g. Crisis: sudden return to normal
   h. Fever of unknown origin (FUO): temperature >100.9 °F that lasts for 3 weeks in adults and 1 week in children without a known related diagnosis
9. Equipment: thermometer: device used to measure body temperature
   a. Electronic: consists of a battery-powered unit and a probe covered by a disposable plastic cover; temperature is displayed digitally; unit has blue (oral) and red (rectal) probes
   b. Tympanic (aural): handheld processor unit with a tympanic probe covered by a disposable cover: picks up infrared energy from the tympanic membrane: proper technique is important for correct results
   c. Temporal artery: electronic device consisting of a probe attached to a portable unit: probe slowly moved across the patient's forehead: sensor picks up infrared heat given off by the temporal artery
   d. Chemical, single-use: contain chemicals that are heat sensitive; dots containing chemicals change color in response to body heat; placed under the tongue
   e. Temperature sensitive strips: reusable plastic strip that contains heat-sensitive liquid crystals that change color; strip is pressed onto the forehead

10. Charting
    a. Record the patient's temperature within the patient chart
    b. Indicate (after the number) whether the patient's temperature was recorded by oral (O), rectal (R), axillary (A), tympanic (T), or temporal artery (TA)
11. Procedure
    a. Oral: place the thermometer under the patient's tongue; instruct the patient to keep the lips closed around the thermometer and to breathe through the nose
    b. Axillary: wipe the axilla dry; place the thermometer under the patient's arm
    c. Rectal: apply lubricating jelly to the thermometer; insert into the rectum approximately 1 inch
    d. Tympanic (see Figure 15-1)
       1) For adult: gently pull the pinna up and back; insert the probe into the ear canal
       2) For child: gently pull the pinna down and back; insert the probe into the ear canal

FIGURE 15-1 Positioning the ear for temperature taking. (Bonewit-West K: *Clinical procedures for medical assistants*, ed 7, St Louis, 2008, Saunders.)

C. **Pulse**
1. Palpable beat of arteries as they expand with the beat of the heart
2. Pulse in any artery will usually be the same as the heartbeat
3. Rate and characteristics can give information about the cardiovascular system
4. Factors affecting pulse
   a. Increased pulse rate: pain, fever, infection, and hyperthyroidism
   b. Decreased pulse rate: chronic pain, central nervous system disorders, and hypothyroidism
5. Characteristics
   a. Rate: number of beats per minute (bpm)
   b. Rhythm: time between beats
   c. Volume: force of beats
   d. Condition of the arterial wall: springy, resilient, and elastic
6. Normal ranges
   a. Birth: 70 to 190 bpm
   b. 1 to 4 years: 80 to 120 bpm
   c. 6 to 12 years: 70 to 110 bpm
   d. 12 to 16 years: 75 to 90 bpm
   e. Adult: 60 to 80 bpm
7. Pulse sites (see Figure 15-2)
   a. Radial: most common; located on the thumb side of the wrist
   b. Carotid: located in the groove of the neck between the larynx and the sternocleidomastoid muscle; used in emergencies and during cardiopulmonary resuscitation (CPR)
   c. Brachial: located in the antecubital space; reference for BP
   d. Femoral: located in the groin
   e. Temporal: located over the temporal bone
   f. Popliteal: located at the back of the knee
   g. Dorsalis pedis: located on the top of the foot
   h. Apical: located just below the left nipple on the left side of the chest; taken with a stethoscope for 1 full minute; used for infants, young children, and cardiac patients
8. Procedure
   a. Radial pulse
      1) Have the patient in a sitting or lying position
      2) Gently press on the radial artery until the pulse is felt
      3) Count the beat for 30 seconds and multiply by 2; if the beat is irregular, then count for the full minute
      4) Chart the pulse; note the rate, rhythm, and strength
   b. Apical pulse
      1) Have the patient in a sitting or lying position
      2) Place the stethoscope below the patient's left nipple at the fifth intercostal space midclavicular line (apex of the heart)

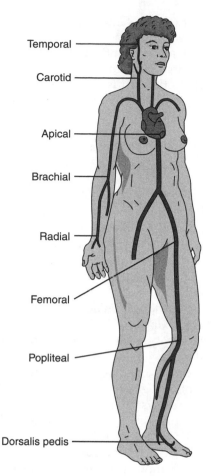

Temporal

Carotid

Apical

Brachial

Radial

Femoral

Popliteal

Dorsalis pedis

FIGURE 15-2 Pulse sites. (Young AP, Kennedy DB: *Kinn's the medical assistant: an applied learning approach*, ed 10, St Louis, 2007, Saunders.)

3) Count for 1 full minute
4) Chart the pulse; note the rate, rhythm, and strength and indicate that the pulse was taken apically (A)

D. Respiration

1. Involves the exchange of oxygen and carbon dioxide in lungs
2. Cycle consists of one inspiration and one expiration
3. Controlled by the medulla oblongata; the breathing rate is determined by the carbon dioxide level in the blood
4. Factors affecting respiration
   a. Disease
   b. Age
   c. Physical activity
   d. Emotional status
   e. Medications and drugs
   f. Body position
5. Characteristics
   a. Rate: number of respirations per minute
   b. Rhythm: breathing pattern
   c. Depth: amount of air being inhaled

6. Normal ranges (respirations per minute)
   a. Newborn: 30 to 40 breaths/min
   b. 1 to 6 years: 20 to 40 breaths/min
   c. 7 to 14 years: 15 to 25 breaths/min
   d. Adult: 16 to 20 breaths/min
7. Breathing patterns
   a. Eupnea: normal breathing
   b. Dyspnea: difficult, painful, or labored breathing
   c. Apnea: absence of breathing; temporary condition
   d. Orthopnea: difficulty breathing while lying down
   e. Hyperpnea: increased rate of breathing
   f. Tachypnea: excessively rapid breathing
   g. Rales: gurgling sounds caused by secretions
   h. Rhonchi: rattling sounds
   i. Cheyne-Stokes respirations: alternating periods of apnea and tachypnea; can indicate impending death
8. Procedure
   a. Respiration can be consciously controlled; the respiration rate should be counted without the patient's knowledge so that the patient is unaware of your respiration count; continue to act as if you are taking the pulse
   b. Watch the rise and fall of the patient's chest; count one inhalation and one exhalation as one respiration
   c. Count for 30 seconds and multiply by 2; if irregular, then count for a full minute
   d. Chart the respiration; note the rate, depth, and rhythm; note any irregularities

E. Blood Pressure

1. Measurement of the pressure of the blood against the walls of the arteries
2. Two readings
   a. Systolic pressure (systole): highest pressure; occurs when the heart contracts
   b. Diastolic pressure (diastole): lowest pressure; occurs when the heart relaxes
3. Systole + diastole = one cardiac cycle
4. Measured in millimeters of mercury (mm Hg)
5. Recorded as a fraction: systolic/diastolic
6. Factors affecting BP
   a. Age: BP increases with age
   b. Activity: BP increases with physical activity
   c. Gender
   d. Diurnal variation: BP is lower in the morning than it is at other times of the day
   e. Stress
   f. Disease state
   g. Medication
7. Normal ranges
   a. Newborn: 50/30 mm Hg
   b. 1 to 6 years: 95/65 mm Hg

c. 6 to 12 years: 100/65 mm Hg

d. 16 to adult: 118/75 mm Hg

e. Adult: 120/80 mm Hg (average); normally ranges from 90/60 to <140/90 mm Hg

f. Older adults: 140/90 mm Hg

8. Characteristics

a. Hypertension (HTN): high BP

1) BP >140/90 mm Hg

2) Essential HTN: unknown cause

3) Secondary HTN: associated with other disease processes

4) Malignant: life-threatening severe form of hypertension

b. Hypotension: low BP: <90/60 mm Hg

c. Orthostatic hypotension: temporary fall in BP that occurs when the patient rapidly changes from a lying or sitting position to a standing position

d. Pulse pressure

1) Difference between systolic and diastolic pressure

2) Average is 40 mm Hg

9. Equipment

a. Sphygmomanometer: consists of an inflatable cuff (various sizes for sizes of patient) with an inflation bulb (with control valve) and pressure gauge (mercury column or aneroid dial)

b. Stethoscope; instrument used to listen to pulse

10. Procedure (see Figure 15-3)

a. Objective

1) Use of the inflatable cuff causes circulation in the artery to disappear

2) As the cuff is slowly deflated, blood flow resumes, and cardiac cycle sounds are heard through the stethoscope

3) Gauge readings are taken when the first sound is heard (systolic) and when the last sound is heard (diastolic)

b. Palpate the brachial artery in the antecubital space

c. Place the cuff snugly around the patient's arm approximately 1 to 2 inches above the arm fold, with the arrow on the cuff pointing to the brachial artery

d. Place the stethoscope over the brachial artery

e. Close the valve and inflate the cuff to approximately 200 mm Hg

f. Slowly release the valve to deflate the cuff; the gauge needle should drop 2 mm Hg per second for proper release rate

g. Note the gauge reading when the first beat is heard (systolic)

h. Continue deflating the cuff until the last beat is heard (diastolic)

i. Fully release the bulb valve, deflate the cuff, and remove it from the patient

FIGURE 15-3 Measurement of blood pressure. (Applegate EJ: *The anatomy and physiology learning system*, ed 3, St Louis, 2006, Saunders.)

j. Record the result in the patient's chart; indicate which arm was used for reading (R or L); may also indicate the patient's position (sitting, standing, lying)

11. Korotkoff sounds: sounds heard during the measurement of BP
    a. Phase I: first sound heard as the cuff deflates; systolic reading
    b. Phase II: swishing sound; blood is flowing through the artery, and sounds may completely disappear and reappear later (auscultatory gap)
    c. Phase III: sharp, tapping sounds return and continue rhythmically
    d. Phase IV: soft tapping sound that becomes muffled and begins to grow fainter; may be recorded as the fading sound and recorded between the systolic and diastolic (e.g., 130/85/70 mm Hg)
    e. Phase V: sounds disappear; last sound heard; diastolic reading

II. PAIN

A. Definition
1. Unpleasant sensory and emotional experience arising from actual or potential tissue damage
2. Approximately one half of patients seek medical attention due to pain
3. Can arise from any organ system
4. Subjective and personal
5. Can reveal tremendous amount about the health status of the patient

B. Effects of Pain
1. Disturbs sleep patterns
2. Affects eating patterns and appetite
3. Affects activity patterns
4. Affects mood and emotions
5. Can affect family relations
6. Can alter physical appearance, sexual function, and energy levels

C. Factors That Influence Pain Experience
1. Nature of the illness or injury
2. Physical and emotional health of the patient
3. Whether the symptoms are acute or chronic

4. Social status or cultural upbringing of the patient
5. Memory and personality of the patient

D. Symptoms and Diagnosis (COLDER)
1. C: character of the pain
2. O: onset of the pain
3. L: location of the pain
4. D: duration of the pain
5. E: what exacerbates the pain
6. R: what relieves the pain

E. Assessment Tools (see Figure 15-4)
1. Wong-Baker Faces Pain Rating Scale
2. Numerical pain scale
   a. Scale of 1 to 10 (0 represents no pain, 10 represents the worst pain imaginable)

F. Pain Management
1. Analgesic medication
2. Tactile stimulation
3. Relaxation techniques
4. Diversion

III. ANTHROPOMETRIC MEASUREMENT

A. General
1. Deals with the measurement of size, weight, and proportion of the human body
2. Often included with vital signs

B. Weight
1. May be measured in pounds or kilograms
   a. Place a paper towel on the base of the scale if the patient removes his or her shoes; the patient should be weighed consistently with or without shoes, depending on office procedure
   b. Have the patient stand erect in the center of the base of the scale
   c. Move the large weight to the 50-lb notch nearest to, but under, the patient's weight
   d. Move the smaller weight to the right until the balance needle is in the middle of the frame
   e. Add the large and small weights together; record the result, in pounds, on the patient's chart to the nearest ¼ lb
   f. Return both weights to zero after the patient leaves the scale
   g. 1 kg = 2.2 lb; 1 lb = 0.45 kg

0
No hurt

1
Hurts little bit

2
Hurts little more

3
Hurts even more

4
Hurts whole lot

5
Hurts worst

FIGURE 15-4 Wong-Baker Faces Pain Rating Scale. (Hockenberry MJ: *Wong's clinical manual of pediatric nursing,* ed 6, St Louis, 2004, Mosby.)

C. Height

1. May be measured in inches or centimeters
   a. Place a paper towel on the base of the scale if the patient removes his or her shoes (as previously described)
   b. Have the patient stand erect in the center of the base of the scale
   c. Lower the height bar until it rests on the top of the patient's head
   d. Note the height indicated on the height bar; record the result, in inches, on the patient's chart to the nearest ¼ inch
   e. Return the height bar to the lowest position
   f. 1 inch = 2.54 cm; 1 cm = 0.39 inch

D. Body Fat

1. Measures percentage of body fat; percentage of body fat may be an indicator of cardiovascular disease, health, vitality, and appearance
2. Three methods:
   a. Body density measurement method
      1) Patient is submerged under water
      2) Most accurate and most difficult
   b. Electroimpedance method
      1) Electrodes are placed on the patient
      2) Computer determines body fat percentage on an impedance monitor
   c. Caliper method
      1) Measures the thickness of a fold of fat tissue
      2) Measurements are taken in three to four sites on the body; most common are
         a) Triceps
         b) Biceps
         c) Subscapular
         d) Suprailiac
      3) Indicates total percentage of body fat
      4) Normal range for men is 15% to 19%
      5) Normal range for women is 22% to 25%

I. GENERAL

A. Preparation

1. The medical assistant prepares the patient for examination by gowning, positioning and draping
2. The medical assistant prepares the examination room by setting out the correct equipment/supplies

II. GOWNING

A. General

1. Patient must undress and put on a gown; makes performing the procedure easier for the health care provider
2. Principle of gowning: expose only the body part that needs to be examined or exposed

B. Considerations of Gowning

1. Patient's need for privacy and comfort
2. Type of examination or procedure to be performed
3. Patient's age and gender
4. Accessibility of the body part to be examined or exposed

C. Types of Gowns

1. Usually all patient clothing is removed under the gown
2. Gown will have an opening either in back or in front
   a. Full gown
      1) Knee length
      2) Opening extends the full length of the gown
      3) Closures of Velcro or ties
      4) Can be paper or cloth material
   b. Partial gown
      1) Covers only the chest, back, and shoulders
      2) Opening extends the full length of the gown
      3) Can be paper or cloth material

III. POSITIONING AND DRAPING

A. General

1. Patient is generally positioned on an examination table
2. Table should be long and wide enough to support any size patient
3. Table covered with a paper covering or cloth sheet; the covering is changed after each patient

B. Positions (see Figure 16-1, A-I)

1. Erect
   a. Standing
   b. Patient is upright with arms at sides
   c. Used to examine musculoskeletal system and nervous system
2. Sitting (part A)
   a. Patient sits upright on the table with legs dangling over the edge of the table
   b. Used to examine the head, chest, heart, lungs, breasts, axilla, and upper extremities
   c. Draping: drape the sheet across the lap
3. Supine (part B)
   a. Patient lies flat on the back with arms at the sides
   b. Used to examine the chest, abdominal area, heart, and extremities
   c. Draping: the drape sheet extends from under the arms
4. Dorsal recumbent (part C)
   a. Patient is supine with legs bent at the knees and feet flat on the table
   b. Used to examine the genital and rectal areas
   c. Draping: drape sheet is placed over that patient in a diamond-shaped fashion with side corners wrapped around each leg; upper and lower corners cover the chest, abdominal, and pubic areas

FIGURE 16-1 Positions for examination. (Young AP, Proctor DB: *Kinn's the medical assistant: an applied learning approach*, ed 10, St Louis, 2007, Saunders.)

(Continued)

FIGURE 16-1—cont'd

5. Lithotomy (part D)
   a. Patient is in dorsal recumbent position, except that the feet are placed in stirrups; knees are bent; buttocks are moved to the end of the table
   b. Used for vaginal examination, pelvic examination, and Papanicolaou (Pap) smear procedure
   c. Draping: same as for dorsal recumbent
6. Sims' (part E)
   a. Lateral position
   b. Patient lies on the left side with the left arm behind the body and the right arm forward; both legs are flexed at the knees, but the right leg is sharply bent and positioned next to the left leg
   c. Used to examine the rectal area, perform enemas and douches, and insert suppositories
   d. Draping: drape sheet covers the patient from the shoulders to the toes; adjust to expose the necessary area
7. Prone (part F)
   a. Patient lies flat on the abdomen with the head turned to the side; arms are positioned above the head or at the sides of the body

   b. Used to examine the back, spine, and lower extremities
   c. Draping: drape sheet covers the patient from the waist to the knees; adjust to expose the necessary area
8. Knee-chest (part G)
   a. Genupectoral
   b. Patient assumes a kneeling position with the buttocks elevated, with head and chest on the table
   c. Used for proctologic examinations
   d. Draping: drape sheet covers the buttocks; adjust to expose the necessary area
9. Proctologic
   a. Knee-chest position facilitated by the use of a special table
   b. Used for a proctologic examination
   c. Draping: same as for knee-chest
10. Fowler's
   a. Patient sits on the examination table with the back supported at a 90-degree angle
   b. Used for examination and treatment of the head, neck, and chest; helpful for patients with breathing difficulties
   c. Draping: drape sheet covers the patient from the shoulders down; adjust to expose the necessary area

11. Semi-Fowler's (part H)
    a. Modification of Fowler's; back supported at a 45-degree angle
    b. Used for postsurgical examinations and for patients with head trauma or head pain
    c. Draping: same as for Fowler's
12. Trendelenburg (part I)
    a. Patient is supine with the foot of the table elevated 45 degrees (head lower than feet)
    b. Used for shock or abdominal surgery
    c. Draping: drape sheet covers the patient from underarms to below the knees; neck, head, and hands are left uncovered

C. General Considerations
1. Expose only the body part being examined or treated
2. Keep the patient as comfortable as possible
3. Provide a blanket for comfort and warmth
4. Modify the position to accommodate a weak or painful body part
5. Prevent the patient from falling from the table
6. Medical assistant should be present when a male physician examines a female patient

IV. COMPLETE PHYSICAL EXAMINATIONS

A. General
1. Normally performed on new patients to assess their health status and to establish the patient's baseline
2. Also performed on established patients for health maintenance
3. Medical assistant must be familiar with the process, principles, and methods to prepare the patient and to assist the provider

B. Methods of Examination
1. Inspection
    a. Process of visual observation
    b. Includes looking for abnormalities in size, shape, color, continuity, symmetry, or position
2. Palpation
    a. Process of touching and feeling
    b. Can detect abnormalities of size, shape, texture, and tenderness
3. Percussion
    a. Process of tapping or striking the body
    b. Done with fingers or small hammer
    c. Aids in determination of size, position, or density of an organ or body cavity
4. Manipulation
    a. Forceful passive movement of a joint to determine range of motion
5. Auscultation
    a. Process of listening to the body using a stethoscope

6. Mensuration
    a. Process of measurement

C. Commonly Used Equipment (see Figure 16-2)
1. Ophthalmoscope
    a. Instrument used to illuminate the internal eye for visual inspection
    b. Runs off power source (battery or wall unit)
2. Otoscope
    a. Instrument used to illuminate the external and internal ear for visual examination
    b. Runs off power source (battery or wall unit)
3. Pocket flashlight or headlight
    a. Instrument used to illuminate the mouth, throat, and nose for visual examination
4. Tape measure
    a. Instrument used to measure body structures
5. Tongue depressor
    a. Instrument used to control tongue movement while examining the mouth and throat
    b. Disposable; nonsterile
6. Stethoscope
    a. Instrument used to listen to the sounds of the body
7. Gloves and lubricant
    a. Used for rectal and/or pelvic examinations
8. Vaginal speculum
    a. Instrument inserted into the patient's vagina to allow visualization of the cervix and vagina
9. Percussion hammer
    a. Rubber-tipped hammer used to test patient's reflexes
10. Tuning fork
    a. Instrument used to test the patient's hearing; vibrates when struck to produce sound

FIGURE 16-2 Physical examination instruments. (Young AP, Proctor DB: *Kinn's the medical assistant: an applied learning approach*, ed 10, St Louis, 2007, Saunders.)

11. Miscellaneous
    a. Cotton-tipped applicators
    b. 2-inch × 2-inch gauze squares
    c. Glass slides
    d. Specimen and slide fixative
    e. Tissues

D. Sequence of Events
1. Patient health history
2. Vital signs and anthropometric measurements
3. Physical examination
4. Specimen collection
    a. Includes urine, blood, or other body fluids
    b. Examination may be more comfortable if the patient's bladder is empty
5. Diagnostic tests
    a. Includes electrocardiogram, x-ray, spirometry, and immunizations
6. Patient consultation or discussion with provider

V. PHYSICAL EXAMINATION SEQUENCE

A. Presenting Appearance (Patient's General Appearance)
1. General assessment of patient's state of health
2. Includes:
    a. Signs of distress
    b. Appearance of skin
    c. Posture, gait, and motor activity
    d. General grooming
    e. Presence of odors
    f. Speech patterns
    g. Body language and facial expressions

B. Head—Patient in Sitting Position
1. Hair, scalp, and face
2. Eyes: ophthalmoscope used to visually examine the retina and vessels
3. Ears: otoscope used to examine the external ear and tympanic membrane
4. Nose and sinuses: otoscope or nasal speculum used to examine the nares and sinus cavities
5. Mouth and throat
    a. Lips, gums, teeth, and tongue
    b. Light source, tongue depressor (blade), and laryngeal mirror used to visually examine the throat
6. Neck: inspect and palpate the thyroid, trachea, and lymph nodes

C. Thorax—Patient in Sitting Position
1. Back
    a. Spine and muscles of the back are visually inspected
    b. Lungs are auscultated with a stethoscope
2. Chest
    a. Visually inspected for symmetry and expansion
    b. Inspirations auscultated
    c. Axillary nodes palpated

3. Heart
    a. Stethoscope used to listen to heart sounds
    b. Complete silence in the examination room is necessary to interpret the sounds
4. Breasts
    a. Examined for masses, tenderness, and discharge
    b. May also be examined with the patient in supine position

D. Abdomen—Patient in Supine Position
1. Auscultated for the presence or absence of bowel sounds
2. Visually inspected for symmetry and contour
3. Manipulated and palpated for contours of the organs
4. Area needs to be relaxed for proper examination

E. Genital and Rectal—Patient in Supine Position
1. Inguinal area: palpated for lymph nodes and hernias
2. Male genital and rectal: penis, scrotum, prostate, and anus palpated and inspected
3. Female genital and rectal—patient in the lithotomy position
    a. External genitalia, vagina, cervix, and anus inspected
    b. Pelvic examination
        1) Speculum inserted into the vagina to visualize the vaginal wall and cervix
        2) Bimanual examination done with a gloved hand inserted into the vagina and the other hand palpating the external abdomen to examine the uterus, ovaries, and fallopian tubes

F. Legs—Patient in Standing Position
1. Inspected for pulse and varicosities

VI. DIAGNOSIS (See Figure 16-3)

A. Symptoms
1. Conditions and feelings experienced by the patient

B. Signs
1. Observable characteristics by health care providers
2. May also be noticed by patient

C. Differential Diagnosis
1. Comparing certain diseases with others that have similar signs and symptoms
2. Process of ruling out (R/O)

D. Impression
1. Working diagnosis
2. Subject to change as the provider adds data from other diagnostic tools

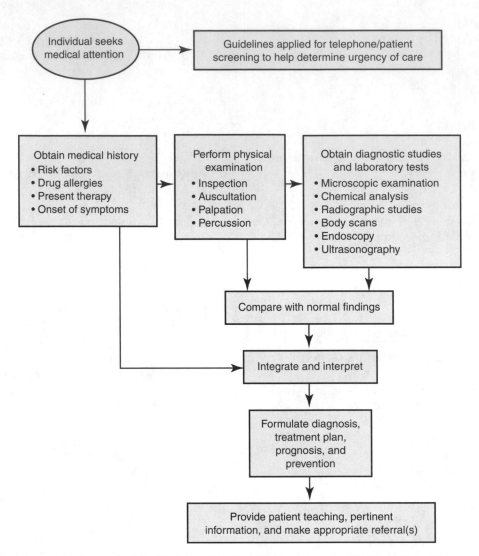

FIGURE 16-3 Essential steps in diagnosis. (Modified from Frazier MS, Drzymkowski JW: *Essentials of human diseases and conditions*, ed 4, St Louis, 2008, Saunders.)

E. Diagnostic Tools
1. Patient history
2. Physical examination
3. Vital signs
4. Laboratory and diagnostic tests

5. Patient's communications
6. Physician's perceptions

F. Final Diagnosis
1. The provider's final conclusion

I. DERMATOLOGY

A. General
1. Deals with disorders of the skin, hair, glands, nails, and subcutaneous tissue
2. Specialized physician: dermatologist

B. Common Symptoms of Skin Disorders
1. Lesions and/or eruptions
2. Pruritus/hives
3. Inflammation
4. Edema
5. Discomfort
6. Erythema

C. General Examination
1. Skin, hair, and nails
2. Examine for:
   a. Color
   b. Consistency and texture
   c. Eruptions, lesions, growths
   d. Tenderness
   e. Irregularities

D. Diagnostic Procedures
1. Fungal, bacterial, and viral cultures: tissue scrapings, purulent material, and exudate sent to the laboratory to identify pathogenic organisms
2. Potassium hydroxide (KOH) smears: skin scrapings immersed in 20% KOH; sample examined for fungus
3. Biopsy
   a. Excisional: removal of the entire section of tissue for microscopic examination
   b. Incisional: removal of a portion of the tissue for microscopic examination
   c. Punch: use of an instrument (dermal punch) to remove only a small amount of tissue for microscopic examination
4. Allergy testing
   a. Patch test: a small piece of gauze with a small amount of allergen is placed on the skin; a positive reaction occurs if the skin becomes red or blistered after 48 hours
   b. Scratch test: a minute amount of allergen is placed, by scratch, in the skin; a positive reaction occurs if the scratch becomes red and swollen
   c. Intradermal: a small amount of allergen is injected intradermally; a positive reaction is determined by measuring the size of the wheals produced
5. Wood's light examination: detects fluorescent characteristics of certain fungi; the skin is viewed in a darkened room under ultraviolet light that is filtered through Wood's glass
6. Antinuclear antibody (ANA) titer: blood test used to screen for cutaneous lupus erythematosus and similar connective tissue diseases
7. Tuberculin (TB) skin testing: tests patient for tuberculosis antibodies
   a. Mantoux: intradermal injection using purified protein derivative (PPD)
   b. Tine: multipuncture method using a small plastic device

E. Treatment Procedures
1. Cryosurgery: use of extreme cold (liquid nitrogen) to freeze and destroy unwanted tissue
2. Curettage: removal of the surface of the skin or a lesion by scraping with a sharp, spoon-shaped instrument (curette)
3. Dermabrasion: removal of scars or lesions by the use of mechanical or chemical abrasives
4. Electrodesiccation: destruction of growths, warts, or unwanted areas of tissue with electric current (diathermy)
5. Mohs' surgery: removal and microscopic examination of layers of malignant growth

F. Medications
1. Antiacneics
   a. Used to treat acne
   b. Examples: Accutane, Retin-A, Cleocin, Persa-Gel
2. Antifungals
   a. Used to treat fungal infections
   b. Examples: Lotrimin, Monistat, Nizoral

3. Antihistamines
   a. Used to decrease allergic reactions
   b. Examples: Atarax, Benadryl
4. Antiinfectives
   a. Used to kill microorganisms
   b. Examples: Erythromycin, Keflex, Mycolog, Sumycin
5. Antivirals
   a. Used to inhibit viruses
   b. Example: Zovirax
6. Scabicides and pediculicides
   a. Used to kill scabies and lice
   b. Examples: Lindane, Kwell
7. Topical steroids
   a. Used externally to decrease inflammation
   b. Examples: Aristocort, Medrol, Topicort, Kenalog

II. ORTHOPEDICS

A. General
1. Deals with disorders of the musculoskeletal systems
2. Specialized physician: orthopedist, orthopod

B. Common Symptoms of Musculoskeletal Disorders
1. Joint stiffness, pain, inflammation, swelling
2. Weight loss
3. Bone mass loss; deformation of bones
4. Fatigue, malaise, weakness, fever
5. Tenderness and swelling of joints and bones
6. Loss of motion, immobility

C. General Examination
1. Observes for:
   a. Decreased range of motion (ROM)
   b. Tenderness and swelling
   c. Unequal or decreased strength
   d. Deformities or growths

D. Diagnostic Procedures
1. Arthrocentesis: removal of joint fluid with a needle for analysis of fluid
2. Arthroscopy: examination of a joint with a viewing scope (arthroscope)
3. Electromyography: recording the strength of muscle contraction as a result of electrical stimulation
4. Muscle biopsy: removal of muscle tissue for examination
5. Bone scan: use of a machine to measure the uptake of a radioactive substance injected intravenously
6. Computed tomography (CT) scan: computer-assisted x-ray technique used to distinguish pathologic conditions such as tumors or fractures; a noninvasive method of viewing inside the body
7. Magnetic resonance imaging (MRI): production of detailed pictures of internal structures, using magnetism and computers; a noninvasive method of viewing inside the body
8. Skeletal x-ray: plain x-ray of the appropriate body part
9. Erythrocyte sedimentation rate (ESR; sed rate): blood test that determines whether inflammation is present within the patient's body
10. Latex fixation: test for the presence of rheumatoid factor present in rheumatoid arthritis

E. Treatment Procedures
1. Wrap or splint: cloth or elastic material or rigid material used to immobilize limbs or joints
2. Cast: application of material (plaster, resin, fiberglass) molded to the affected limb and allowed to harden; holds the affected limb or joint in a fixed position until healing is complete
3. Arthroscopic surgery: surgical procedures performed on joints using an arthroscope
4. Reduction: restoration of a fracture to normal position
   a. Closed reduction: manipulation without an incision
   b. Open reduction: incision is made at the fracture site
5. Physical therapy: use of exercise, heat, cold, and other physical means to reduce pain and swelling, to increase movement and circulation, and to promote healing

F. Medications
1. Analgesics
   a. Used to reduce pain
   b. Examples: aspirin, Tylenol
2. Narcotic analgesics
   a. Used to reduce pain with narcotics
   b. Examples: Darvon, Lortab, Percodan
3. Antibiotics
   a. Used to kill microorganisms
   b. Examples: Cipro, Keflex
4. Nonsteroidal antiinflammatory drugs (NSAIDs)
   a. Used to reduce inflammation without the use of steroids
   b. Examples: Advil, Motrin, Naprosyn, Indocin, Clinoril
5. Muscle relaxants
   a. Used to relax skeletal muscles
   b. Examples: Flexeril, Valium

III. CARDIOLOGY

A. General
1. Deals with diseases and disorders of the heart and vessels
2. Specialized physician: cardiologist

B. Common Symptoms of Cardiovascular System Disorders
1. Chest pain
2. Dyspnea
3. Fatigue, weakness
4. Palpitations, tachycardia
5. Bradycardia
6. Pallor, cyanosis
7. Edema
8. Syncope
9. Unusual sweating
10. Nausea, vomiting, anorexia
11. Headache
12. Anxiety

C. General Examination
1. Listening to the heart with a stethoscope, noting heart sounds, rate, and rhythm

D. Diagnostic Procedures
1. Cardiac catheterization
   a. Intensive study of the heart
   b. Uses catheters to perform angiocardiography or pressure-and-flow measurements
   c. Can determine the severity of heart disease and/or vessel blockage
   d. Medical assistant would schedule this procedure at the hospital
2. Echocardiogram: graphic recording of ultrasound waves from the heart
3. Electrocardiogram (ECG) (see details later): recording of the electrical activity of the heart
4. Holter monitor (see Figure 17-1)
   a. Portable ambulatory monitoring system
   b. Monitors ECG activity over a 24-hour period
   c. Designed so that the patient is able to maintain usual daily activities with minimal inconvenience while being monitored

   d. Device is connected to the patient by electrodes placed on the patient's chest and a special portable magnetic tape recorder that continually monitors the heart's activity
   e. Recorder is in a protective case that is either worn on a belt around the patient's waist or hung over the shoulder by a strap
   f. Patient completes an activity diary; all activities and emotional states are recorded along with any symptoms experienced (chest pain, vertigo, palpitations)
   g. Monitor is removed from patient after a 24-hour period, and the tape is evaluated and analyzed
   h. Electrodes (floating electrodes) are placed as follows:
      1) Right border of the sternum (manubrium)
      2) Left border of the sternum (manubrium)
      3) Right sternal border at the level of the fifth rib
      4) Fifth rib space at the left anterior axillary line
      5) Fifth rib space at the right anterior axillary line
5. Treadmill: motorized machine that allows patient to walk in place; allows evaluation of the patient's heart function while exercising
6. Angiography: x-ray of blood vessels after an injection of radiopaque material
7. Arterial blood gases (ABGs): measures oxygen, carbon dioxide, and metabolic balance in an arterial blood sample
8. Cardiac enzymes
   a. Creatine phosphokinase (CPK): enzyme released into the blood when the heart or skeletal muscles are injured
   b. Aspartate aminotransferase (AST) (formerly serum glutamic-oxaloacetic transaminase [SGOT]): found in high concentration in heart muscle and in the liver
   c. Lactic dehydrogenase (LDH): enzyme found in heart muscle, skeletal muscles, kidneys, liver, and red blood cells
9. Prothrombin time (PT): tests coagulation of blood

E. Treatment Procedures
1. Angioplasty: surgical repair of a blood vessel
2. Defibrillation (cardioversion): brief charges of electricity applied to the chest to stop cardiac arrhythmia
3. Coronary artery bypass: open-heart surgery for the purpose of bypassing an obstructed coronary artery
4. Endarterectomy: removal of the interior portion of an artery and occluding fatty deposits
5. Phlebotomy: opening into a vein; venipuncture
6. Vein stripping: removal of a diseased portion of a vein

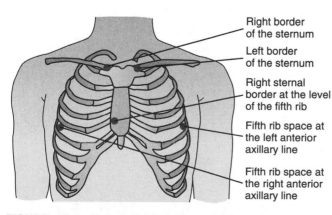

Right border of the sternum

Left border of the sternum

Right sternal border at the level of the fifth rib

Fifth rib space at the left anterior axillary line

Fifth rib space at the right anterior axillary line

FIGURE 17-1 Holter monitor electrode positions. (Bonewit-West K: *Clinical procedures for medical assistants*, ed 7, St Louis, 2008, Saunders.)

F. Medications
1. Diuretics
   a. Promote urination; decrease blood pressure
   b. Examples: Bumex, Dyazide, Lasix, Hydro-Diuril
2. Antihypertensives
   a. Decrease blood pressure
   b. Examples: Inderal, Lanoxin, Procardia, Tenormin, Minipress
3. Antilipemics
   a. Decrease cholesterol levels in blood
   b. Examples: Loped, Mevacor, Crestor, Lipitor
4. Antianginals
   a. Decrease chest pain
   b. Examples: Nitrostat, Transderm-Nitro

G. Electrocardiogram (see Figure 17-2)
1. Cardiac electrical activity is generated, spreads through the heart, and creates an electrical wave
2. This electrical wave is measured as an ECG
   a. Electrical system of the heart
      1) Sinoatrial (SA) node (pacemaker)
      2) Atrioventricular (AV) node
      3) Bundle of His
      4) Right and left bundle branches
      5) Purkinje fibers

   b. Electrical states of the heart
      1) Polarization: cardiac muscle cells are resting
      2) Depolarization: cardiac muscle cells contract
      3) Repolarization: cardiac muscle cells transform from active to resting state for recharging
   c. Normal ECG (see Figure 17-3): all heartbeats appear as a pattern, consisting of:
      1) P-wave: impulse starting in the atria
      2) QRS complex: impulse going through ventricles
      3) T-wave: repolarization of ventricles
   d. ECG leads (see Figure 17-4)
      1) Externally applied electrodes
      2) Relative to an axis (a direct line) between two poles
      3) Each lead makes up one positive pole, one negative pole, and one ground
      4) Leads give an electrical picture of the heart from different angles
      5) ECG uses 10 electrodes (four limb electrodes and six chest electrodes) to give 12 leads

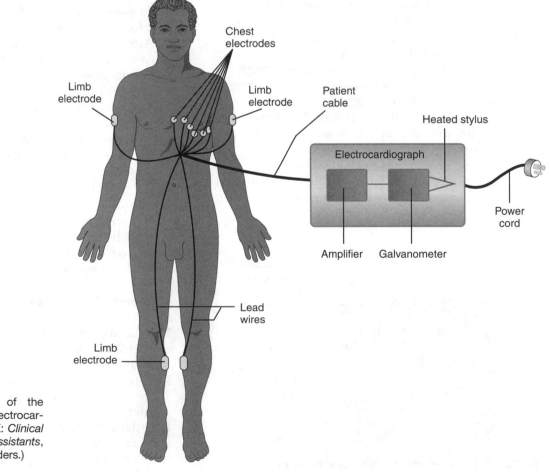

FIGURE 17-2 Diagram of the basic components of the electrocardiograph. (Bonewit-West K: *Clinical procedures for medical assistants*, ed 7, St Louis, 2008, Saunders.)

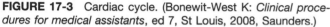

FIGURE 17-3 Cardiac cycle. (Bonewit-West K: *Clinical procedures for medical assistants*, ed 7, St Louis, 2008, Saunders.)

a) Bipolar (standard) limb leads
   (1) Six of the 12 leads
   (2) Electrodes are placed on the patient's extremities (upper arms and inside of calves)
   (3) Measures cardiac electrical activity between two extremities (negative and positive poles)
   (4) Right electrode is used for the ground
     (a) Lead I: measures activity from right arm to left arm (RA to LA)
     (b) Lead II: measures activity from right arm to left leg (RA to LL)
     (c) Lead III: measures activity from left arm to left leg (LA to LL)
b) Unipolar (augmented) limb leads (see Figure 17-5): measures cardiac electrical activity between the heart and one extremity
   (1) aVR: right side
   (2) aVL: left side
   (3) aVF: left foot
c) Precordial (chest) leads (see Figure 17-6)
   (1) Provide points of reference across the chest wall
   (2) Differentiate left- and right-sided heart events
     (a) Lead V1: electrode placed at the fourth intercostal space to the right of the sternum
     (b) Lead V2: electrode placed at the fourth intercostal space to the left of the sternum

     (c) Lead V3: electrode placed midway between leads V2 and V4
     (d) Lead V4: electrode placed left-midclavicular line in the fifth intercostal space
     (e) Lead V5: electrode placed at the level of V4 at axillary line
     (f) Lead V6: electrode placed at the level of V5 at the midaxillary line
d) Leads in relation to the anatomy of the heart
   (1) Right side of the heart: V1, aVR
   (2) Left side of the heart: V5, V6, I, aVL
   (3) Transition from right to left sides of the heart: V2, V3, V4
   (4) Inferior heart: II, III, aVF
e. ECG equipment
 1) Paper (see Figure 17-7)
   a) Records visible record of the heart's electrical activity
   b) Paper is heat-sensitive
   c) Heated stylus on the machine traces the heart activity onto the paper
   d) Composed of 1-mm squares: every fifth line is darkened, creating large blocks five squares wide and five squares high
   e) Cardiac voltage is measured on the vertical scale; time is measured on the horizontal scale
   f) Horizontally, each large block represents 0.2 second
   g) Vertically, each large block represents 0.5 millivolt of electricity
   h) Paper moves continuously through the machine at the rate of 1 inch per second on the standard machine setting
 2) Controls
   a) Main power switch: turns the machine on and off
   b) RUN/STOP: activates (or stops) the amplifier so that the stylus can react to the heartbeat
   c) Run-25: moves the paper 25 mm (1 inch) per second (standard speed)
   d) Run-50: doubles the paper's speed to 50 mm (2 inches) per second
   e) Sensitivity control: regulates the output of the amplifier
   f) Standard (STD) button: manually checks the machine's calibration (stylus should deflect 10 mm, or two large squares)
   g) Lead selector: changes leads
   h) Marker button: allows manual identification of leads; uses codes of dots or dashes

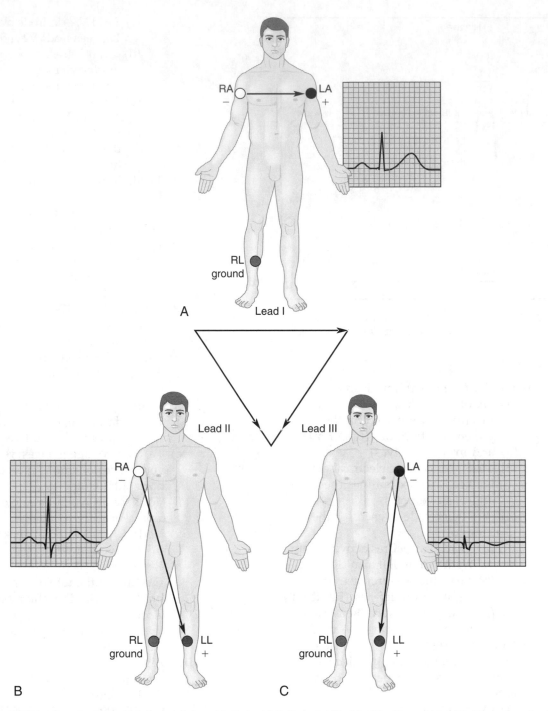

FIGURE 17-4 ECG leads, wires, and tracings. **A,** Lead I. **B,** Lead II. **C,** Lead III. (Modified from Hunt SA: *Saunders fundamentals of medical assisting*, Philadelphia, 2002, Saunders.)

3) Artifacts: abnormal ECG tracings not caused by heart activity
   a) Somatic tremor: caused by the patient's muscle movement
   b) Alternating current (AC) interference: caused by nearby operation of electrical equipment
   c) Wandering baseline: caused by electrodes applied too loosely or too tightly

IV. HEMATOLOGY

A. General
   1. Deals with blood disorders, bone marrow, and coagulation
   2. Specialized physician: hematologist

B. Common Symptoms of Blood Disorders
   1. Cold, numb extremities
   2. Fatigue
   3. Dyspnea

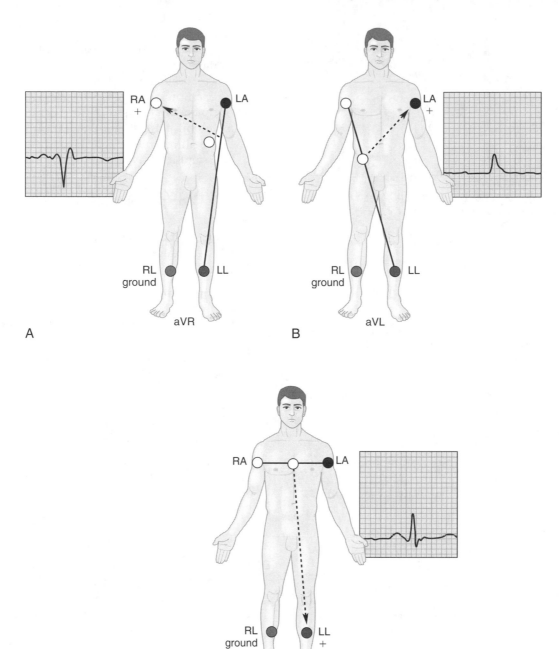

FIGURE 17-5 Augmented (unipolar) ECG leads and tracings. (Modified from Hunt SA: *Saunders fundamentals of medical assisting*, Philadelphia, 2002, Saunders.)

4. Headache
5. Anorexia
6. Edema
7. Pallor
8. Syncope
9. Bone pain
10. Easy bleeding, bruising

C. General Examination
1. Obtain blood or bone marrow samples for testing
2. Palpation of spleen and liver

D. Diagnostic Procedures
1. Bone marrow aspiration: insertion of a large needle into the sternum or iliac crest to remove bone marrow for testing
2. Blood cell counts (red blood cell [RBC] and white blood cell [WBC]): blood test to determine the number of RBCs and WBCs per cubic millimeter of blood
3. Differential: blood smear on glass slide; stain is applied to the smear; the smear is studied under a microscope to differentiate the types of WBCs

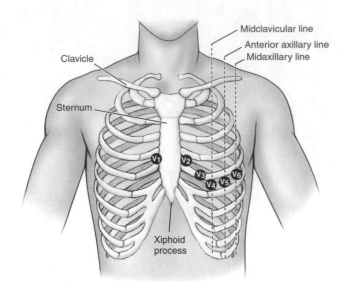

FIGURE 17-6 Precordial (chest) ECG leads: V_1 to V_6. (Modified from Hunt SA: *Saunders fundamentals of medical assisting*, Philadelphia, 2002, Saunders.)

4. Hematocrit (HCT): measures the percentage of RBCs in volume of blood
5. Hemoglobin (Hgb): measures the grams of hemoglobin in volume of blood
6. Platelet count: estimates the number of platelets in volume of blood
7. Prothrombin time (PT): measures coagulation time of blood

E. Medications
1. Anticoagulants
   a. Prevent blood from clotting
   b. Examples: Coumadin, Heparin
2. Stimulating factors
   a. Stimulate production of blood cells
   b. Examples: Neupogen, Leukine
3. Thrombolytic agents
   a. Dissolve clots
   b. Examples: Abbokinase, Streptase
4. Antianemics
   a. Treat anemias
   b. Examples: Epogen, Slow-Fe, vitamin B_{12}
5. Antiplatelet agents
   a. Inhibit platelet aggregation; prolonged bleeding time
   b. Example: Plavix

V. PULMONOLOGY

A. General
1. Deals with diseases and disorders of the lungs and respiratory system
2. Specialized physician: pulmonologist

B. Common Symptoms of Respiratory System Disorders
1. Pain in respiratory tract including chest pain, sore throat
2. Dyspnea, wheezing, rales, cyanosis
3. Cough, productive or nonproductive
4. Dysphonia
5. Fatigue, malaise
6. Chills, fever, headache
7. Hemoptysis, epistaxis

C. General Examination
1. Inspection of the nose, face, and throat
2. Examination of the mucous membranes
3. Inspection and palpation of the sinuses, neck, and lymph nodes
4. Auscultation of the lungs

D. Diagnostic Procedures
1. Bronchoscopy: visualization of the bronchi through a bronchoscope
2. Spirometry: measurement of the breathing capacity of the lungs
3. Lung biopsy: biopsy of tissue taken from the lungs

FIGURE 17-7 ECG paper. (Bonewit-West K: *Clinical procedures for medical assistants*, ed 7, St Louis, 2008, Saunders.)

4. Pulmonary function test (PFT): evaluates how the patient breathes; determines lung volumes, pulmonary gas exchange, and flow rates
5. Thoracentesis: puncture of the chest wall with a needle to obtain fluid for testing
6. Tracheostomy: emergency or elective procedure that creates an opening through the neck into the trachea
7. Chest x-ray: full view of the lungs from the back (posteroanterior [PA]) and sides (lateral)
8. Sputum culture: collection of a sputum sample and testing it for microorganisms
9. Arterial blood gases (ABGs): measurement of hydrogen, carbon dioxide, pH, and oxygen pressure from an arterial blood sample

E. Treatment Procedures
1. Endotracheal intubation: a procedure that establishes an airway by inserting a tube through the nose, pharynx, and larynx into the trachea
2. Thoracotomy: surgical insertion of a tube into the chest to drain fluid or air
3. Nebulizer: machine that produces a fine mist of water and medication; the patient receives the medication by inhaling the mist

F. Medications
1. Antibiotics
   a. Kill microorganisms
   b. Examples: Amoxil, ampicillin, Biaxin, Ceclor, Keflex
2. Antihistamines
   a. Counteract the effects of histamine
   b. Examples: Benadryl, Phenergan, Seldane
3. Bronchodilators
   a. Dilate bronchial tubes
   b. Examples: Albuterol, Proventil, Ventolin, aminophylline
4. Expectorants
   a. Produce productive cough
   b. Example: Humibid
5. Decongestants
   a. Decrease congestion in the nose and nasal passages
   b. Examples: Entex, Afrin, Sudafed

VI. GASTROENTEROLOGY

A. General
1. Treats diseases and disorders of the digestive tract
2. Specialized physician: gastroenterologist

B. Common Symptoms of Gastrointestinal Disorders
1. Anorexia, weight loss
2. Abdominal pain
3. Nausea, vomiting
4. Change in bowel habits
5. Flatulence
6. Blood, mucus in feces
7. Fever
8. Heartburn, indigestion, difficulty swallowing
9. Diaphoresis

C. General Examination
1. Examination of the mouth
2. Palpation of the abdomen and intestines
3. Inspection of the rectum (can be accomplished with a scope)

D. Diagnostic Procedures
1. Colonoscopy: visual examination of the colon using a lighted scope
2. Liver biopsy: removal of a tissue sample from the liver for microscopic examination
3. Proctoscopy (sigmoidoscopy): visual examination of the anus, the rectum, and part of the sigmoid colon
4. Barium enema (BE): infusion of barium into the rectum for visualization by x-ray
5. Cholecystogram: x-ray examination of the gallbladder
6. Upper gastrointestinal (GI) series: x-ray study of the esophagus, stomach, and duodenum; contrast medium is orally administered
7. Gastric analysis: aspiration of the stomach contents by a tube placed into the stomach, through the nose; contents analyzed
8. Occult blood (guaiac) test: test for hidden blood in the stool; Hemoccult
9. Ova and parasites (O&P): analysis of a stool sample for the presence of eggs and parasites
10. Liver function tests: tests performed to diagnose liver-related diseases or disorders

E. Treatment Procedures
1. Appendectomy: removal of the appendix
2. Cholecystectomy: removal of the gallbladder
3. Colostomy: creation of an opening between the colon and the body surface
4. Hemorrhoid ligation: removal of hemorrhoids by using tying off (ligating)
5. Lithotripsy: crushing of stones
6. Hemorrhoidectomy: excision of hemorrhoids
7. Vagotomy: surgical transection of the vagus nerve to decrease stomach acid secretion in patients with ulcers

F. Medications
1. Antihelmintics
   a. Kill helminths (worms)
   b. Example: Vermox

2. Antibiotics
   a. Kill microorganisms
   b. Examples: Sumycin, Flagyl
3. Antispasmodics
   a. Decrease spasms of the GI tract
   b. Examples: Bentyl, Librax, Donnatal
4. Antidiarrheals
   a. Decrease or slow diarrhea
   b. Examples: Imodium, Lomotil, Pepto-Bismol
5. H$_2$ antagonists
   a. Decrease stomach acids
   b. Examples: Tagamet, Zantac, Axid, Pepcid
6. Laxatives
   a. Encourage bowel movements
   b. Examples: Colace, Dulcolax, Ex-Lax, Milk of Magnesia

VII. UROLOGY

A. General
1. Treats diseases and disorders of the male and female urinary systems and the male reproductive system
2. Specialized physician: urologist

B. Common Symptoms of Urinary System Disorders
1. Anorexia, nausea, vomiting
2. Malaise, fatigue, lethargy
3. Nocturia, hematuria, pyuria, proteinuria
4. Dysuria, urgency, frequency, incontinence
5. Pain in lumbar region or flank
6. Edema, ascites
7. Hypertension, shortness of breath

C. General Examination
1. Palpation of the kidneys and bladder
2. Inspection of the external genitalia
3. Palpation of the prostate gland through the rectum

D. Diagnostic Procedures
1. Cystoscopy: visual examination of the bladder with a cystoscope
2. Retrograde pyelogram: x-ray of the kidney after introducing a contrast medium through the ureter
3. Intravenous pyelogram (IVP): study of the kidney using an intravenous contrast medium
4. Renal ultrasound: ultrasound of the kidneys
5. X-ray of the kidney, ureter, and bladder (KUB): x-ray done without injection of air or contrast medium; shows the size and location of the organs
6. Urinalysis (UA): analysis of urine to determine its physical, chemical, and microscopic properties

7. Blood urea nitrogen (BUN): measures the amount of urea in the blood; kidney function test
8. Semen analysis: measures the quantity and motility of sperm
9. Prostate specific antigen (PSA): blood test to check for the presence of prostate cancer

E. Treatment Procedures
1. Dialysis: artificial means of removing waste products from the blood when the kidneys have failed
2. Lithotripsy: procedure to crush or break up stones in the urinary tract
3. Catheterization: introduction of a flexible tube through the urethra into the urinary bladder
4. Circumcision: removal of the foreskin of the penis
5. Prostatectomy: removal of the prostate
6. Transurethral resection of the prostate (TURP): prostatic tissue removed through an endoscope introduced through the urethra
7. Vasectomy: removal of a segment of the vas deferens; male sterilization technique

F. Medications
1. Antibiotics
   a. Destroy microorganisms
   b. Examples: Bactrim, Furadantin, Gantrisin, Rocephin
2. Analgesics
   a. Reduce pain
   b. Example: Pyridium
3. Gonadotropins
   a. Stimulate gonads
   b. Example: Pergonal
4. For impotence
   a. Example: Viagra

VIII. OBSTETRICS AND GYNECOLOGY

A. General
1. Diagnosis and treatment of diseases and disorders of the female reproductive system and pregnancy
2. Specialized physician: obstetrician (pregnancy and childbirth) or gynecologist (female reproductive system)

B. Common Symptoms of Female Reproduction System Disorders
1. Sexually transmitted diseases/sexually transmitted infections (STDs/STIs)
   a. Pelvic or genital pain
   b. Dysuria, hematuria, purulent discharge
   c. Burning or itching on urination
   d. Urinary frequency, incontinence
   e. Dyspareunia

f. Fever, malaise
g. Lesions in genital area
2. Infertility
   a. Abnormal pregnancies
   b. Endometriosis
   c. Congenital malformations
   d. Decreased sperm count
3. Specific to female reproductive system
   a. Fever
   b. Abnormal vaginal discharge and/or itching
   c. Pain in lower abdomen or pelvic region

C. General Examination

1. Inspection and palpation of the breasts
2. Inspection of the external genitalia, vagina, and cervix
3. Palpation of the uterus, ovaries, and fallopian tubes
4. Prenatal: includes initial general examination, as well as periodic examinations to monitor fetal growth and development

D. Diagnostic Procedures

1. Amniocentesis
   a. Puncture of the amniotic sac with a needle to withdraw amniotic fluid for analysis
   b. Can detect genetic disorders
2. Cervical biopsy: removal of tissue to evaluate the presence of abnormalities
3. Colposcopy: examination of the cervix with a scope
4. Dilation and curettage (D&C): expansion of the cervix so that the uterine wall can be scraped
5. Fetal monitoring: recording of the fetal heart rate
6. Laparoscopy: examination of the abdomen by insertion of a laparoscope through the abdominal wall
7. Human chorionic gonadotropin (HCG)
   a. Hormone produced by the placenta during pregnancy
   b. Basis for pregnancy testing
   c. Testing performed on blood or urine
8. Chorionic villi sampling (CVS)
   a. Use of ultrasound to guide a needle into the uterine wall to obtain a sample of chorion
   b. Can detect chromosomal abnormalities
9. Endovaginal ultrasound: sound probe placed in the vagina for a closer, sharper look within the pelvis
10. Hysterosalpingography: x-ray of the uterus and fallopian tubes, using radiopaque material
11. Pelvimetry: measurement of the dimensions of the pelvis

12. Pap (Papanicolaou) smear (ThinPrep)
    a. Scrapings from the cervix used to detect tissue changes
    b. Screening test for cervical cancer

E. Treatment Procedures

1. Abortion
   a. Premature termination of pregnancy
   b. May be spontaneous or therapeutic
2. Cauterization: use of heat to destroy abnormal tissue
3. Cesarean section (C-section): birth of an infant through a surgical incision into uterus
4. Conization: removal of a cone-shaped wedge of tissue from the cervix for examination
5. Cryosurgery: use of cold to destroy abnormal tissue
6. Hysterectomy: surgical removal of the uterus through the abdominal wall or vagina
7. Hysteroscopy: insertion of a scope into the uterus to view the endometrial cavity
8. Kegel exercises: simple exercises to strengthen the pubococcygeal muscles
9. Tubal ligation
   a. Tying off the fallopian tubes
   b. Female sterilization procedure

F. MEDICATIONS

1. Hormone replacement
   a. Examples: Premarin, Depo-Provera, Ogen
2. Ovulation stimulants
   a. Example: Clomid
3. Oral contraceptives
   a. Prevent pregnancy
   b. Examples: Triphasil, Ovral, Ortho-Novum, Ortho Tri-Cyclen
4. Supplements
   a. Vitamins and iron
   b. Examples: Ferro-Sequels, Natalins
5. Antifungals
   a. Treat fungal or yeast infections
   b. Examples: Monistat, Gyne-Lotrimin

G. Contraception

1. Prevents fertilization of ovum
2. Commonly referred to as birth control
3. No method is 100% effective
4. Variety of methods
   a. Hormonal
      1) Prevents ovulation
      2) Can be in the form of oral contraceptives (pills); injection (Depo-Provera); intrauterine device/intrauterine contraceptive (Mirena); vaginal ring (NuvaRing); long-acting implants (Implanon)

b. Nonhormonal/barrier
   1) Blocks entrance of sperm into the uterus
   2) Can be in the form of condoms (male and female); cervical cap with spermicide; diaphragm with spermicide; spermicidal creams, foams, suppositories
c. Surgical
   1) Permanent
   2) Vasectomy: performed on the male vas deferens; results in no sperm in seminal fluid
   3) Tubal ligation: performed on the female fallopian tubes; results in no eggs reaching the tubes
d. Behavioral
   1) Abstinence: no intercourse
   2) Rhythm: avoidance of intercourse for several days near the time of ovulation
   3) Withdrawal (coitus interruptus): penis withdrawn before ejaculation

IX. ENDOCRINOLOGY

A. General
1. Diagnosis and treatment of diseases and disorders of the endocrine system
2. Specialized physician: endocrinologist

B. Common Symptoms of Endocrine System Disorders
1. Mental deviations
2. Changes in energy levels
3. Growth abnormalities
4. Skin, hair, nail changes
5. Muscle weakness, atrophy
6. Emotional disturbances
7. Edema
8. Changes in blood pressure, heart irregularities
9. Sexual irregularities
10. Changes in urinary output

C. General Examination
1. Complete physical examination

D. Diagnostic Procedures
1. Radioactive iodine uptake: measures the uptake of a dose of radioactive iodine by the thyroid gland
2. Thyroid scan
   a. Administration of a radioactive compound to visualize the thyroid gland
   b. Used to detect tumors and nodules
3. CT scans
   a. Can visualize the endocrine glands
   b. Can detect disease processes and masses
4. Ultrasonography: use of sound waves to obtain images

5. Blood tests
   a. Used to diagnose and manage endocrine disorders
   b. Blood tests for:
      1) Adrenocorticotropic hormone (ACTH): from the pituitary
      2) Aldosterone: from the adrenal cortex
      3) Thyroxin: from the thyroid
      4) Calcium: from the parathyroid
      5) Cortisol: from the adrenal cortex
      6) Electrolytes (sodium, potassium, and chloride): from the adrenal cortex
      7) Estradiol: from the ovaries
      8) Follicle-stimulating hormone (FSH): from the pituitary
      9) Growth hormone (GH): from the pituitary
      10) Glucose: from the pancreas
      11) Insulin: from the pancreas
      12) Luteinizing hormone (LH): from the pituitary
      13) Parathyroid hormone: from the parathyroid
      14) Triiodothyronine (T_3) and thyroxine (tetraiodothyronine [T_4]): from the thyroid
      15) Testosterone: from the testes
6. Basal metabolic rate (BMR)
   a. Not an often-ordered test
   b. Measures the energy exchange rate of the body in a state of rest
7. Glucose tolerance test (GTT)
   a. Blood is tested at specific intervals after the patient ingests a measured amount of glucose

E. Treatment Procedures
1. Oophorectomy: surgical removal of the ovaries
2. Orchiectomy: surgical removal of the testes
3. Thyroidectomy: total or partial removal of thyroid gland

F. Medications
1. Thyroid medications
   a. Replace thyroid hormones
   b. Examples: Synthroid, Euthroid
2. Corticosteroids
   a. decrease inflammation
   b. Examples: Cortisone, Aristocort, Kenalog, Medrol, Decadron
3. GH
   a. stimulates growth
   b. Example: Humatrope
4. Antidiuretic hormones
   a. Reduces urine volume; treat diabetes insipidus
   b. Example: Pitressin; vasopressin
5. Labor inducers
   a. Initiate or improve uterine contractions
   b. Example: Pitocin

6. Oral antidiabetics
   a. Lower blood glucose levels in type 2 diabetes
   b. Examples: Orinase, Glucotrol, Diabinese, Glucophage
7. Insulin
   a. lower blood glucose levels by increasing glucose uptake
   b. Examples: Humulin, Novolin

X. NEUROLOGY

A. General
1. Diagnosis and treatment of diseases and disorders of the nervous system
2. Specialized physician: neurologist

B. Common Symptoms of Nervous System Disorders
1. Headaches
2. Nausea, vomiting
3. Weakness, motor disturbances
4. Mood swings, memory impairment
5. Drowsiness, stupor, coma
6. Seizures, paralysis, convulsions, numbness
7. Muscle rigidity, flaccidity
8. Disturbances in speech, vision, hearing, taste
9. Tremors
10. Radiating pain

C. General Examination
1. Mental status: includes assessment of intelligence; assessment of memory; orientation to person, place, and time; and general appearance
2. Evaluation of all cranial nerves
3. Motor nerves: includes coordination, strength, Romberg test, walking, and finger-to-nose exercise
4. Sensory nervous system
5. Reflexes

D. Diagnostic Procedures
1. Electroencephalogram (EEG)
   a. Study of the electrical activity of the brain
   b. Uses electrodes attached to the scalp
2. Electromyogram (EMG): study of the contraction of a muscle as a result of electrical stimulation
3. Lumbar puncture: procedure for removal of cerebrospinal fluid (CSF) for analysis
4. Brain scan: procedure that uses radioactive chemicals and specialized machines to record the passage through, and absorption into, brain lesions
5. Myelography: x-ray of the spinal cord
6. Skull series: standard x-ray views of the skull
7. Cervical, thoracic, and lumbosacral spine series: standard x-ray views of specific portions of the spine

E. Treatment Procedures
1. Craniotomy: surgical opening into the cranium
2. Laminectomy: removal of laminae to decompress pinched spinal nerve roots
3. Halo traction: traction device for neck stability

F. Medications
1. Anticonvulsants
   a. Decrease seizure activity
   b. Examples: Depakote, Dilantin, Tegretol
2. Antiemetics (antivertigo agents)
   a. Decrease vomiting, dizziness
   b. Examples: Antivert, Compazine, Dramamine
3. Anti-Parkinson's agents
   a. Decrease symptoms of Parkinson's disease
   b. Examples: Artane, Cogentin, Sinemet
4. Antidepressants
   a. Counteract depression
   b. Examples: Paxil, Prozac, Celexa

XI. OPHTHALMOLOGY

A. General
1. Diagnosis and treatment of diseases and disorders of the eye
2. Specialized physician: ophthalmologist

B. Common Symptoms of Eye Disorders
1. Visual disturbances
2. Redness
3. Pain/burning around the eye

C. General Examination
1. Inspection and measurement of the external eye, eyelids, and accessory structures
2. Measurement of eye movements and pupillary distance

D. Diagnostic Procedures
1. Keratometry (K-readings): measurement of the steepness of the cornea
2. Ophthalmoscopy: visual examination of the interior eye using an ophthalmoscope
3. Visual acuity
   a. Determines the amount of myopia, hyperopia, or astigmatism
   b. Uses the Snellen eye chart
4. Slit lamp examination: examines the cornea, conjunctiva, iris, lens, and vitreous humor using a slit light and biomicroscope
5. Tonometry
   a. Measures intraocular tension
   b. May indicate the presence of glaucoma
6. Ishihara color vision test: tests color vision

E. Treatment Procedures
1. Blepharoplasty: surgical repair of the eyelids
2. Cataract extraction: removal of the lens of the eye

3. Enucleation: removal of the eye from the socket
4. Glaucoma operation: procedure that relieves increased intraocular pressure

F. Medications
1. Antibiotics
   a. treatment of bacterial infections
   b. Examples: Tobrex, Bacitracin Opthalmic
2. Corticosteroids
   a. reduces inflammation
   b. Examples: Decadron, Opticrom
3. Glaucoma treatment
   a. reduces intraocular pressure
   b. Examples: Timoptic, Propine, Betagan

XII. OTORHINOLARYNGOLOGY (ENT)

A. General
1. Diagnosis and treatment of diseases and disorders of the ear, nose, and throat
2. Specialized physician: otorhinolaryngologist

B. Common Symptoms of Ear, Nose, and Throat Disorders
1. Loss of hearing
2. Vertigo, dizziness
3. Tinnitus
4. Earache, increased ear pressure
5. Sore throat
6. Fever, malaise, headache
7. Epistaxis
8. Nasal congestion, rhinorrhea

C. General Examination
1. Examination of the ear with an otoscope
2. Examination of the nasal structures, throat, and sinuses

D. Diagnostic Procedures
1. Audiometry
   a. Use of an audiometer to deliver sound frequencies
   b. Determines the patient's hearing threshold
2. Laryngoscopy: visual examination of the larynx with a laryngoscope
3. Otoscopy: visual examination of the ear with an otoscope
4. Throat culture: inflamed areas of the throat are swabbed and analyzed for various pathogens
5. Nasal smear: removal of a specimen and analysis for pathogens
6. Skull, mastoid, sinus, and chest x-rays: standard views of specific body parts
7. Rapid strep test: test for beta-hemolytic *Streptococcus*

E. Treatment Procedures
1. Adenoidectomy: surgical excision of adenoids
2. Myringotomy: incision into the eardrum

3. Myringotomy with tubes: incision into the eardrum with placement of ventilation tubes
4. Rhinoplasty: reconstruction or plastic surgery of the nose
5. Tonsillectomy: surgical excision of tonsils
6. Tonsilloadenoidectomy (T&A): surgical removal of the tonsils and adenoids
7. Ear irrigation: irrigation (washing) of external ear canal

F. Medications
1. Antibiotics
   a. Kills or inhibits the growth of microorganisms
   b. Examples: Amoxil, Ceclor, Erythromycin, Keflex
2. Otics
   a. Treat otitis externa
   b. Examples: Cipro HC, Ciprodex, Floxin Otic

XIII. PEDIATRICS

A. General
1. Diagnosis and treatment of diseases and disorders associated with childhood and health maintenance for infants, children, and adolescents
2. Specialized physician: pediatrician

B. General Examination
1. Similar to a complete physical examination for an adult
2. Examinations fall into two general categories:
   a. Well-child (well-baby) visit
      1) Evaluates the child's growth and development
      2) Physical examination is performed at this time
      3) Necessary immunizations are administered
   b. Sick-child (sick-baby) visit
      1) Child shows signs and symptoms of a disease process or injury
      2) Provider diagnoses and prescribes treatment

C. Growth Chart
1. Chart used to plot the physical growth pattern of a child
2. Includes height, weight, and head circumference
3. Identifies the percentile the child's growth falls into, as compared with the measurements listed on the standardized chart
4. Should be plotted at each well-baby visit
5. Separate charts
   a. Girls, 2 to 20 years (see Figure 17-8)
   b. Boys, birth to 36 months (see Figure 17-9)
   c. Girls, birth to 36 months
   d. Boys, 2 to 18 years

2 to 20 years: Girls
Stature-for-age and Weight-for-age percentiles

NAME _____

RECORD # _____

Published May 30, 2000 (modified 11/21/00).
SOURCE: Developed by the National Center for Health Statistics in collaboration with
the National Center for Chronic Disease Prevention and Health Promotion (2000).
http://www.cdc.gov/growthcharts

FIGURE 17-8 Growth rate graph: girls (2 to 20 years). (Developed by the National Center for Health Statistics in collaboration with the National Center for Chronic Disease Prevention and Health Promotion [2000]. Available at: http://www.cdc.gov/growthcharts. Published May 30, 2000.)

Birth to 36 months: Boys
Length-for-age and Weight-for-age percentiles

NAME _____

RECORD # _____

Published May 30, 2000 (modified 4/20/01).

SOURCE: Developed by the National Center for Health Statistics in collaboration with
the National Center for Chronic Disease Prevention and Health Promotion (2000).
http://www.cdc.gov/growthcharts

FIGURE 17-9 Growth rate graph: males (birth to 36 months). (Developed by the National Center for Health Statistics in collaboration with the National Center for Chronic Disease Prevention and Health Promotion [2000]. Available at: http://www.cdc.gov/growthcharts. Published May 30, 2000 [modified 4/20/01].)

D. Common Pediatric Diseases and Disorders

1. Colic: abdominal distress
2. Diarrhea: loose stools; two or more watery or abnormal stools within 24 hours
3. Failure to thrive: infant or young child whose weight is consistently below the third percentile on growth charts; medical and social factors must be evaluated
4. Obesity: BMI-for-age is between 85th and 95th percentile
5. Common cold: highly contagious viral disease spread through droplets
6. Otitis media: infection or inflammation of the middle ear; can be serous or suppurative
7. Croup: viral inflammation of the larynx and trachea causing edema and spasms of the vocal cords
8. Bronchiolitis: viral infection of the small bronchi and bronchioles
9. Asthma: result of bronchospasm and inflammation
10. Influenza: highly contagious viral infection of the respiratory tract
11. Conjunctivitis: "pink eye"; highly contagious bacterial infection that affects the conjunctiva
12. Tonsillitis: inflammation of the tonsils most frequently caused by *Streptococcus* A
13. Fifth disease: *erythema infectiosum*; "slapped cheek disease"; caused by parvovirus B19
14. Varicella: chickenpox; viral disease caused by a herpesvirus; transmitted by droplets; vaccine available for protection
15. Meningitis: inflammation of the membranes that cover the brain and spinal cord; can be caused by bacteria, fungi, or viruses; vaccine available (Hib) for protection
16. Hepatitis B: viral infection that can be transmitted across the placenta or during birth process if the mother is infected; vaccine available for protection
17. Reye's syndrome: cause unknown; linked to use of aspirin during a viral illness

E. Immunizations (see Figure 17-10)

1. Always refer to the Centers for Disease Control and Prevention (CDC) guidelines for current schedule
    a. Childhood diphtheria-tetanus-acellular pertussis vaccine (DtaP)
       1) Total of five doses required by law between 2 months and 6 years of age
       2) Administer: 0.5 mL intramuscularly (IM)
    b. Adolescent tetanus-diphtheria toxoids vaccine (Td): 11 and 12 years of age, Td booster
    c. Adult tetanus vaccine (Td)
       1) Given as a booster from age 7 through adult
       2) Adults are given one dose each 10 years for life
       3) For severe or dirty wounds, a booster is given if the last normal dose was more than 5 years ago
       4) For minor or clean wounds, a booster is given if the last normal dose was given 10 or more years ago
    d. *Haemophilus influenzae* type b (Hib)
       1) Four doses administered between 2 months and 18 months of age
       2) Administer: 0.5 mL IM
       3) Vaccine consists of killed virus grown in chicken embryo tissue
    e. Inactivated poliovirus (poliomyelitis) vaccine (IPV)
       1) Four doses administered between 2 months and 4 to 6 years of age
       2) Administer: 0.5 mL IM or SC
    f. Hepatitis B vaccine (HepB)
       1) Three doses administered between birth and 18 months of age
       2) Administer: 0.5 mL IM
       3) Two doses of Recombivax HB (Merck) 1 mL may be given to 11- to 15-year-olds
    g. Mumps, measles, and rubella (MMR) vaccine
       1) Two doses administered between 12 months and 11 to 12 years of age
       2) Administer: 0.5 mL subcutaneously (SC)
       3) Vaccine consists of attenuated measles, mumps, and rubella virus
    h. Varicella vaccine (Var; chickenpox)
       1) Administered after 12 months of age
       2) Administer: 0.5 mL SC
    i. Pneumococcal vaccine (PCV)
       1) Three doses administered before age 12 months; last dose given after 12 months and before age 5
       2) Administer 0.5 mL IM or SC
    j. Human papillomavirus (HPV)
       1) Three doses over a 6-month period to female patients ages 9 to 26 years
       2) Administer: 0.5 mL IM
    k. Influenza, live attenuated (LAIV)
       1) One dose yearly up to age 50
       2) Administer: 0.2 mL intranasal spray
    l. Influenza, trivalent inactivated (TIV)
       1) One dose yearly
       2) Administer: for 6-35 mos 0.25 mL IM; for >3 yrs 0.5 mL IM
    m. Hepatitis A (Hep A)
       1) Two doses 6 months apart
       2) Administer: for <18 yrs 0.5 mL IM; for >19 yrs 1.0mL IM
    n. Rotavirus
       1) Two doses between ages 2 and 6 mos
       2) Administer: 0.5 mL IM

Recommended Immunization Schedule for Persons Aged 0 Through 6 Years—United States • 2010
For those who fall behind or start late, see the catch-up schedule

Vaccine ▼ Age ▶	Birth	1 month	2 months	4 months	6 months	12 months	15 months	18 months	19–23 months	2–3 years	4–6 years
Hepatitis B[1]	HepB	HepB			HepB						
Rotavirus[2]			RV	RV	RV[2]						
Diphtheria, Tetanus, Pertussis[3]			DTaP	DTaP	DTaP	see footnote[3]	DTaP				DTaP
Haemophilus influenzae type b[4]			Hib	Hib	Hib[4]	Hib					
Pneumococcal[5]			PCV	PCV	PCV	PCV				PPSV	
Inactivated Poliovirus[6]			IPV	IPV		IPV					IPV
Influenza[7]						Influenza (Yearly)					
Measles, Mumps, Rubella[8]						MMR		see footnote[8]			MMR
Varicella[9]						Varicella		see footnote[9]			Varicella
Hepatitis A[10]						HepA (2 doses)				HepA Series	
Meningococcal[11]										MCV	

Range of recommended ages for all children except certain high-risk groups

Range of recommended ages for certain high-risk groups

This schedule includes recommendations in effect as of December 15, 2009. Any dose not administered at the recommended age should be administered at a subsequent visit, when indicated and feasible. The use of a combination vaccine generally is preferred over separate injections of its equivalent component vaccines. Considerations should include provider assessment, patient preference, and the potential for adverse events. Providers should consult the relevant Advisory Committee on Immunization Practices statement for detailed recommendations: **http://www.cdc.gov/vaccines/pubs/acip-list.htm**. Clinically significant adverse events that follow immunization should be reported to the Vaccine Adverse Event Reporting System (VAERS) at **http://www.vaers.hhs.gov** or by telephone, **800-822-7967.**

Recommended Immunization Schedule for Persons Aged 7 Through 18 Years—United States • 2010
For those who fall behind or start late, see the schedule below and the catch-up schedule

Vaccine ▼ Age ▶	7–10 years	11–12 years	13–18 years
Tetanus, Diphtheria, Pertussis[1]		Tdap	Tdap
Human Papillomavirus[2]	see footnote 2	HPV (3 doses)	HPV series
Meningococcal[3]	MCV	MCV	MCV
Influenza[4]	Influenza (Yearly)		
Pneumococcal[5]	PPSV		
Hepatitis A[6]	HepA Series		
Hepatitis B[7]	Hep B Series		
Inactivated Poliovirus[8]	IPV Series		
Measles, Mumps, Rubella[9]	MMR Series		
Varicella[10]	Varicella Series		

Range of recommended ages for all children except certain high-risk groups

Range of recommended ages for catch-up immunization

Range of recommended ages for certain high-risk groups

This schedule includes recommendations in effect as of December 15, 2009. Any dose not administered at the recommended age should be administered at a subsequent visit, when indicated and feasible. The use of a combination vaccine generally is preferred over separate injections of its equivalent component vaccines. Considerations should include provider assessment, patient preference, and the potential for adverse events. Providers should consult the relevant Advisory Committee on Immunization Practices statement for detailed recommendations: **http://www.cdc.gov/vaccines/pubs/acip-list.htm**. Clinically significant adverse events that follow immunization should be reported to the Vaccine Adverse Event Reporting System (VAERS) at **http://www.vaers.hhs.gov** or by telephone, **800-822-7967.**

CS207330-A

The Recommended Immunization Schedules for Persons Aged 0 through 18 Years are approved by the Advisory Committee on Immunization Practices (**http://www.cdc.gov/vaccines/recs/acip**), the American Academy of Pediatrics (**http://www.aap.org**), and the American Academy of Family Physicians (**http://www.aafp.org**). Department of Health and Human Services • Centers for Disease Control and Prevention

FIGURE 17-10   Immunization schedule. (From U.S. Department of Health and Human Services, Centers for Disease Control and Prevention.)

2. Combination vaccines
   1) DTaP + HepB + IPV (Pediarix): 0.5 mL IM
   2) DTaP + Hib + IPV (Pentacel) : 0.5 mL IM
   3) DTaP + Hib (Trihibit): 0.5 mL IM
   4) DTaP + IPV (Kinrix) : 0.5 mL IM
   5) Hib + HepB (Comvax): 0.5 mL IM
   6) MMR + Var (ProQuad): younger than 12 yrs 0.5 mL SC
   7) HepA + HepB (Twinrix): older than 18 yrs 1 mL IM

XIV. GERIATRICS

A. General
1. Treatment of older adults
2. Specialized physician: gerontologist and internist

B. Aging
1. Complex physiologic, psychological, and social process
2. Aging is not an illness; it is a normal life process
3. Changes occur in the patient's
   a. Appearance
   b. Abilities
   c. Vision
   d. Hearing
   e. Taste
   f. Smell

C. Caring for the Older Patient
1. Speak slowly and distinctly if the person is hearing impaired
2. Use indirect lighting in examination rooms to decrease glare
3. Do not carry on conversations with the patient where a large amount of background noise is present
4. Do not patronize the older patient
5. Touch the older patient as you would any other patient
6. Touch the older patient politely and affectionately, not in a controlling manner
7. Use eye contact when conversing with the older patient
8. Offer assistance to the older patient as needed
9. Treat the older patient as an individual
10. Reinforce treatment instructions by writing them down
11. Never approach a visually impaired person without making your presence known; identify yourself and others in the room

D. Problems Associated with Aging
1. Inability to perform personal care, including bathing, dressing, eating, getting out of bed, and using the toilet
2. Inability to live independently, including preparing meals, shopping, managing money, using the telephone, and doing housework
3. Functioning such as walking, climbing the stairs, lifting, and standing for periods of time

XV. PSYCHIATRY

A. General
1. Deals with the diagnosis, prevention, and treatment of mental illness
2. Specialized physician: psychiatrist
3. Psychologist: nonmedical person trained in methods of therapy

B. Common Signs and Symptoms of Mental Disorders
1. Stress, anxiety, depression
2. Withdrawal from society
3. Disorganized thinking, hallucinations
4. Inappropriate or violent behavior
5. Crying, mood swings
6. Sleep disturbances, fatigue, agitation
7. Loss of concentration
8. Inability to experience pleasure
9. Forgetfulness
10. Inability to place self in environment, person, place
11. Paranoia

C. Psychiatric Disorders
1. Anxiety disorders
   a. Characterized by anxiety (unpleasant tension, distress, troubled feelings, avoidance behavior)
      1) Panic disorder
      2) Phobic disorders
      3) Obsessive-compulsive disorder (OCD)
      4) Posttraumatic stress disorder (PTSD)
2. Delirium and dementia
   a. Abnormal cognition (mental processes of thinking, perception, reasoning, judgment)
      1) Delirium
      2) Dementia
3. Dissociative disorders
   a. Chronic or sudden disturbances of memory, identity, consciousness, perception of environment
      1) Not caused by direct effects of brain damage, drug abuse
      2) Dissociative identity disorder
      3) Dissociative amnesia
      4) Dissociative fugue
4. Eating disorders
   a. Disturbances in eating behavior
      1) Anorexia nervosa
      2) Bulimia nervosa
5. Mood disorders
   a. Prolonged emotion that dominates person's entire mental life

1) Bipolar I
2) Bipolar II
3) Depressive disorder
4) Seasonal affective disorder (SAD)

6. Personality disorders
   a. inflexible and rigid personality traits causing impairment of functioning, distress, conflict with others
      1) Antisocial
      2) Histrionic
      3) Narcissistic
      4) Paranoid
      5) Schizoid

7. Schizophrenia
   a. Characterized by withdrawal from reality into an inner world of conflict and disorganized thinking
   b. Symptoms
      1) Delusions
      2) Hallucinations
      3) Disorganized thinking
      4) Flat affect
      5) Impaired interpersonal functioning, relationships

8. Sexual and gender identity disorders
   a. Sexual disorders
      1) Paraphilias: recurrent intense sexual urges, fantasies, behaviors
      2) Sexual dysfunctions: disturbances in sexual desire, response
   b. Gender identity disorders
      1) Strong, persistent cross-gender identification with opposite sex

9. Somatoform disorders
   a. Patient's mental conflicts expressed as physical symptoms
      1) Conversion disorder
      2) Hypochondriasis

10. Substance-related disorders
    a. Symptoms, behavioral changes associated with regular use of substances that affect the central nervous system
    b. Prolonged use produces dependence
       1) Alcohol
       2) Amphetamines
       3) Cannabis
       4) Cocaine
       5) Hallucinogens
       6) Opioids
       7) Sedatives
    c. Common signs and symptoms of substance abuse
       1) Changes in weight, sleep habits
       2) Impaired memory
       3) Illogical thinking
       4) Mood swings, irritability, depression, anger
       5) Anxiety, overreaction to difficult situations
       6) Changes in vital signs
       7) Runny nose, nasal stuffiness, bloodshot eyes, sweating
       8) Changes in friends, appearance

D. Therapeutic Techniques
   1. Psychotherapy
      a. Treatment of emotional problems using psychological techniques
   2. Cognitive behavior therapy
   3. Family therapy
   4. Group therapy
   5. Hypnosis
   6. Play therapy
   7. Psychoanalysis
   8. Sex therapy
   9. Supportive psychotherapy
   10. Electroconvulsive therapy (ECT)
       a. Electric current applied to brain while patient is anesthetized and ventilated
       b. Used mainly for serious depression and bipolar disorder
   11. Drug therapy
       a. Use of medications to treat psychiatric disorders
          1) Antianxiety agents: lessen anxiety, tension, agitation
             a) Examples: Xanax, Valium, Buspar, Paxil, Ativan
          2) Antidepressants: reverse depressive symptoms; produce feelings of well-being
             a) Examples: Prozac, Paxil, Elavil, Wellbutrin, Celexa
          3) Antiobsessive-compulsive agents: relieve symptoms of OCD
             a) Examples: Anafranil, Zoloft
          4) Antipsychotics: modify psychotic symptoms, behavior
             a) Examples: Haldol, Zyprexa, Risperdol
          5) Hypnotics: produce sleep
             a) Examples: Ambien, Restoril, Halcion
          6) Mood stabilizers: treat manic episodes of bipolar illness
             a) Examples: Eskalith, Tegretol, Lithium, Lamictal
          7) Stimulants: prescribed for attention deficit and hyperactivity disorder in children
             a) Examples: Ritalin, Cyclert

XVI. ONCOLOGY

A. General
   1. Care and treatment of persons with tumors or cancer
   2. Specialized physician: oncologist

B. Common Signs and Symptoms of Cancer (CAUTION)
1. Change in bowel and bladder habits
2. A sore that does not heal
3. Unusual bleeding or discharge
4. Thickening or lump in a breast or elsewhere
5. Indigestion or difficulty swallowing
6. Obvious change in a wart or mole
7. Nagging cough or hoarseness

C. Tumors
1. Malignant: cancerous tumor
   a. Cells multiply rapidly
   b. Invasive
   c. Undifferentiated
   d. Metastatic
2. Benign: noncancerous tumor
   a. Slow growing
   b. Encapsulated, noninvasive
   c. Well-differentiated
   d. Nonmetastatic
3. Carcinoma: malignant tumor derived from epithelial tissue (skin, glands)
4. Sarcoma: malignant tumor derived from connective tissue (bone, muscle, fat)
5. Lymphoma: malignant tumor that develops in lymphatic tissue
6. Leukemia: malignancy of the bone marrow
7. Myeloma: malignant tumor of the plasma cells in bone marrow
8. Mixed tumors: combination of cells
9. Carcinoma in situ (CIS): cancer cells have not invaded the organ of origin

D. Staging and Grading Tumors
1. Provider must determine severity of cancer (grade) and size and spread (stage) in order to treat
2. Grading
   a. Grade I: tumors well differentiated
   b. Grade II: moderately/poorly differentiated
   c. Grade III: moderately/poorly differentiated
   d. Grade IV: Undifferentiated
3. Staging
   a. TNM System
      1) T: size of the tumor
      2) N: number of lymph nodes involved
      3) M: presence of distant metastasis
      4) Numbers after the letters denote size and degree of involvement (0-4)

E. Diagnosis
1. Patient history
2. Tumor markers
3. Biopsy
4. Imaging
5. Self-detection

F. Treatment
1. Surgery
   a. Cautery: burning of tissue to destroy it
   b. Cryosurgery: use of cold to destroy tissue
   c. En bloc resection: tumor and large amount of surrounding tissue removed
   d. Excisional biopsy: removal of tumor and margin of normal tissue
   e. Incisional biopsy: piece of tumor removed for examination to determine diagnosis
2. Radiation therapy (radiation oncology)
   a. Goal: deliver maximum dose of radiation to the tumor and minimal dose to surrounding tissue
   b. Can produce undesirable side effects
      1) Alopecia
      2) Nausea and vomiting
      3) Xerostomia (dry mouth)
      4) Myelosuppression
      5) Mucositis
3. Chemotherapy
   a. Treatment of cancer using chemicals/drugs
      1) Alkylating agents
      2) Antibiotics
      3) Antimetabolites
      4) Antimitotics
      5) Hormonal agents

G. Clinical Procedures
1. Used to detect, treat malignancies
   a. Bone marrow biopsy
   b. Bone marrow/stem cell transplant
   c. Fiberoptic colonoscopy
   d. Cytology
   e. Laparoscopy
   f. Mammography
   g. Needle biopsy

18 Nutrition

I. NUTRITION

A. Definition
1. All processes involved in the intake and use of nutrients
2. Can indicate the condition of the body resulting from the use of nutrients
3. Good health is a state of emotional and physical well-being that can be mostly determined by diet and lifestyle factors
4. "We are what we eat"

B. Nutrients
1. Organic and inorganic chemicals in foods
2. Supply the energy and raw materials for cellular activities
3. Include:
   a. Carbohydrates
   b. Fats
   c. Proteins
   d. Vitamins
   e. Minerals
   f. Water
4. Perform one or more of three basic functions in the body:
   a. Provide a source of fuel or energy
   b. Supply material for growth and repair of tissues
   c. Regulate metabolic processes

C. Health Problems Related to Poor Nutrition and Lifestyle Choices
1. Anemia: low iron or folate intake
2. Cancers: high-fat, low-fiber diet; high alcohol and sodium intake; sedentary lifestyle; tobacco use
3. Constipation: low fiber, inadequate fluids; high-fat diet; sedentary lifestyle
4. Type 2 diabetes: high-calorie, high-fat diet; obesity; sedentary lifestyle
5. Hypercholesterolemia and atherosclerosis: high-fat, low-fiber diet; high sugar and alcohol intake; tobacco use; sedentary lifestyle
6. Hypertension: high-calorie, high-fat diet; high sodium intake; sedentary lifestyle; obesity; stress
7. Osteoporosis: low calcium intake; inadequate vitamin D; high alcohol intake; sedentary lifestyle; tobacco use
8. Stroke: high-fat, low-fiber diet; high alcohol intake; tobacco use; stress

D. Reasons for Food Choices
1. Convenience
2. Cost
3. Emotional comfort
4. Routine
5. Positive experiences
6. Ethnic and regional influences
7. Health and weight

II. COMPONENTS OF NUTRIENTS

A. Carbohydrates (CHO)
1. Organic compounds primarily from plants
2. Supply fuel for energy and all basic cellular functions
3. Three groups:
   a. Simple sugars (table sugar, molasses, candy, milk): easily digested and absorbed
   b. Complex carbohydrates (whole grains, cereal, pasta, rice, vegetables): easily digested and absorbed
   c. Dietary fiber (bran, oatmeal, beans, vegetables, seeds): indigestible, passing through the digestive tract unchanged
4. Recommended consumption (per the U.S. Food and Drug Administration)
   a. 55% to 57% of total calories per day

B. Fats
1. Storage form of fuel; backup for carbohydrates as energy source
2. Provide essential fatty acids for absorption of fat-soluble vitamins
3. Support and protect vital organs
4. Help regulate body temperature
5. Protect nerve fibers and help relay nerve impulses
6. Crucial to cell membrane development
7. Stored in adipose (fat) tissue

8. Cholesterol: nonessential nutrient that plays a vital role in metabolic activities
   a. Manufactured in the liver
   b. Found only in animal tissues, not plants
   c. High-density lipoproteins (HDL): "good" fat; carry cholesterol from body tissues to liver for metabolism and excretion
   d. Low-density lipoproteins (LDL): "bad" fat; carry cholesterol to the cells; can collect as plaques on blood vessel walls
9. Recommended consumption (per the U.S. Food and Drug Administration)
   a. 20% to 35% of total calories per day

C. Protein
1. Large molecules made up of amino acids
2. Builds and repairs body tissue including new tissue, blood, and hormones
3. Aids in the body's defense mechanisms against disease
4. Regulates fluid and electrolyte balance
5. Provides energy when carbohydrates and fat stores are depleted
6. Found in meat, fish, poultry, eggs
7. Recommended protein consumption
   a. No more than 18% of total calories per day

D. Vitamins (see Table 18-1)
1. Organic substances that occur in minute quantities in plant and animal tissue
2. Function as catalysts to help/allow metabolic reactions
3. Regulate synthesis of bone, skin, glands, nerves, blood
4. Aid in the metabolism of protein, carbohydrates, fats
5. Prevent nutritional deficiency diseases
6. Provide for good health at all ages
7. Do not cure diseases
8. Two groups:
   a. Fat-soluble: A, D, E, K
   b. Water-soluble: B complex, C

E. Minerals (see Table 18-2)
1. Electrolytes
2. Required in small amounts
3. Supplied through food or supplements
4. Contribute to body's water balance and acid-base balance
5. Essential components of enzymes

F. Water
1. Body can survive longer without food than without water
2. Part of almost every vital body function
3. Plays a key role in maintenance of body temperature
4. Solvent and medium for biochemical reactions
5. Vehicle to transport substances such as nutrients, hormones, antibodies, wastes
6. Acts as lubricant for joints and mucous membranes
7. Lost from the body in urine, feces, sweat, expiration

III. FOOD GUIDE PYRAMID (See Figure 18-1)

A. General
1. Developed by USDA to explain dietary guidelines
2. Good nutrition is a balance among:
   a. Carbohydrates
   b. Protein
   c. Vitamins
   d. Minerals
   e. Fiber
   f. Water
   g. Exercise
3. Explaining the Food Pyramid to patients encourages healthy eating habits

IV. THERAPEUTIC NUTRITION (DIETS)

A. General
1. Some illnesses and diseases can be cured and recovery can be facilitated with special diets
2. Consider patient's lifestyle, cultural influences, and background
3. Normal diet is modified to create the therapeutic diet by either restricting or increasing needed nutrients

B. Liquid Diet
1. Two types:
   a. Clear liquid: broth, tea, gelatin
   b. Full liquid: all foods on a clear diet plus milk, custard, strained cream soup, milkshakes, all juices
2. Indicated for preparation for certain diagnostic tests and postoperatively

C. Soft Diet
1. Foods with roughage (fiber) are eliminated
2. Eliminate raw fruits/vegetables; strongly flavored/gas-forming vegetables (onions, beans, broccoli, cauliflower)
3. Indicated postoperatively; certain gastrointestinal (GI) disorders

D. Mechanical Soft Diet
1. Regular diet in which foods are ground, chopped, or pureed
2. Indicated after oral surgery and for patients who have difficulty chewing/swallowing

E. Bland Diet
1. Restricts components that are GI irritants
2. Chemically irritating agents:
   a. Caffeine
   b. Pepper
   c. Chili
   d. Alcohol

TABLE 18-1 Vitamins

Vitamin	U.S. RDA*	Best Sources	Functions	Deficiency Symptoms†	Toxic?	Processing Tips	Did You Know?
A (carotene)	5000 IU/day	Yellow or orange fruits and vegetables, green leafy vegetables, fortified oatmeal, liver, dairy products	Formation and maintenance of skin, hair, and mucous membranes; helps vision in dim light; bone and tooth growth.	Night blindness, dry and scaly skin, frequent fatigue	Yes, in high doses, but beta-carotene is nontoxic	Serve fruits and vegetables raw and keep covered and refrigerated; steam vegetables; broil, bake, or braise meats	Low-fat and skim milks are often fortified with vitamin A, which was removed with the fat.
B₁ (thiamine)	1.5 mg/day	Fortified cereals and oatmeals, meats, rice and pasta, whole grains, liver	Helps body release energy from carbohydrates during metabolism; growth and muscle tone.	Heart irregularity, fatigue, nerve disorders, mental confusion	No, high doses are excreted by the kidneys	Do not rinse rice or pasta before and after cooking. Cook in minimal water.	Pasta and breads made of refined flours have B₁ added because it is lost in the milling process.
B₂ (riboflavin)	1.7 mg/day	Whole grains, green leafy vegetables, organ meats, milk and eggs	Helps body release energy from protein, fat, and carbohydrates during metabolism.	Cracks in corners of mouth, rash, anemia	No toxic effects reported	Store food in containers that light cannot enter; cook vegetables in minimal water; roast or broil meats.	Most ready-to-eat cereals are fortified with 25% of the U.S. RDA for B₂.
B₆ (pyridoxine)	2 mg/day	Fish, poultry, lean meats, bananas, prunes, dried beans, whole grains, avocados	Helps build body tissue and aids in metabolism of protein.	Convulsions, dermatitis, muscular weakness, skin cracks, anemia	Long-term megadoses may cause nerve damage in hands and feet	Serve fruits raw or cook for shortest time in little water; roast or broil meats.	Because B₆ aids in use of protein in the body, the need for B₆ increases with protein intake.
B₁₂ (cobalamin)	6 μg/day	Meats, milk products, seafood	Aids cell development, functioning of the nervous system, and the metabolism of protein and fat.	Anemia, nervousness, fatigue, and, in some cases, neuritis and brain degeneration	No toxic effects reported	Roast or broil meat and fish.	Vegetarians who do not eat any animal products may need a supplement.
Biotin	0.3 mg/day	Cereal/grain products, yeast, legumes, liver	Involved in metabolism of protein, fats, and carbohydrates.	Nausea, vomiting, depression, hair loss, dry scaly skin	No toxic effects reported	Storage, processing, and cooking do not appear to affect this vitamin.	Biotin deficiency is extremely rare in the United States.
Folate (folacin, folic acid)	0.4 mg/day	Green leafy vegetables, organ meats, dried peas, beans, and lentils	Aids in genetic material development and involved in red blood cell production.	Gastrointestinal disorders, anemia, cracks on lips	Some evidence of toxicity in high doses	Store vegetables in refrigerator and steam, boil, or simmer in minimal water.	Deficiencies can occur in premature infants and pregnant women.
Niacin	20 mg/day	Meat, poultry, fish, enriched cereals, peanuts, potatoes, dairy products, eggs	Involved in carbohydrate, protein, and fat metabolism.	Skin disorders, diarrhea, indigestion, general fatigue	Nicotinic acid form should be taken only under physician's care	Roast or broil beef, veal, lamb, and poultry. Cook potatoes in minimal water.	Niacin is formed in the body by converting an amino acid found in proteins.

Vitamin	Amount	Sources	Functions	Deficiency symptoms	Toxic effects	Storage/preparation	Comments
Pantothenic acid	10 mg/day	Lean meats, whole grains, legumes, vegetables, fruits	Helps in the release of energy from fats and carbohydrates.	Fatigue, vomiting, stomach stress, infections, muscle cramps	No toxic effects reported	Eat fruits and vegetables raw.	It is believed some pantothenic acid is produced in the gastrointestinal tract.
C (ascorbic acid)	60 mg/day	Citrus fruits, berries, and vegetables—especially peppers	Essential for structure of bones, cartilage, muscle, and blood vessels; also helps maintain capillaries and gums and aids in absorption of iron.	Swollen or bleeding gums, slow wound healing, fatigue/depression, poor digestion	Intakes of 1 g or more can cause nausea, cramps, and diarrhea.	Do not store or soak fruits and vegetables in water; refrigerate juices and store only 2 to 3 days.	Smokers may benefit from an increased intake of vitamin C.
D	400 IU/day	Fortified milk, sunlight, fish, eggs, butter, fortified margarine	Aids in bone and tooth formation; helps maintain heart action and nervous system.	In children: rickets and other bone deformities. In adults: calcium loss from bones.	High intakes may cause diarrhea and weight loss.	Storage, processing, and cooking do not appear to affect this vitamin.	Sunlight starts vitamin D production in the skin.
E	30 IU/day	Fortified and multigrain cereals, nuts, wheat germ, vegetable oils, green leafy vegetables	Protects blood cells, body tissue, and essential fatty acids from harmful destruction in the body.	Muscular wasting, nerve damage, anemia, reproductive failure	Relatively nontoxic.	Store in air-tight containers away from light.	Most fortified cereals have 40% of the FDA requirements.
K	—‡	Green leafy vegetables, fruit, dairy, and grain products	Essential for blood clotting functions.	Bleeding disorders in newborns and those on blood-thinning medications	Not toxic as found in food.	Store in containers away from light.	Vitamin K is also formed by bacteria in the colon.

*For adults and children older than 4.
†Many of the symptoms outlined under this heading can also be attributed to problems other than vitamin deficiency. If you have these symptoms and they persist, consult your physician.
‡There is no U.S. RDA for vitamin K; however, the Recommended Dietary Allowance is 1 μg/kg of body weight.
Information for this chart was obtained from the Food and Drug Administration, the American Institute for Cancer Research, and the United States Department of Agriculture/Human Nutrition Information Service. Vitamins A, D, E, and K are fat soluble; the other vitamins in this table are water-soluble.
From Young AP, Proctor DB: Kinn's the medical assistant, ec 10, St Louis, 2007, Saunders.

TABLE 18-2   Minerals

Functions	Sources	Deficiency Symptoms	Toxicity Symptoms
MINERAL AND ELEMENTAL SYMBOL: CALCIUM (Ca^{2+})			
Helps muscles to contract and relax, thereby helping to regulate heartbeat Plays a role in the normal functioning of the nervous system Aids in blood coagulation and the functioning of some enzymes Helps build strong bones and teeth	Primarily found in milk and milk products; also found in dark green, leafy vegetables, tofu and other soy products, sardines, salmon with bones, and hard water	Poor bone growth and tooth development, leading to stunted growth and increased risk of dental caries, rickets (bowing of legs) in children, osteomalacia (soft bones) and osteoporosis (brittle bones) in adults, poor blood clotting, and possible hypertension	Kidney stones
MINERAL AND ELEMENTAL SYMBOL: CHLORIDE (Cl^-)			
Involved in the maintenance of fluid and acid-base balance Provides an acid medium, in the form of hydrochloric acid, for activation of gastric enzymes	Major source is table salt (sodium chloride); also found in fish and vegetables	Disturbances in acid-base balance, with possible growth retardation, psychomotor defects, memory loss	Disturbances in acid-base balance
MINERAL AND ELEMENTAL SYMBOL: MAGNESIUM (Mg^{2+})			
Helps build strong bones and teeth Activates many enzymes Participates in protein synthesis and lipid metabolism Helps regulate heartbeat	Raw, dark green vegetables, nuts and soybeans, whole grains and wheat bran, bananas and apricots, seafood and coffee, tea, cocoa, and hard water	Rare but in disease states may lead to central nervous system problems (confusion, apathy, hallucinations, poor memory) and neuromuscular problems (muscle weakness, cramps, tremor, cardiac arrhythmia)	Drowsiness, weakness, and lethargy and in severe toxicity skeletal paralysis, central nervous system depression, respiratory depression, and ultimately coma and death
MINERAL AND ELEMENTAL SYMBOL: PHOSPHORUS (PO_4^-)			
Helps build strong bones and teeth Present in the nuclei of all cells Helps in the oxidation of fats and carbohydrates (energy metabolism) Aids in maintaining the body's acid-base balance	Milk and milk products, eggs, meats, legumes, whole grains, soft drinks (used to make the "fizz")	Rare but with malabsorption can cause anorexia, weakness, stiff joints, and fragile bones	Hypocalcemic tetany (muscle spasms)
MINERAL AND ELEMENTAL SYMBOL: POTASSIUM (K^+)			
Plays a key role in fluid and acid-base balance Transmits nerve impulses, helps control muscle contractions, and promotes regular heartbeat Needed foe enzyme reactions	Apricots, bananas, oranges, grapefruit, raisins, green beans, broccoli, carrots, greens, potatoes, meats, milk and milk products, peanut butter and legumes, molasses, coffee, tea, cocoa	May cause impaired growth, hypertension, bone fragility, central nervous system changes, renal hypertrophy, diminished heart rate, and death	Hyperkalemia (excess potassium in the blood) with cardiac function disturbances
MINERAL AND ELEMENTAL SYMBOL: SODIUM (Na^+)			
Plays a key role in the maintenance of acid-base balance Transmits nerve impulses and helps control muscle contractions Regulates cell membrane permeability	Salt (sodium chloride) is the major dietary source; minor sources occur naturally in foods such as milk and milk products and several vegetables	Hyponatremia (too little sodium in the blood)	May cause hypertension, which can lead to cardiovascular diseases and renal (kidney) disease, in the form of salt tablets, can cause gastric irritation

Continued

TABLE 18-2	Minerals—cont'd		
Functions	**Sources**	**Deficiency Symptoms**	**Toxicity Symptoms**
MINERAL AND ELEMENTAL SYMBOL: CHROMIUM (Cr^{3+})			
Activates several enzymes Enhances the removal of glucose from the blood	Liver and other meats, whole grains, cheese, legumes, and brewer's yeast	Weight loss, abnormalities of the central nervous system, and possible aggravation of diabetes mellitus	Inhibited insulin activity
MINERAL AND ELEMENTAL SYMBOL: COPPER (Cu^{2+})			
Aids in the production and survival of red blood cells Parts of many enzymes involved in respiration Plays a role in normal lipid metabolism	Shellfish – especially oysters – Liver, nuts and seeds, raisins, whole grains, and chocolate	Anemia, central nervous system problems, abnormal electrocardiograms, bone fragility, impaired immune response; may be a factor in failure to thrive in premature infants	In Wilson's disease and Huntington's chorea (both hereditary diseases), copper accumulation causes neuron and liver cell damage
MINERAL AND ELEMENTAL SYMBOL: FLUORINE (F^-)			
Helps the formation of solid bones and teeth, thereby reducing incidence of dental caries, and may help prevent osteoporosis	Fluoridated water (and foods cooked in fluoridated water), fish, tea, gelatin	Increased susceptibility to dental caries	Fluorosis and mottling of teeth
MINERAL AND ELEMENTAL SYMBOL: IODINE (I^-)			
Helps regulate energy metabolism through being part of thyroid hormones Essential for normal cell functioning, helps to keep skin, hair, and nails healthy	Primarily from iodized salt, also found in saltwater fish, seaweed products, vegetables grown in iodine-rich soils	Goiter, cretinism in infants born to iodine-deficient mothers, with accompanying mental retardation; diffuse central nervous system abnormalities	Little toxic effect in individuals with normal thyroid gland functioning
MINERAL AND ELEMENTAL SYMBOL: IRON (Fe^{3+})			
Essential to the formation of hemoglobin, which is important for tissue respiration and ultimately growth and development Part of several enzymes and proteins in the body	Heme sources: organ meats—especially liver, red meats, and other meats Nonheme sources: iron-fortified cereals, dark green leafy vegetables, legumes, whole grains, blackstrap molasses, dried fruit, and foods cooked in iron pans	Iron-deficiency anemia and possible alterations that impair behavior	Idiopathic hemochromatosis, which can lead to cirrhosis, diabetes mellitus, skin pigmentation, arthralgias (joint pain), and cardiomyopathy
MINERAL AND ELEMENTAL SYMBOL: MANGANESE (Mn^{2+})			
Needed for normal bone structure, reproduction, normal functioning of cells and the central nervous system A component of some enzymes	Protein-rich foods (meat, eggs; milk), whole grains, seafood, liver and other meats, and garlic	Keshan disease (a human cardiomyopathy) and Kashin-Bek disease (an endemic human osteoarthropathy)	Physical defects of the fingernails and toenails and hair loss
MINERAL AND ELEMENTAL SYMBOL: ZINC (Zn^{2+})			
Plays a role in protein synthesis Essential for normal growth and sexual development, wound healing, immune function, cell division and differentiation, and small acuity	Whole grains, wheat germ, crabmeat, oyster, liver and other meats, brewer's yeast	Depressed immune function, poor growth, dwarfism, impaired skeletal growth and delayed sexual maturation, acrodermatitis	Severe anemia, nausea, vomiting, abdominal cramps, diarrhea, fever, hypocupremia (low blood serum copper), malaise, fatigue

From Young AP, Proctor DB: *Kinn's the medical assistant*, ed 10, St Louis, 2007, Saunders; charts based on Poleman CM, Peckenpaugh NJ: *Nutrition essentials and diet therapy*, ed 6, Philadelphia, WB Saunders, 1991, pp 128-129; Garrison RH, Somer E: *The nutrition desk reference*, New Canaan, CT, 1985, Keats Publishing; and Griffeth HW: *Complete guide to vitamins, minerals and supplements*, Tucson, AZ, 1988, Fisher Books.

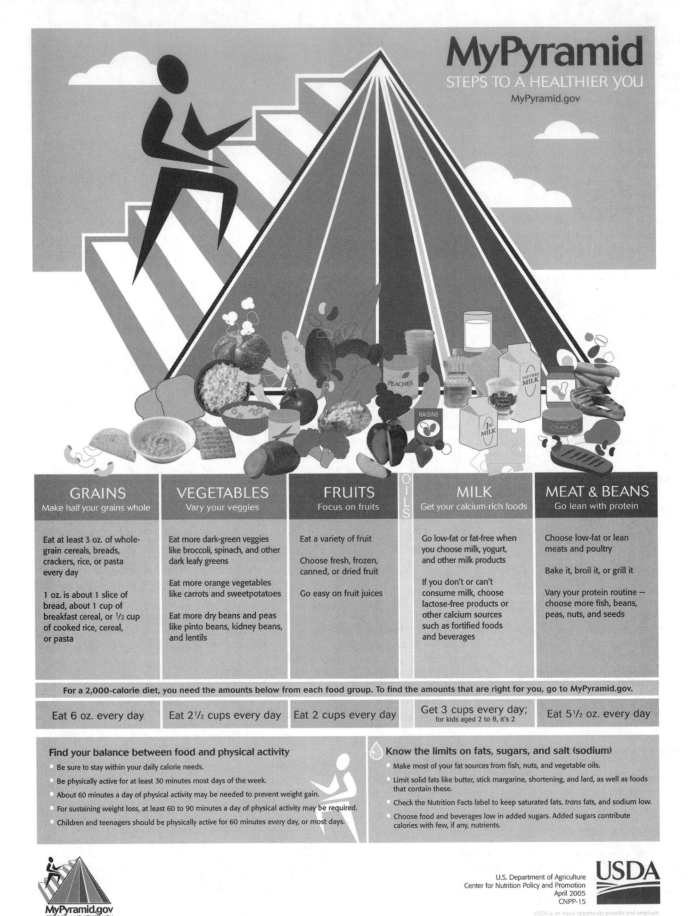

FIGURE 18-1 USDA Food Guide Pyramid. (From Klieger DM: *Essentials of medical assisting*, ed 2, 2010, St Louis, Saunders.)

3. Mechanically irritating agents:
   a. High-fiber foods
4. Eliminate fried foods and highly concentrated sweets
5. Indicated for GI problems

F. Elimination Diet
1. Eliminates certain foods in order to treat allergies
2. Types
   a. Simple elimination diet: removes only one or two foods
   b. Rowe elimination diet: more extensive diet; begins with few hypoallergenic foods (rice cereal, apples, pears, carrots, sweet potatoes, lamb, milk substitutes); if no allergic reaction, single food groups are introduced about every 10 days

G. High- or Low-Fiber Diet
1. Fiber in the diet is either increased or decreased depending on the specific disorder
2. Low-fiber diets indicated for GI disorders such as diverticulitis
3. High-fiber diets indicated for hypercholesterolemia, diabetes mellitus, prevention of certain cancers

H. Diabetic Diet
1. Basic goal is to control blood-glucose levels
2. Based on an exchange list; objective is to achieve balance of carbohydrates, proteins, fats
3. Diet plan is individual; must take into consideration weight control, patient preferences, exercise patterns, lifestyle
4. Glycemic index places carbohydrate foods on a scale from slowest to fastest effects on blood glucose levels

I. Heart-Healthy Diet
1. Goals of diet are to eat foods that reduce cholesterol, decrease LDLs, increase HDLs, keep blood pressure within normal limits
2. Includes exercise

V. FOOD LABELS

A. General
1. FDA requires all food products to carry a nutritional fact label
   a. Found on back or side of package
   b. Source of nutrition information and nutrients within the package
   c. Mandatory components and order in which they must appear:
      1) Serving size
      2) Calories per serving
      3) Calories from fat per serving
      4) Grams of total fat
      5) Milligrams of cholesterol
      6) Milligrams of sodium
      7) Milligrams of potassium
      8) Grams of total carbohydrates
      9) Grams of dietary fiber
      10) Grams of sugars
      11) Grams of protein
      12) Percent of daily values of vitamins A and C
      13) Percent of daily values of calcium and iron

B. Use of Label Information
1. Tells amount of nutrients in each serving size
2. Tells about the foods eaten
3. Ingredients listed in descending order of weight (proportion of ingredients)

VI. EATING DISORDERS

A. Definition
1. Any eating behavior pattern that can lead to a health problem
2. Can damage all body systems and lead to death

B. Anorexia Nervosa
1. Characterized by self-induced starvation
2. Patient is typically adolescent who is sensitive to failure and criticism and a perfectionist
3. Patient uses avoidance of food as a way of controlling feelings
4. Patient loses 15% to 60% of normal body weight resulting in malnutrition
5. Patient has distorted body image
6. Patient requires psychotherapy to alleviate depression, deal with emotional issues, form positive self-image

C. Bulimia
1. Characterized by cycles of bingeing and purging
2. Patient believes self-worth is related to being thin
3. Intake during binge period can be as high as 20,000 calories
4. Purge period can include vomiting, use of laxatives and enemas, excessive exercise, food abstinence
5. Treatment is combination of medication, psychotherapy, nutritional counseling to establish healthy eating patterns and improve self-image

D. Obesity
1. Affects more than 60% of population
2. Obese patients are at risk for hypertension, type 2 diabetes, coronary artery disease, stroke, gallbladder diseases, osteoarthritis, sleep apnea, certain types of cancer
3. Assessment includes body mass index
4. Treatment can be surgical (bariatric surgery) or by medication (appetite suppressants, lipase inhibitors)

Therapeutic Modalities and Physical Agents to Promote Tissue Healing

I. THERAPEUTIC MODALITIES

A. General
1. Use of heat, cold, massage, water, exercise, or electricity to restore normal function to injured tissues
2. Physical therapy program may be prescribed by the provider and implemented by a physical therapist

B. Objectives
1. Relieve pain
2. Increase or improve circulation
3. Increase or restore muscle function
4. Improve strength, range of motion, and joint mobility

II. HEAT APPLICATION (THERMOTHERAPY)

A. General
1. Relieves pain, inflammation, and congestion
2. Promotes muscle relaxation
3. Local effects
   a. Dilation of blood vessels, resulting in increased blood supply and tissue metabolism
   b. Increases nutrients and oxygen to area and eliminates waste products

B. Heat Therapy
1. Infrared therapy
   a. Administered by a heat lamp
   b. Lamp is placed 2 to 4 feet from the affected area for 15 to 20 minutes
2. Diathermy
   a. Electrical field that produces deep heat penetration
   b. Commonly used for muscular injuries and inflammation in joints
   c. Types
      1) Microwave: electromagnetic radiation
      2) Shortwave: high-frequency current
      3) Ultrasound: high-frequency sound waves
3. Ultrasound
   a. High-frequency sound waves used as deep-heating agent
   b. Used for strains, sprains, arthritis, edema, and dislocation
   c. Coupling agent (oil or gel) is used to increase conductivity
   d. Ordered by intensity of sound waves per unit of time
4. Paraffin wax
   a. Wax is melted and heated to approximately 125 °F
   b. Affected part is immersed in the melted wax and lifted out
   c. Wax hardens and holds in the heat
   d. Relieves arthritis, increases circulation, and reduces stiffness
5. Hot water bag
   a. Rubber bag filled approximately one-half full with hot water (115 °F to 125 °F)
   b. Bag is applied to the affected body part for the prescribed period
   c. Place some sort of covering (towel, blanket) over the body part before positioning the hot water bag
6. Hot soaks
   a. Basin is filled with a warmed solution (105 °F to 110 °F)
   b. Body part is immersed in the basin for the prescribed period
   c. As the solution cools, replace it with more warmed solution
7. Hot compress
   a. Immerse cloth or gauze squares in warm solution (105 °F to 110 °F)
   b. Wring out excess fluid, and place the material over the affected body part
   c. Replace the hot compress every 2 to 3 minutes for the prescribed time

III. COLD APPLICATION (CRYOTHERAPY)

A. General
1. Prevents edema by constricting vessels
2. Applied immediately after the trauma
3. Relieves pain by numbing
4. Local effects: vascular constriction, which leads to decreased blood supply to the area, decreased tissue metabolism, and decreased accumulation of wastes

B. Types of Cold Therapies
1. Ice bag
   a. Ice bag is filled one-half to two-thirds full of ice
   b. Applied to the affected area for the prescribed time
   c. Place some sort of covering (towel, blanket) over the body part before positioning ice bag
   d. Check for pallor, numbness, or cyanosis, and report any of these signs immediately
2. Cold compress
   a. Immerse cloth or gauze squares in a basin filled with cold water and ice
   b. Wring out excess fluid, and place the material over the affected body part
   c. Replace the cold compress every 2 to 3 minutes for the prescribed time

IV. HYDROTHERAPY

A. General
1. Use of external water applications for therapeutic purposes
2. Used for:
   a. Relaxation
   b. Increased circulation
   c. Improved mobility

B. Types of Hydrotherapies
1. Whirlpool: moist heat with massage action
2. Contrast baths: patient moves affected part from hot, to cold, to hot baths
3. Underwater exercise: buoyant effect of water facilitates exercise

V. ULTRAVIOLET THERAPY

A. General
1. Produced by the sun and sunlamps
2. Capable of killing bacteria
3. Activates the formation of vitamin D in skin
4. Used to treat acne, psoriasis, wound applications, and pressure sores
5. Cover eyes when using ultraviolet (UV) therapy

B. Types of Ultraviolet Therapy
1. Exposure to natural sunlight
2. Exposure to UVB rays for prescribed amounts of time in a light box

VI. EXERCISE THERAPY

A. General
1. Use of body motion to help the patient regain function
2. Dose must be constantly adjusted for the patient to benefit
3. Types
   a. Active: patient performs the exercise
   b. Passive: exercises are performed on the patient by someone else
   c. Aided: active exercise helped by a physical aid (such as a pool)
   d. Active resistance: counterpressure is applied
   e. Range of motion: active or passive joint mobility

VII. MASSAGE

A. General
1. Manipulation of external body tissues to promote healing
2. Patient must be relaxed to receive benefit
3. Lubricating oil or cream should be used
4. Approaches
   a. Stroking: systematic movement of the hand across the patient's skin
   b. Compression: squeezing, kneading, or pressing the patient's soft tissues
   c. Percussion: thumping or striking the patient's skin with the hand
   d. Effleurage: stroking movement
   e. Friction: deep stroking or rubbing that involves the deeper tissues
   f. Pétrissage: kneading or rolling type of motion
   g. Tapotement: rapidly repeated light percussion or tapping

VIII. DEVICES TO ASSIST PATIENT MOBILITY

A. Crutches
1. Wood or aluminum devices that serve as aids for walking
2. Patient's weight is transferred from the legs to the arms
3. Types
   a. Axillary crutches
      1) Crutch that extends from the patient's axillary region to the ground
      2) Used for temporary assistance
      3) Measured to fit for each individual patient
   b. Lofstrand crutches
      1) Cuff and handgrip that extend from the patient's forearm to the ground
      2) Used by patients who require permanent walking assistance

4. Crutch gaits
   a. Four-point gait
      1) Patient must be able to bear own weight on both legs
      2) Used for muscle weakness
      3) Right crutch moves forward, left foot moves to the level of the left crutch; left crutch moves forward, and right foot moves to the level of the right crutch
   b. Three-point gait
      1) Used when the patient cannot bear his or her own weight on one leg
      2) Move both crutches and weak leg forward, then move the strong leg forward while balancing on both crutches
   c. Two-point gait
      1) Similar to four-point gait
      2) Move the right crutch and left foot forward simultaneously, then move the left crutch and right foot forward simultaneously
   d. Swing gait
      1) Used by patients with lower extremity paralysis
      2) Patient moves both crutches forward simultaneously then swings both legs through

B. **Canes**
   1. Wood or aluminum pole with a handle or handgrip
   2. Provides a balance point and/or support to the patient with leg weakness on one side
   3. Used on the side of the strong leg
   4. Measured so that the handle is level with the greater trochanter; the elbow should be flexed at 25 to 30 degrees
   5. Types
      a. Standard cane: the least amount of support; used by patients who require slight assistance
      b. Tripod cane: three legs and a bent shaft; provides greater stability because of wider support base
      c. Quad cane: four legs and a bent shaft; provides the same support as a tripod
   6. Gait
      a. Cane is held on the strong side; move the cane forward 12 inches, move the weak leg to the level of the cane, move the strong leg ahead of the weak leg and the cane
      b. Patient needs to stand erect and not lean on the cane to ensure good balance and support

C. **Walkers**
   1. Aluminum frame consisting of handgrips for both of the patient's hands and four squarely placed legs
   2. Provides optimum balance for patients with balance problems
   3. Gait: pick up the walker and move it forward 6 inches, move the right foot, then the left foot forward into the walker, then move the walker again

D. **Wheelchairs**
   1. Lock the wheels so the chair cannot move
   2. Fold back the foot rests
   3. Patient should back into the chair using the arm rests
   4. To leave the chair, lock the chair
   5. Patient should place unaffected foot or feet flat on floor and lift her or his body, supporting him or herself on the arm rests

E. **Casts**
   1. Stiff cylindrical synthetic or plaster casing
   2. Used to immobilize body part
      a. Broken bones
      b. Support and stabilize weak/dislocated joints
      c. Promote healing after surgical correction
      d. Aid non-surgical correction of deformities
   3. Plaster casts
      a. Bandage roll must be soaked in water; becomes pliable to mold to the body
   4. Synthetic casts
      a. Made of fiberglass, polyester, and cotton or plastic

F. **Splints and Braces**
   1. Used to assist in treatment of fractures
   2. Splint: rigid removable device used to support and immobilize; can be used for sprains and strains; molded to fit body part
   3. Brace: designed to support body part in its correct position for functioning while healing takes place

Radiography and Diagnostic Imaging 20

(Depending on the location, a medical assistant may or may not be legally permitted to perform x-ray procedures.)

I. INTRODUCTION TO RADIOGRAPHY

A. General
1. High-energy, invisible, electromagnetic waves
2. Have the ability to penetrate body structures
3. Discovered by Wilhelm Konrad Roentgen in 1895
4. X-ray images called *radiographs*
5. Some states may require a limited radiography license to take films

II. FUNCTIONS

A. Reveals the presence of fractures and/or abnormalities of bones

B. Reveals the size and shape of organs

C. Reveals the presence and position of foreign bodies

D. Destroys pathological cells

III. EQUIPMENT

A. Table
1. Supports the patient's body
2. Contains grids and Bucky mechanism for film placement

B. X-ray Tube
1. Glass vacuum tube that produces, focuses, and transmits the x-rays

C. Collimator
1. Apparatus below the tube that permits the radiographer to vary the size of the radiation field

D. Control Panel
1. Allows control of x-ray emissions
2. Regulates the machine
3. Should be located behind lead-lined wall so that the operator is protected from the rays
   a. Main switch: turns machine on and off
   b. Milliamperes (MA) setting: sets the amount of radiation that comes from the tube
   c. Time switch: number of seconds the patient is exposed to the x-rays
   d. Kilovolts peak (kVp) setting: penetrating power of the x-ray beam
   e. Bucky switch: turns on the Bucky mechanism
   f. Exposure switch: exposes the patient to the x-rays

E. Grid
1. Absorbs the scattered radiation
2. Prevents blurring of the film
3. Placed between the patient and the film to reduce secondary wave interference

F. Potter-Bucky Diaphragm (Bucky)
1. Framelike structure under the table
2. Holds the grid above the film
3. Used when thicker body parts are exposed to x-rays

G. Cassette
1. Device that holds the film

H. Intensifying Screen
1. Special plates located within the cassette
2. Reduces the amount of exposure required, which reduces the time the patient is exposed to radiation

I. X-ray Film
1. Coated with special material that is sensitive to x-rays
2. Creates a visible record for viewing and archives
3. Film that receives x-ray appears black and gray; film that does not receive x-ray appears white; the more dense the object, the lighter the image is on the film
4. Use only under safety light in a darkroom to avoid exposure
5. Common sizes are 5×7, 8×10, 10×12, 11×14, and 14×17

J. View Box
1. Lighted box for viewing the developed x-ray film

K. Caliper
1. Measures the thickness of body parts
2. Used to calculate the amount of x-ray exposure

IV. SAFETY

A. Hazards
1. Radiation has a cumulative effect on the body
2. Exposure damages body cells, especially gametes and the developing fetus
3. Eye exposure can cause cataracts
4. Exposure over a long period may cause cancer, sterility, or genetic defects
5. High exposure over a short period may cause radiation sickness (nausea, vomiting, diarrhea, and hair loss)

B. Precautions
1. Keep appropriate equipment in good condition
2. Prevent exposure to gonads by using lead shields or lead aprons on both patients and operators
3. Always ask women of childbearing age whether any chance exists that they are pregnant; if so, the physician must approve the x-ray procedure
4. Wear a dosimeter (x-ray badge containing reactive material that is sensitive to radiation); must be checked periodically to measure the technician's exposure level
5. Wear the lead shield or lead apron

V. PATIENT POSITIONING (See Figures 20-1 Through 20-4)

A. Body Positioning
1. The body part nearest the film gives the greatest detail
2. Anteroposterior (AP): x-ray beam enters the anterior of the body surface and exits the posterior of the body surface before it hits the film
3. Posteroanterior (PA): x-ray beam enters the posterior of the body surface and exits the anterior of the body surface before it hits the film

FIGURE 20-1 Anteroposterior view. (Long BW et al: *Radiography essentials for limited practice*, ed 3, St Louis, 2010, Saunders.)

FIGURE 20-2 Posteroanterior view. (Long BW et al: *Radiography essentials for limited practice*, ed 3, St Louis, 2010, Saunders.)

4. Lateral: x-ray beam passes from one side to the other side before hitting the film; this x-ray order may be right lateral (from the right to the left side) or left lateral (from the left to the right)
5. Oblique: x-ray beam passes through the body part at an angle

VI. DARKROOM

A. General
1. Location where film is handled and developed
2. Lit by a safety light
3. Developer may be manual or automatic
4. Film is handled by the edges only
5. After film is dried, put in storage envelope or file
6. Undeveloped film is kept in a lead-lined vault

VII. SPECIAL X-RAY STUDIES

A. Angiogram
1. Contrast medium is injected intravenously
2. Can determine cardiovascular disease

B. Arteriogram
1. Similar to angiogram but specifically studies the arteries

C. Barium Enema, Lower Gastrointestinal (GI) Series
1. Contrast medium is instilled by enema into the colon
2. Used to visualize the lower intestines

D. Barium Meal (Upper GI Series)
1. Orally administered contrast medium
2. Used to visualize the esophagus, stomach, and duodenum

E. Bronchogram
1. Contrast medium administered through trachea and into the bronchial tree
2. Detects cancer and other lung disorders

F. Cholecystogram
1. Tablet form of contrast medium is ingested the night before the procedure
2. Gallbladder is observed on film

Left lateral   Right lateral

FIGURE 20-3 Lateral view. (Long BW et al: *Radiography essentials for limited practice*, ed 3, St Louis, 2010, Saunders.)

A   B

C   D

FIGURE 20-4 Oblique projections. **A,** right anterior oblique (RAO). **B,** left anterior oblique (LAO). **C,** Left posterior oblique (LPO). **D,** Right posterior oblique (RPO). (Long BW et al: *Radiography essentials for limited practice*, ed 3, St Louis, 2010, Saunders.)

G. Hysterosalpingogram
1. Contrast medium is injected into the fallopian tubes
2. Detects patency of the tubes

H. Kidney, Ureter, Bladder (KUB)
1. Basic flat x-ray of the abdominal area
2. Shows size, shape, location, malformation of kidneys and bladder
3. Used to visualize calculi (stones)

I. Intravenous Pyelogram (IVP)
1. Contrast medium (dye) is injected intravenously
2. Pathway of contrast medium is observed as it is excreted through the kidneys
3. Films obtained at intervals until contrast medium is completely excreted
4. Used to visualize outline of ureters and bladder
5. Used to diagnose tumors, calculi, obstructions, congenital abnormalities

J. Mammogram
1. X-ray of the breast
2. Detects abnormalities, masses, and breast cancer

VIII. DIAGNOSTIC IMAGING MODALITIES

A. Computed Tomography (CT)
1. Radiographic technique that produces a picture that represents a detailed cross section of tissue structures
2. More sensitive than x-rays
3. Wide range of applications including scans of the brain, spine, abdomen, chest, neck, pelvis, sinuses
4. Also used with contrast media

B. Magnetic Resonance Imaging (MRI)
1. Combines radio waves and magnetic field to produce images of soft tissues
2. Noninvasive
3. Images can be managed in a computer database
4. Used for diagnosis of intracranial/spinal lesions, aneurysms, heart defects, soft tissue abnormalities

C. Fluoroscopy
1. X-ray examination that permits visualization of internal body structures; contrast medium is used
2. Motion of a body part can be observed

D. Sonography
1. Diagnostic ultrasound
2. Not a radiologic procedure
3. Permits visualization of internal structures by the use of high-frequency sound waves
4. Sound waves echo off the body part and are displayed on a screen
5. Useful for observation of obstetric and soft tissue (brain, eye, breast, reproductive organs)

E. DEXA Scan
1. Dual energy x-ray absorptiometry
2. Measures bone density

F. PET Scan
1. Positron emission tomography
2. Use of radionuclides to reconstruct brain sections
3. Can be used to assist diagnosis of Alzheimer's disease, stroke

21 Pharmacology, Medication Administration, and Intravenous Therapy

I. DEFINITION

A. Pharmacology
1. Science that deals with the study of drugs and their actions, uses, properties, and origins

II. DRUGS

A. General
1. Any substances that cause a change in body functions or structure

B. Uses
1. Therapeutic
   a. Treats diseases
   b. Relieves symptoms
   c. Replaces a necessary body substance
2. Prophylactic: prevents disease
3. Diagnostic: helps diagnose diseases and disorders

C. Sources
1. Plant
   a. Naturally occurring substance from plants
   b. Parts used include roots, leaves, and fruits
2. Animal
   a. Substances obtained from animals
   b. Includes glands, organs, and tissues
3. Mineral: naturally occurring substances obtained from the earth or soil
4. Synthetic
   a. Artificially prepared substances
   b. Prepared using chemicals and techniques in a laboratory

D. Names
1. Chemical name: drug's chemical formula that identifies its molecular structure
2. Generic name
   a. Official name of the drug
   b. Not capitalized
3. Trade name
   a. Brand name
   b. Name owned by the manufacturer and copyrighted (uses registered trademark [®])
   c. Always capitalized

E. Drug References
1. *Physicians' Desk Reference* (PDR)
   a. Common reference book
   b. Provides information on uses, precautions, indications, and doses for a variety of drugs
   c. Organized in color-coded sections
      1) Section 1 (white)
         a) Manufacturer's Index
         b) Lists manufacturers who have given product information for use in the book
      2) Section 2 (pink)
         a) Product Name Index
         b) Gives trade and generic names alphabetically
      3) Section 3 (blue)
         a) Product Category Index
         b) Drugs are listed according to their classification
      4) Section 4 (yellow)
         a) Generic and Chemical Name Index
         b) Lists drugs alphabetically according to the main ingredient
      5) Section 5 (noncolored pages)
         a) Product Identification
         b) Color photographs of the drugs on plain-color pages
      6) Section 6 (white)
         a) Product Information
         b) Detailed descriptions of the drugs
2. Product insert
   a. Folded sheet of paper within the drug container or box
   b. Contains information similar to the information on the drug contained in the PDR
3. United States Pharmacopoeia/National Formulary (USP/NF)
   a. Published every 5 years
   b. All drugs listed have met federal governmental standards
4. *Physicians' Desk Reference for Nonprescription Drugs and Dietary Supplements:* similar to PDR but for over-the-counter medications

F. Forms of Drugs

1. Syrup: drug is dissolved in water, mixed with sugar and flavoring
2. Solution: liquid preparation containing one or more solutes dissolved in a solvent
3. Suspension: drug that does not dissolve evenly in a liquid; must be shaken to mix before administration
4. Emulsion: mixture of water and oil; must be shaken to mix before administration
5. Tincture: drug is dissolved in alcohol
6. Elixir: drug is dissolved in a mixture of water, alcohol, and sugar
7. Lotion
   a. Topical preparation that is nongreasy
   b. Contains suspended particles of the drug mixed in an aqueous solution
8. Liniment
   a. Drug is mixed with soap, oil, or water
   b. Applied topically to produce a feeling of heat and warmth
9. Aerosol: drug is suspended in a liquid and administered in a spray or aerosol form
10. Capsule: powdered or liquid drug within a gelatin capsule
11. Gelcap: drug contained within gelatin-coated capsule
12. Spansule
    a. Granulated drug is enclosed within a capsule
    b. Designed to release the drug at various times after ingestion
13. Tablet
    a. Powdered medication is compressed into a disk shape
    b. May be scored for breaking into halves or quarters
    c. May be enteric-coated for dissolution in intestines instead of stomach
14. Caplet: capsule-shaped tablet
15. Geltab: gelatin-coated tablet
16. Suppository
    a. Drug is mixed with a base of fat or wax
    b. Shaped into a cone or cylinder
    c. Made to be inserted into the rectum, vagina, or urethra
    d. Suppository dissolves at body temperature
17. Ointment
    a. Semisolid preparation
    b. Drug is combined with oil or fat; topically applied
18. Lozenge (troche): medicine is mixed within a candylike base made to be dissolved within the mouth
19. Patch: transdermal administration of a medication
20. Time-release tablets, capsules, patches: medication dissolves or is administered over a period

G. Transactions

1. Prescribe: an order for a medication by a practitioner
2. Administer: to give a medication that has been prescribed
3. Dispense: to prepare and give out to a patient
4. All practitioners who prescribe, administer, or dispense controlled substances *must* register with the Drug Enforcement Administration (DEA)
   a. Practitioner receives a DEA registration number that is valid for 3 years
   b. All controlled substances *must* be stored separately from other medications within the office; *must* be kept locked
   c. Separate records *must* be kept of all controlled substances
   d. Controlled substance inventory *must* be counted and recorded daily
   e. Discarded liquid controlled substances must be poured down the sink drains
   f. Discarded solid controlled substances must be crushed and flushed down the toilet

H. Drug Regulations and Controls

1. Controlled Substances Act of 1970
   a. Federal legislation designed to control dispensing of drugs that have a high potential for abuse
   b. Five schedules, based on medical usefulness and potential for abuse:
      1) Schedule I
         a) Drugs with a high potential for abuse and no acceptable medical use
         b) Examples: heroin and LSD (D-lysergic acid diethylamide)
      2) Schedule II
         a) Drugs with some accepted medical use but high potential for abuse
         b) Examples: morphine and cocaine
      3) Schedule III
         a) Drugs with moderate abuse potential; require prescription with refills limited to five within 6 months
         b) Example: Tylenol with codeine
      4) Schedule IV
         a) Drugs with low abuse potential; prescription is limited to five refills within 6 months
         b) Example: Valium, Darvon, and Librium
      5) Schedule V
         a) Low abuse potential; may include drug mixtures with a limited amount of narcotics
         b) Examples: cough medicines with codeine, Lomotil

2. Federal Food, Drug, and Cosmetic Act: allows U.S. Food and Drug Administration (FDA) to protect the public by requiring rigid standards for drug development
3. DEA: responsible for controlling narcotics abuse and illegal sales of drugs

I. Pharmacokinetics

1. Study of how drugs are used within the body
2. Process includes:
   a. Absorption
      1) How a drug enters the body
      2) Depends on how the drug is administered
   b. Distribution: how a drug is transported from the site of administration to the site or sites of action
   c. Action: changes that the drug causes when it reaches the site or sites of action
   d. Biotransformation
      1) How the drug is inactivated
      2) Usually occurs within the liver
   e. Elimination: route by which the drug is eliminated from the body

III. PRESCRIPTIONS (See Figure 21-1)

A. General

1. An order written by the practitioner for the compounding, dispensing, and administration of a particular drug for a particular patient
2. A prescription is a legal document
3. Using common or accepted abbreviations is acceptable when writing a prescription; check with the agency for approved abbreviations

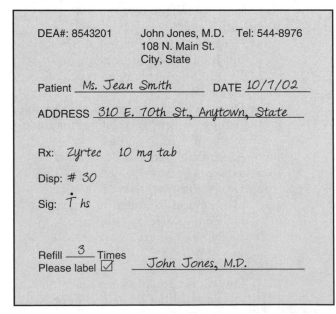

DEA#: 8543201   John Jones, M.D.   Tel: 544-8976
                  108 N. Main St.
                  City, State

Patient *Ms. Jean Smith*   DATE *10/1/02*

ADDRESS *310 E. 70th St., Anytown, State*

Rx: *Zyrtec   10 mg tab*

Disp: *# 30*

Sig: *ī hs*

Refill __*3*__ Times
Please label ☑   *John Jones, M.D.*

FIGURE 21-1 A sample prescription. (Young AP, Kennedy DB: *Kinn's the medical assistant: an applied learning approach,* ed 10, St Louis, 2007, Saunders.)

B. Parts of a Prescription

1. Preprinted physician's name, address, telephone number, and DEA number
2. Date the prescription was written
   a. Prescriptions must be filled within 12 months of writing or may be refilled for 12 months after initial filling
3. Patient's name, address, telephone number, and age (if a child)
4. Superscription: symbol R*x*
   a. Means "take thou" or "recipe"
5. Inscription: name, form, quantity, and strength of drug prescribed
   a. Active ingredient shown in milligrams in each dosage form
6. Subscription
   a. Practitioner's instructions to the pharmacist
   b. Includes the number of doses prescribed and special preparations
7. Signature
   a. *Sig* (label)
   b. Patient instructions for taking the drug
8. Refill information: number of refills allowed for the prescription, if any
   a. Enter "0" or "none" if there are no refills allowed; do not leave blank
9. Practitioner's handwritten signature

C. Prescription Pads

1. Keep locked up except when being used
2. *Never* presign blank prescription forms
3. *Never* use blank prescription forms for scratch paper
4. *Never* leave blank pads in examination rooms

IV. DRUG CLASSIFICATIONS

A. Anti-Infectives

1. Antibiotic: destroys or inhibits the growth of microorganisms
2. Antifungal: kills or prevents the growth of fungi and yeast
3. Antiviral: prevents or treats viral infections
4. Antiparasitic: prevents or treats parasitic infections
5. Antiretroviral: manages HIV infections

B. Dermatologic Agents

1. Antiacneic: treats acne vulgaris
2. Antiseptic: kills or inhibits the growth of microorganisms
3. Antipruritic: relieves itching
4. Anesthetic: causes loss of sensation and local numbing
5. Emollient: soothes skin and mucous membranes
6. Keratolytic: causes sloughing of hardened skin

C. **Musculoskeletal Agents**
 1. Antiarthritic: treats arthritis
 2. Antigout: treats gout (gouty arthritis)
 3. Antiinflammatory: decreases inflammation
 4. Antispasmodic: relieves or prevents spasms from musculoskeletal injury or inflammation
 5. Muscle relaxant: aids in the relaxation of skeletal muscles
 6. Osteoporosis agent: inhibits bone reabsorption or promotes use of calcium

D. **Cardiovascular Agents**
 1. Adrenergic blocking agent: controls hypertension
 2. Angiotensin-converting enzyme (ACE) inhibitor: decreases blood pressure
 3. Antianginal: reduces chest pain
 4. Antiarrhythmic: regulates the heart rhythm and rate
 5. Anticoagulant: prevents or delays blood clotting
 6. Antihyperlipidemic: decreases blood cholesterol levels
 7. Antihypertensive: decreases blood pressure
 8. Beta blocker: decreases blood pressure
 9. Calcium channel blocker: decreases blood pressure
 10. Cardiotonic: increases heart muscle strength
 11. Hematenic: increases blood iron levels
 12. Hemostatic: controls or stops bleeding
 13. Hematopoietic: promotes RBC production
 14. Vasoconstrictor: constricts blood vessels, raises blood pressure
 15. Vasodilator: dilates blood vessels, lowers blood pressure

E. **Endocrine Agents**
 1. Hypoglycemic: lowers blood glucose levels
 2. Thyroid: replaces thyroid hormones
 3. Hormone replacement therapy (HRT): replaces hormones or compensates for deficiencies

F. **Nervous System Agents**
 1. Anesthetic: produces insensibility to pain; can be local or general
 2. Central nervous system (CNS) stimulant: increases brain and body activity
 3. CNS depressant: decreases brain and body activity
 4. Analgesic: relieves pain
    a. Narcotic agents: highly addictive
    b. Nonnarcotic agents
 5. Antipyretic: reduces fever
 6. Anticonvulsant: controls seizure activity
 7. Antidepressant: relieves depression
 8. Tranquilizer: reduces anxiety; calms the patient
 9. Sedative: produces relaxation
 10. Hypnotic: induces sleep
 11. Antianxiety: reduces anxiety and tension
 12. Antiparkinsonian: treats Parkinson's disease

G. **Respiratory Agents**
 1. Antihistamine: relieves allergic symptoms; reduces secretions
 2. Antitubercular: treats tuberculosis
 3. Antitussive: suppresses cough
 4. Bronchodilator: opens air passages (bronchi)
 5. Decongestant: relieves congestion in respiratory tract
 6. Expectorant: liquefies mucus; helps expel secretions
 7. Mucolytic: breaks up thick mucus in the respiratory tract

H. **Gastrointestinal (GI) Agents**
 1. Antacid: neutralizes stomach acid
 2. Antiemetic: prevents nausea and vomiting
 3. Antidiarrheal: controls or stops diarrhea
 4. Cathartic, laxative: relieves constipation
 5. Emetic: induces vomiting
 6. Antispasmodic: prevents, controls spasms of the GI tract
 7. Antiulcer: treats gastric or duodenal ulcers
 8. Antiflatulant: relieves discomfort of gas

I. **Urinary Agents**
 1. Alpha-adrenergic inhibitor: relaxes smooth muscles in prostate
 2. Diuretic: promotes or increases urination

J. **Cancer Agents**
 1. Antineoplastic: inhibits growth of malignant cells

K. **Reproductive Agents**
 1. Abortifacient: terminates a pregnancy
 2. Anti-impotence: alleviates erectile dysfunction
 3. Contraceptive: inhibits conception
 4. Emergency contraceptive: prevents pregnancy after unprotected intercourse
 5. Ovulation stimulant: triggers ovulation
 6. Spermicide: kills sperm

V. 50 MOST PRESCRIBED DRUGS OF 2009

A. **Lipitor**
 1. Generic: atorvastatin calcium
 2. Classification: antilipemic
 3. Indication: high cholesterol

B. **Hydrocodone with APAP**
 1. *N*-acetyl-para-amino-phenol (acetaminophen)
 2. Generic: same
 3. Classification: analgesic
 4. Indication: pain

C. **Synthroid**
 1. Generic: levothyroxine sodium
 2. Classification: hormone replacement
 3. Indication: hypothyroidism

D. Amoxil
1. Generic: amoxicillin
2. Classification: antiinfective
3. Indication: upper respiratory infection, urinary tract infection

E. Zestril
1. Generic: lisinopril
2. Classification: antihypertensive
3. Indication: hypertension

F. Nexium
1. Generic: esomeprazole magnesium
2. Classification: proton pump inhibitor
3. Indication: heartburn, gastroesophageal reflux disease

G. Lexapro
1. Generic: escitalopram oxalate
2. Classification: selective serotonin reuptake inhibitor (SSRI)
3. Indication: depression

H. Singulair
1. Generic: montelukast sodium
2. Classification: antiasthmatic
3. Indication: asthma

I. Plavix
1. Generic: clopidogrel bisulfate
2. Classification: antiplatelet drug
3. Indication: myocardial infarction (MI), stroke, peripheral artery disease

J. Zocor
1. Generic: simvastatin
2. Classification: antilipemic
3. Indication: high cholesterol

K. Hydrochlorothiazide (HCTZ)
1. Generic: same
2. Classification: diuretic
3. Indication: edema, hypertension

L. Norvasc
1. Generic: amlodipine
2. Classification: antianginal
3. Indication: angina

M. Zithromax (Z-Pak)
1. Generic: azithromycin
2. Classification: anti-infective
3. Indication: infections

N. Coumadin
1. Generic: warfarin sodium
2. Classification: anticoagulant
3. Indication: embolism, MI

O. Lasix
1. Generic: furosemide
2. Classification: diuretic
3. Indication: edema, hypertension

P. Advair Diskus
1. Generic: fluticasone propionate/salmeterol
2. Classification: bronchodilator (inhalation powder)
3. Indication: asthma

Q. Toprol-XL
1. Generic: metoprolol
2. Classification: antihypertensive
3. Indication: hypertension

R. Diovan
1. Generic: valsartan
2. Classification: antihypertensive
3. Indication: hypertension

S. Effexor XR
1. Generic: venlafaxine hydrochloride
2. Classification: antidepressant
3. Indication: depression

T. Crestor
1. Generic: rosuvastatin
2. Classification: antilipemic
3. Indication: high cholesterol

U. OxyContin
1. Generic: oxycodone hydrochloride
2. Classification: analgesic (narcotic)
3. Indication: high cholesterol

V. Cephalexin
1. Generic: cephalexin monohydrate
2. Classification: antiinfective
3. Indication: infections

W. ProAir HFA (inhaler)
1. Generic: albuterol sulfate
2. Classification: bronchodilator
3. Indication: asthma

X. Glucophage
1. Generic: metformin
2. Classification: antidiabetic
3. Indication: type 2 diabetes

Y. Vytorin
1. Generic: ezetimibe simvastatin
2. Classification: antihyperlipidemic
3. Indication: high cholesterol

Z. Prevacid
1. Generic: lansoprazole
2. Classification: proton pump inhibitor
3. Indication: duodenal ulcers

AA. Seroquel
1. Generic: quetiapine fumarate
2. Classification: antipsychotic
3. Indication: bipolar disorder

BB. Cymbalta
1. Generic: duloxetine hydrochloride
2. Classification: antidepressant
3. Indication: depression

CC. **Zoloft**
1. Generic: sertraline
2. Classification: antidepressant
3. Indication: depression

DD. **Levaquin**
1. Generic: levofloxacin
2. Classification: antiinfective
3. Indication: staphylococcal infections

EE. **Flomax**
1. Generic: tamsulosin
2. Classification: selective alpha-andrenergic blocker
3. Indication: benign prostatic hypertrophy

FF. **Actos**
1. Generic: ploglitazone hydrochloride
2. Classification: antidiabetic
3. Indication: type 2 diabetes

GG. **Xanax**
1. Generic: alprazolam
2. Classification: antianxiety
3. Indication: anxiety

HH. **Zetia**
1. Generic: enzetimibe
2. Classification: antilipemic
3. Indications: high cholesterol

II. **Prozac**
1. Generic: fluoxetine
2. Classification: antidepressant
3. Indication: depression

JJ. **Tenormin**
1. Generic: atenolol
2. Classification: antihypertensive
3. Indication: hypertension

KK. **Celebrex**
1. Generic: celecoxib
2. Classification: NSAID
3. Indication: pain

LL. **Lantus**
1. Generic: insulin glargine
2. Classification: antidiabetic
3. Indication: type 1 diabetes

MM. **Ambien**
1. Generic: zolpidem tartrate
2. Classification: sedative-hypnotic
3. Indication: insomnia

NN. **Nasonex**
1. Generic: mometasone furoate monohydrate
2. Classification: corticosteroid
3. Indication: allergic rhinitis

OO. **Prednisone**
1. Generic: prednisone
2. Classification: antiinflammatory
3. Indication: severe inflammation, immunosuppression

PP. **Darvon**
1. Generic: propoxyphene
2. Classification: analgesic (narcotic)
3. Indication: pain

QQ. **Albuterol**
1. Generic: salbutamol
2. Classification: bronchodilator
3. Indication: asthma

RR. **Ibuprofen**
1. Generic: same
2. Classification: nonsteroidal antiinflammatory drug (NSAID)
3. Indication: inflammation, pain

SS. **Premarin**
1. Generic: conjugated estrogen
2. Classification: hormone replacement
3. Indication: menopause

TT. **Aricept**
1. Generic: donepezil
2. Classification: cholinesterase inhibitor
3. Indication: Alzheimer's disease

UU. **Yaz (Yasmin, Yaz-28)**
1. Generic: none
2. Classification: contraceptive
3. Indication: pregnancy prevention

VV. **Neurontin**
1. Generic: gabapentin
2. Classification: anticonvulsant
3. Indication: pain

WW. **Viagra**
1. Generic: sildenafil
2. Classification: erectile agent
3. Indication: erectile dysfunction

XX. **Allegra**
1. Generic: fexofenadine
2. Classification: antihistamine
3. Indication: allergy

VI. CALCULATION OF DOSES

A. **Metric System**
1. Basic units of measure
   a. Gram (g): used to measure solids
   b. Liter (L): used to measure liquids (volume)
   c. Meter (m): used to measure length

2. Metric conversion
   a. Length
      1) 1 meter = 100 centimeters = 1000 millimeters
      2) 10 millimeters = 1 centimeter
   b. Weight
      1) 1 gram = 1000 milligrams
      2) 1 milligram = 1000 micrograms
      3) 1 kilogram = 1000 grams
   c. Volume for solids
      1) 1000 cubic millimeters = 1 cubic centimeter
      2) 1000 cubic centimeters = 1 cubic decimeter
      3) 1000 cubic decimeters = 1 cubic meter
   d. Volume for fluids
      1) 1 liter = 1000 milliliters
      2) 1 milliliter = 1 cubic centimeter (1 mL = 1 cc)
      3) 10 centimeters = 1 deciliter
      4) 10 deciliters = 1 liter
   e. Weight conversion
      1) 1 kilogram = 2.2 pounds
      2) 1 pound = 16 ounces
      3) 1 ounce = 0.028 kilograms
   f. Temperature conversion
      1) °C = (°F − 32) × 5/9 or 0.5556
      2) °F = (°C) × 9/5 or 1.8 + 32

B. Equivalents

1. 1 cc = 1 mL = 15 drops (gtt)
2. 5 mL = 5 cc = 1 teaspoon (tsp)
3. 15 mL = 15 cc = 1 tablespoon (T or tbsp)
4. 30 mL = 30 cc = 1 ounce (oz)
5. 240 mL = 240 cc = 1 cup = 8 oz
6. 500 mL = 500 cc = 1 pint (pt) = 16 oz
7. 1000 mL = 1000 cc = 1 quart (qt) = 32 oz
8. 1 meter = 39.372 inches (in) = 3.281 feet (ft)
9. 0.914 meters = 3 feet = 1 yard
10. 0.3048 meters = 12 inches = 1 foot
11. 2.54 centimeters = 1 inch

C. Adult Dose Calculation

1. Dose given is dose ordered divided by the available strength times the dose form:

$$\frac{\text{dose ordered}}{\text{available}} \times \text{form} = \text{dose given}$$

   a. Dose given: amount administered to the patient to fill the practitioner's order
   b. Dose ordered: amount of drug the practitioner orders to be given to the patient
   c. Available strength: concentration of medicine on hand
   d. Dose form: number of tablets (or capsules) or amount of liquid that contains the available strength

2. Example:
   Provider orders 500 mg amoxicillin; 250-mg/cap amoxicillin is available

$$\frac{500 \text{ mg}}{250 \text{ mg}} \times 1 = \text{two 250-mg caps administered}$$

D. Pediatric Dose Calculation

1. Young's rule
   a. Used for children younger than 12, based on age
   b. Formula: child's age divided by (child's age + 12) and multiplied by the average adult dose gives the amount administered to the child
2. Fried's rule
   a. Used for infants and children younger than age 2, based on age in months
   b. Formula: infant's age in months divided by 150 and multiplied by the average adult dose gives the amount administered to the child
3. Clark's rule
   a. Used for children under 12, based on weight in pounds
   b. Formula: (child's weight in pounds divided by 150) multiplied by the average adult dose gives the amount administered to the child

VII. ADMINISTRATION OF MEDICATIONS

A. Routes of Administration

1. Buccal: medication is placed between cheek and gum and dissolves
2. Oral: medication is administered by mouth and swallowed
3. Sublingual: medication is placed under the tongue and dissolves
4. Inhalation: medication is delivered to lungs by means of a nebulizer (inhaler unit)
5. Topical: medication is externally applied to skin, eyes, ears, nose, or mucous membranes
6. Vaginal: medication is inserted into, or applied to, the vagina
7. Rectal: medication is inserted into the rectum and absorbed
8. Parenteral: medication is administered through a needle

B. Seven "Rights" of Administration Plus One

1. The right patient
2. The right drug
3. The right dose
4. The right route
5. The right time
6. The right technique
7. The right documentation
8. The right of the patient to refuse

C. Safety

1. Three *"befores"*: read the drug label three times when preparing the medication:
   a. Before removing the medication from storage
   b. Before preparing the medication for administration
   c. Before replacing the medication back in storage
2. Be familiar with the drug; use references
3. Prepare medication in a clean, quiet, well-lit area, away from distractions
4. Do *not* use a medication that does not appear normal (changes in color, odor, or appearance of sediment in the medication)
5. Check the expiration date; *never* administer a date-expired medication
6. Verify the patient's identity before administering (call by name; ask patient his or her name)
7. Always check for allergies
8. Correctly chart the procedure: include date, time, medication, dose, route, patient reactions, and medical assistant's initials

D. Considerations

1. Age: children and older adults require smaller doses than younger adults
2. Gender: women require smaller doses than men
3. Weight: smaller patients require smaller doses than larger persons
4. Tolerance: a patient who has taken this medication over a long period may require a larger dose for required results
5. Condition of the patient: physical and psychological conditions
6. Route: parenteral medications are absorbed more quickly than oral medications
7. Timing: medications are absorbed more quickly on an empty stomach

E. Allergic Reactions

1. Mild reaction: rash, pruritus, and rhinitis
2. Severe reaction: (anaphylaxis): pruritus, edema, dyspnea, cyanosis, and shock; untreated, a severe reaction can lead to coma or death
3. Prevention
   a. Monitor the patient after administration of the drug
   b. Observe the patient for signs and symptoms
   c. Notify the practitioner immediately of any reaction
   d. Be prepared to provide emergency assistance

VIII. PARENTERAL ADMINISTRATION

A. Equipment

1. Syringe (see Figure 21-2)
   a. Parts include:
      1) Barrel: holds medication; calibrated for measuring (cc/mL and minims)

FIGURE 21-2 Parts of a syringe. (Young AP, Kennedy DB: *Kinn's the medical assistant: an applied learning approach,* ed 10, St Louis, 2007, Saunders.)

      2) Flange: rim at the end of the barrel; place to put the fingers while depressing the plunger and keeps the syringe from rolling off a flat surface
      3) Plunger: fits inside the barrel; brings the medication into and out of the barrel
      4) Tip: end of the barrel where the needle attaches
   b. Types include (see Figure 21-3):
      1) Regular hypodermic
         a) Most commonly calibrated in 2 cc, 3 cc, 5 cc, or 10 cc
         b) May be disposable (plastic) or nondisposable (glass)
         c) May come with needle attached or without needle
      2) Tuberculin (TB)
         a) Small syringe calibrated in 0.1 cc
         b) Holds up to a total volume of 1 cc
      3) Insulin
         a) Calibrated in units (U40, U80, U100)
         b) Used for insulin injections
         c) Syringe must correspond to the type of insulin prescribed
      4) Tubex, Carpuject
         a) Closed injection system
         b) Disposable medication cartridge-needle unit fits into a reusable plastic or metal holder

FIGURE 21-3 Various types of syringes used to administer injections. (Young AP, Kennedy DB: *Kinn's the medical assistant: an applied learning approach*, ed 10, St Louis, 2007, Saunders.)

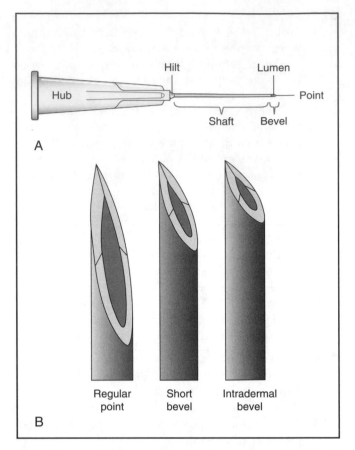

FIGURE 21-4   A, The construction of a hypodermic needle. **B,** Needle points. (**A,** Bonewit-West K: *Clinical procedures for medical assistants*, ed 7, St Louis, 2008, Saunders. **B,** Young AP, Kennedy DB: *Kinn's the medical assistant: an applied learning approach*, ed 10, St Louis, 2007, Saunders.)

2. Needle (see Figure 21-4)
   a. Parts include:
      1) Hub: the part of the needle that connects to the syringe
      2) Shaft: length of the needle; inserted into the body
      3) Point: sharpened end of the shaft
      4) Lumen: inside opening of the shaft
      5) Bevel: slant of the point
   b. Measured by:
      1) Gauge: size of the lumen
         a) The smaller the gauge, the larger the needle
         b) 13G to 27G
      2) Length
         a) Varies according to use
         b) ¼ inch to 6 inch

B. Administration
   1. Intradermal (ID) (See Figures 21-5 and 21-6)
      a. Needle and syringe size
         1) Syringes: TB (1 cc)
         2) Needle gauge: 26G to 27G
         3) Needle length: ⅜ inch to ½ inch
      b. Sites
         1) Anterior forearm
         2) Middle back
      c. Uses of route
         1) Allergy skin testing
         2) TB skin testing medication (Mantoux/ purified protein derivative [PPD])
      d. Injection angle: 10 to 15 degrees (with bevel facing up)
      e. Goal of injection: formation of a wheal
      f. Amount given: 0.01 to 0.2 cc

   2. Intramuscular (IM) (see Figures 21-7 and 21-8)
      a. Needle and syringe size
         1) Syringe: 3 to 5 cc (depending on the amount administered)
         2) Needle gauge: 22G to 25G (depending on the area of the body and the consistency of the medication)
         3) Needle length: ⅝ inch to 2 inches (depending on the size of the patient and the consistency of the medication)
      b. Sites
         1) Deltoid (not for infant or small child)
         2) Dorsogluteal (not for infant or small child)
         3) Vastus lateralis (used for infants and small children)
            a) Rectus femoris (medial to vastus lateralis; self-injection)
            b) Ventrogluteal (side of hip; all patients)
      c. Uses of route
         1) Adult and childhood immunizations (deltoid and vastus)
         2) Thick or oil-based medications (gluteal)

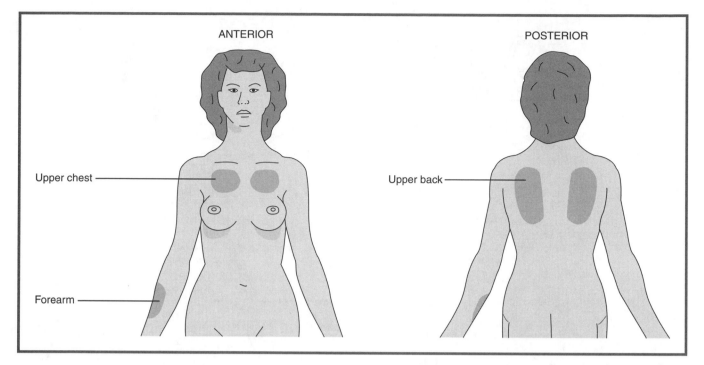

FIGURE 21-5 Sites recommended for intradermal injections. (Young AP, Kennedy DB: *Kinn's the medical assistant: an applied learning approach*, ed 10, St Louis, 2007, Saunders.)

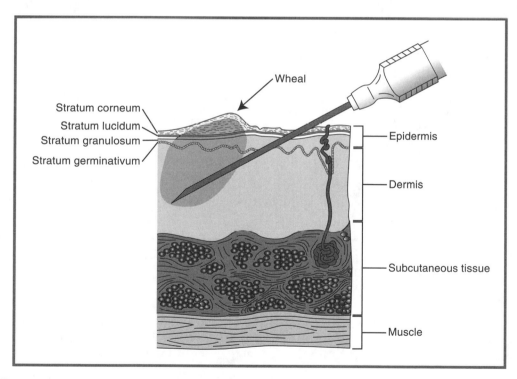

FIGURE 21-6 The intradermal injection is administered just under the epidermis. (Young AP, Kennedy DB: *Kinn's the medical assistant: an applied learning approach*, ed 10, St Louis, 2007, Saunders.)

d. Injection angle: 90 degrees
e. Goal of injection: to deliver medication into muscle tissue
f. Amount given
   1) Less than 2 cc (deltoid and vastus)
   2) 2 to 5 cc (gluteal)

3. Subcutaneous (SC, SQ, subq) (see Figures 21-9 and 21-10)
   a. Needle and syringe size
      1) Syringe: insulin, TB, or 2- to 3-cc syringe
      2) Needle gauge: 25G to 27G
      3) Needle length: 3/8 inch to 5/8 inch

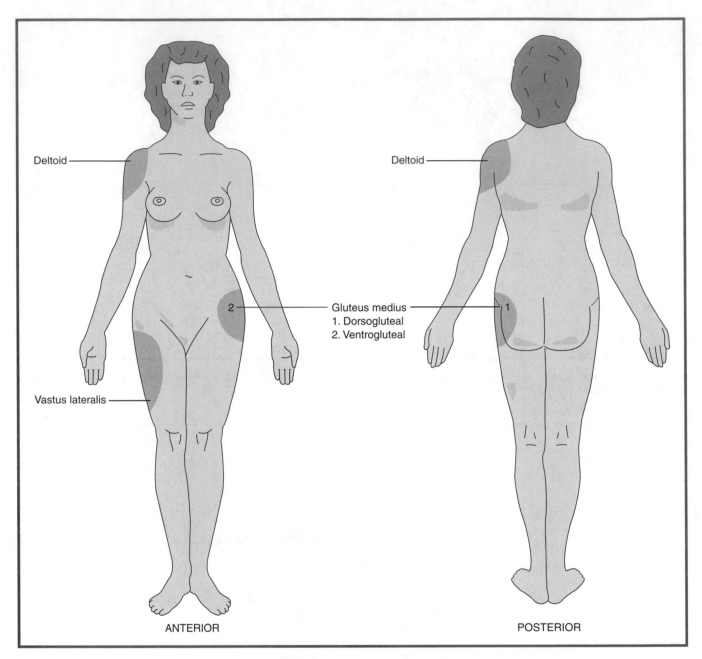

FIGURE 21-7 The muscles commonly used for intramuscular injection. (Young AP, Kennedy DB: *Kinn's the medical assistant: an applied learning approach*, ed 10, St Louis, 2007, Saunders.)

b. Sites
   1) Upper arm (under deltoid, back of arm)
   2) Thigh
   3) Back
   4) Abdomen
   5) Any area where a fat surface exists
c. Uses of route
   1) Insulin
   2) Allergy injections
   3) Mumps, measles, and rubella (MMR) immunization
   4) Epinephrine
d. Injection angle: 45 degrees

e. Goal of injection: delivery of medication into subcutaneous (fatty) tissue
f. Amount given: less than 2 cc

IX. INTRAVENOUS THERAPY

Depending on location, a medical assistant may or may not be permitted to legally administer intravenous (IV) therapy.

A. General
   1. Introduction of therapeutic fluids directly into the venous circulation

Epidermis

Dermis

Subcutaneous tissue

Muscle

FIGURE 21-8 In an intramuscular injection, the needle is inserted at a 90-degree angle, which deposits the medication into the large central part of the muscle. (Young AP, Kennedy DB: *Kinn's the medical assistant: an applied learning approach*, ed 10, St Louis, 2007, Saunders.)

2. Can be used for maintenance therapy, replacement therapy, or restoration therapy
3. Strict aseptic techniques must be used at all times
4. Danger to the patient can be great: the Medical Assistant must be able to follow provider's orders exactly

B. Advantages and Uses of IV Therapy
1. Advantages
   a. Entire amount of a medication is distributed in the bloodstream immediately after administration
   b. No tissue barriers to cross
   c. Route may be indicated for patients who cannot take oral or parenteral medications
   d. Medications are not altered by GI tract
   e. Medications may be given to patients who are unconscious, vomiting, or uncooperative
2. Uses
   a. Maintenance therapy
      1) Provides necessary requirements for water, electrolytes, and nutrition
      2) Amount given depends on patient's age, height, weight, and amount of body fat
      3) Used for patients who have little or no intake of fluids by mouth; require supplements

b. Replacement therapy
   1) Replaces fluid and electrolyte deficits
   2) Indicated for vomiting and diarrhea, starvation, and hemorrhage
   3) Most common in ambulatory care settings
   4) Patient must be carefully monitored
c. Restorative therapy
   1) Daily restoration of fluids and electrolytes
   2) Fluids are physiologically the same as fluids being lost
   3) Several types of fluids are often given
   4) Done more often in in-patient settings

C. Dangers of IV Therapy
1. Possible introduction of microorganisms into the bloodstream
   a. Aseptic technique must be followed
2. Infection at site
   a. Site care and bandaging using medical and surgical asepsis must be used
3. Hypertonic and hypotonic solutions may destroy RBCs
   a. Can cause an embolus
4. Fluid overload
   a. Physician's order for amounts and rate must be carefully followed
5. Introduction of medications into IV fluids cannot be reversed
   a. Medications immediately travel throughout body once administered

D. Types of IV Therapy
1. 0.9% sodium chloride
   a. Normal saline
   b. Isotonic
   c. Maintains body fluid levels
2. Glucose
   a. Dextrose 5% in water (D_5W)
   b. Saline (D_5NS)
   c. Supplies nutritional needs or part of daily caloric requirement
3. Multiple electrolyte solution
   a. Ringer's; lactated Ringer's
   b. Contains sodium, calcium, chloride, and potassium
   c. Usually does not supply calories
4. Hypotonic solution
   a. Causes the flow of water into the cell
   b. Hydrates cells leading to depletion in amount of fluid in circulation
   c. Lowers blood pressure
5. Hypertonic solution
   a. Causes the flow of water out of the cell
   b. Increases blood volume
   c. Used to replace electrolytes
   d. Must be given slowly
6. Isotonic solution
   a. Similar to body fluids
   b. Can cause circulatory overload

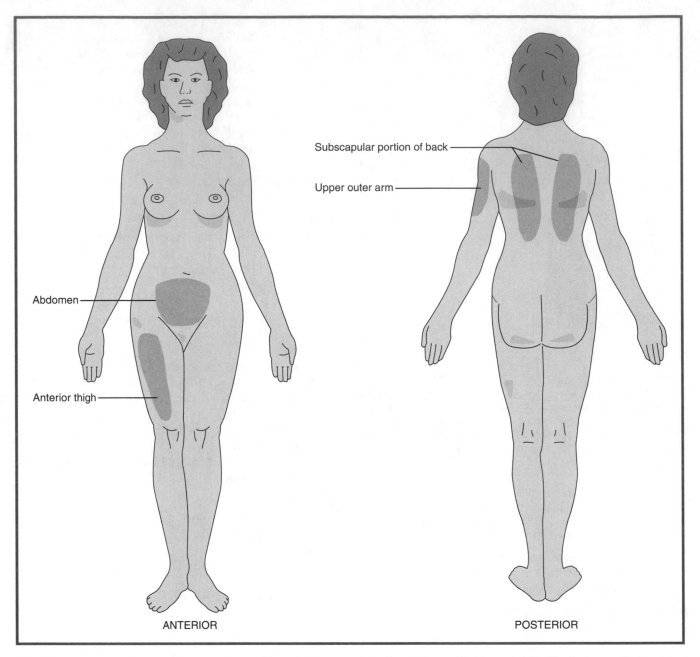

FIGURE 21-9   Areas of the body commonly used for subcutaneous injections. (Young AP, Kennedy DB: *Kinn's the medical assistant: an applied learning approach*, ed 10, St Louis, 2007, Saunders.)

7. Additions
   a. Drugs
   b. Supplements
   c. Fat emulsions
   d. Fluids

E. Equipment
1. Usually found in kits containing all necessary supplies
2. Administration sets
   a. Primary administration sets (see Figure 21-11)
      1) Puts medications directly into bloodstream
      2) Used for infusion in ambulatory care
      3) Gravity or infusion pumps
      4) Macrodrip (8 to 20 drops/mL) and microdrip (50 to 60 drops/mL)
   b. Secondary infusion sets: used to add intermittent medications through secondary tubing
   c. Blood administration sets: used to administer blood and blood products
3. Tubing
   a. Varies in length
   b. Has a sharp spike at the top for insertion into the fluid bag
   c. May have injection port that acts as an access point for the addition of other fluids or secondary infusion sets

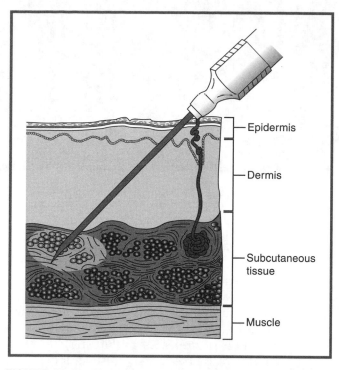

FIGURE 21-10 The subcutaneous needle is administered with a 25- or 26-gauge, ½- or ⅝-inch needle and is injected at a 45-degree angle (or at a 90-degree angle for insulin and heparin). (Young AP, Kennedy DB: *Kinn's the medical assistant: an applied learning approach*, ed 10, St Louis, 2007, Saunders.)

4. Vent
   a. Located under spike
   b. allows air to displace the fluid
5. Drip chamber
   a. Under vent
   b. Holds the fluids before infusion

c. Opening of drip chamber contains the drop orifice, which determines the size and shape of fluid drops

6. Flow control clamp
   a. Compresses the tubing to allow fluid to flow through tubing
   b. Can be a roller or screw
7. Fluid containers
   a. Usually made of plastic
   b. Bag collapses as fluid infuses
8. Needles (see Figure 21-12)
   a. Winged-tip (butterfly)
      1) Used for short-term therapy
      2) Gauge 17 to 25
      3) 0.5 to 1 inch
      4) Patient needs to remain inactive so the tip of the needle does not puncture the vein
   b. Over-the-needle catheters
      1) Plastic sheath covers the distal point of the needle
      2) Needle is used to enter the vein and guide the catheter
      3) After entering the vein, the catheter is threaded off the needle and left in place
      4) Catheter comes in lengths of 0.5 to 2 inches
      5) Gauge 22 to 24

FIGURE 21-11 Intravenous equipment, including tubing, drip chamber, spike, flow-control clamp, and Luer-Lok connector. (Klieger DM: *Saunders essentials of medical assisting*, ed 2, St Louis, 2009, Saunders.)

FIGURE 21-12 Equipment for starting short-term peripheral IV infusions: winged-infusion needle and over-the-needle catheter. (Leahy JM, Kizilay PE: *Foundations of nursing practice: a nursing process approach*, Philadelphia, 1998, Saunders.)

22 *Minor Surgery*

I. SURGICAL PROCEDURES PERFORMED WITHIN THE MEDICAL OFFICE

A. General
1. No general anesthesia
2. Provider explains nature of procedure, risks to patient; answers questions
3. Medical assistant responsible for patient preparation and obtaining signature on consent form

II. COMMON OFFICE SURGICAL PROCEDURES

A. **Sebaceous Cyst Removal**
B. **Incision and Drainage (I&D)**
C. **Needle Biopsy**
D. **Toenail Removal**
E. **Colposcopy**
F. **Cervical/Skin Punch Biopsy**
G. **Cryosurgery**
H. **Mole/Wart Removal**

III. SURGICAL INSTRUMENTS

A. General
1. Have clearly identifiable parts for visual identification
2. Classified according to use

B. Cutting and Dissecting Instruments
1. Scissors (see Figure 22-1)
   a. Used to cut tissue and sutures
   b. Blades touch at the tip; can be curved or straight
   c. Blade combinations include:
      1) Sharp/sharp (S/S)
      2) Blunt/blunt (B/B)
      3) Sharp/blunt (S/B)
   d. Bandage scissors
      1) Blunt probe tip for easy insertion under bandage
      2) Used to remove bandages and dressings
   e. Operating scissors
      1) Metzenbaum scissors: dissects tissues
      2) Mayo scissors: cuts and dissects fascia and muscle
      3) Iris scissors: general use
   f. Gauze shears: used to cut gauze, tubing, and adhesive
   g. Stitch (or suture) scissors (Littauer)
      1) One blade has a hook to slide under sutures
      2) Used to remove sutures
2. Scalpel (see Figure 22-1)
   a. Surgical knife used to make incision
   b. May be reusable or disposable
   c. Parts include:
      1) Handle
         a) Holds the blade
         b) Many sizes and shapes (#3 is standard)
      2) Scalpel blade
         a) Disposable
         b) Fits onto handle
         c) Different sizes and shapes (#15 is standard)

C. Grasping and Clamping Instruments (see Figure 22-1)
1. Used to retract, clamp, hold, or manipulate tissue, other instruments, or sterilized materials
   a. Hemostat forceps (hemostats)
      1) Jaws may or may not be serrated
2. Used to clamp small vessels or hold tissue
   a. Kelly hemostats
   b. Mosquito hemostats
3. Needle holders (needle pushers)
   a. Jaws shorter and look stronger than hemostats
   b. Used to grasp suture needles
4. Splinter forceps
   a. Fine tip for foreign body retrieval or removal
   b. Various designs and construction

5. Thumb forceps (dressing forceps)
   a. Serrated jaws with teeth
   b. Used to insert packing into a wound or to remove objects from cavities
6. Allis tissue forceps
   a. Blunt teeth
   b. Used to grasp tissue, muscle, or skin surrounding a wound
7. Adson thumb forceps (tissue forceps)
   a. Teeth for grasping tissue
   b. Used to grasp tissue and in suturing
8. Bayonet forceps
   a. Smooth-tipped
   b. Used to insert or remove objects from nose and ear
9. Towel clamps (forceps)
   a. Very sharp hooks
   b. Various lengths
   c. Used to hold drapes in place during surgery

10. Transfer forceps
    a. Many sizes and lengths
    b. Sterile forceps used to arrange objects on sterile field

D. **Retracting Instruments (see Figure 22-1)**
   1. Holds tissue away from surgical incision
   2. Rake retractor: has pronged end
   3. Senn retractor
      a. Pronged end may be sharp or dull
      b. Flat end is blunt retractor
   4. Skin hook: sharp point is used to retract small incisions or to secure skin edge for suturing
   5. Ribbon retractor (Crile malleable retractor): used to hold back tissues and organs in large wounds

E. **Probing and Dilating Instruments**
   1. Used for surgery and examinations
   2. Probes search a cavity or wound
   3. Dilators used to stretch a cavity or opening

Scalpels

Operating Scissors (Straight) Blunt-Blunt

Operating Scissors Sharp-Sharp

Operating Scissors Sharp-Blunt

Littauer Suture Scissors Straight

Lister Bandage Scissors

FIGURE 22-1 Instruments used in minor office surgery. (Courtesy Elmed, Addison, Ill.)

Continued

FIGURE 22-1—cont'd

Continued

a. Specula
  1) Most common dilator used
  2) Valves spread apart and dilate the opening
  3) Includes vaginal, nasal, rectal, and ear specula
b. Trocars and obturators
  1) Sharply pointed instrument (trocar) contained within an outer tube
  2) Used to withdraw fluids from cavities or for draining and irrigating with a catheter
c. Probes
  1) Different lengths (from 4 inches to 12 inches)
  2) Used to enter body cavities
d. Sound: long, slender probe

F. Specialty Instruments
  1. Fall into the four main categories (cutting/dissecting, grasping/clamping, retracting, probing/dilating)

  2. Specific for particular examinations in a specialty
    a. Gynecology
      1) Sponge forceps: used the way dressing forceps are used
      2) Uterine dressing forceps
        a) Can reach the cervix and vagina
        b) Used to swab the area or to apply medications
      3) Curettes (endocervical and uterine Sims)
        a) Hollow and spoon-shaped
        b) Used to remove polyps, secretions, and tissue
      4) Schroeder tenaculum forceps
        a) Sharp, pointed tips
        b) Used to hold tissue or cervix while obtaining specimen
      5) Hegar uterine dilators: used to dilate the cervix for dilation and curettage (D&C)

Halsted Mosquito
Hemostatic Forceps
Straight or Curved

Kelly Hemostatic
Forceps
Straight or Curved

Foerster
Sponge Forceps

Rochester-Pean
Hemostatic Forceps
Straight or Curved

Ochsner-Kocher Hemostatic
Forceps Straight or Curved
1 × 2 Teeth

Crile-Wood
Needle Holder

Sharp

Blunt

Volkmann Rake Retractor

Senn-Mueller Retractor

FIGURE 22-1—cont'd

b. Ophthalmology and otolaryngology
   1) Krause nasal snare
      a) Wire loop on tip
      b) Used to remove polyps
   2) Alligator ear forceps: used to remove foreign bodies
   3) Laryngeal mirror
      a) Various sizes
      b) Used to examine larynx and postnasal area
   4) Buck ear curette
      a) Sharp or blunt scraper end
      b) Used to remove foreign matter from ear canals
c. Biopsy
   1) Cervical biopsy forceps: used to obtain specimens
   2) Punch biopsy: used to remove tissue specimens
   3) Biopsy needle: works on the same principle as an obturator
   4) Abscess needle
      a) Used to withdraw fluids or pus from cyst or abscess
      b) Usually disposable
d. Genitourinary: Foley catheter
   1) Manufactured in sizes 8 to 32 (French)
   2) Used as an indwelling catheter
e. Endoscopes
   1) Hollow, cylindrical instruments
   2) Used to visualize the interior of a cavity or opening
      a) Sigmoidoscope: used to visualize the sigmoid colon
      b) Proctoscope: used to visualize the rectum
      c) Anoscope: used to visualize the superficial rectum
      d) Bronchoscope: used to visualize the larynx, trachea, and bronchi
      e) Otoscope: used to visualize the external and middle ear
      f) Cytoscope: used to visualize the urinary bladder
      g) Laparoscope: used to visualize the peritoneal and abdominal cavities

IV. SUTURES AND NEEDLES

A. General
   1. Suture: act of stitching or sewing together
   2. Material used to stitch or sew
   3. May also be used to ligate (tie off)

B. Types
   1. Absorbable
      a. Dissolves and is absorbed by body's enzymes
      b. Includes:
         1) Surgical catgut (surgical gut)
            a) Used in tissues that heal rapidly
            b) Obtained from sheep, cattle, or pig intestines
            c) Packaged in alcohol to keep it pliable
         2) Chromic
            a) Catgut coated with chromic salts
            b) Delayed absorption of up to 80 days
         3) Vicryl
            a) Synthetic suture made of polyglactin
            b) Takes up to 11 weeks to absorb
   2. Nonabsorbable
      a. Left in the body, where it embeds in scar tissue or must be removed when healing is complete
      b. Used frequently in office minor surgeries
      c. Types include:
         1) Silk
            a) Strong
            b) Easy to tie and remove
         2) Cotton: not used much (polyester more common)
         3) Polyester fiber: strongest of all suture material
         4) Stainless steel
            a) Surgical staples
            b) Used on skin, nerves, and blood vessels
            c) Applied with a skin stapler

C. Sizing
   1. Diameter of strand determines the size
   2. Sized from 6-0 (smallest) to 4 (largest)
   3. Lengths of strands are precut (into 18-, 24-, 54-, and 60-inch lengths)
   4. 2-0 to 6-0 most common

D. Suture Removal
   1. Physician determines the length of time sutures remain in place
   2. Must always be left in place long enough for proper healing to take place
   3. General
      a. Skin sutures in head and neck: remove in 3 to 5 days
      b. Skin sutures in other areas: 7 to 10 days

E. Needles
   1. Chosen according to area used
   2. Classified by:
      a. Shape
         1) Straight
         2) Curved (more easily manipulated)
      b. Type of point
         1) Tapered (for delicate tissue)
         2) Cutting (for skin)
      c. Eye
         1) Eyelet (have to thread the needle)
         2) Eyeless (suture material attached to the needle; atraumatic)

F. Adhesive Skin Closures
1. Sterile, nonallergenic tape
2. Available in a variety of widths and lengths
3. Used when not much tension exists on the skin edges
4. Applied transversely across the incision line
5. Eliminate the need for sutures and anesthetic
6. Easily applied and removed
7. Less scarring
8. Example: Steri-Strips

G. Surgical Skin Staples
1. Fastest method of closure for long incisions
2. Reduces trauma to tissue
3. Inserted using a skin-stapling device
4. Removed with a staple remover

H. Skin Glue
1. Special type of medical adhesive that joins the edges of a wound together
2. Can be used for children and adults
3. Usually used for simple cuts or wounds
4. Example: Dermabond

V. DRAPES

A. General
1. Sterile paper or cloth material placed over or around the operative site
2. Used to maintain sterility

B. Types
1. Plain
2. Fenestrated
   a. Contains a precut opening
   b. Opening is placed over the operative site
3. Incisional
   a. Adhesive-backed plastic
   b. Drape adheres directly to skin
   c. Incision is made through the drape

VI. ANESTHESIA

A. General Information
1. Injected into the surgical site to prevent the sensation of pain
2. Medications used for anesthesia end in the suffix -cain(e)
3. Example of anesthesia medication: Xylocaine, lidocaine, novocaine
4. May contain epinephrine
   a. Enhances the effect of the anesthesia
   b. Minimizes bleeding at the operative site
5. Takes effect in 5 to 15 minutes; effective for 1 to 3 hours

B. Types of Local Anesthesia
1. Infiltration: solution is injected under the skin to anesthetize nerve endings
2. Nerve block: solution is injected into an accessible main nerve
3. Topical: solution is painted (or sprayed) directly onto the skin or mucous membranes

VII. SURGICAL ASEPSIS (See Table 22-1)

A. General
1. Destruction of organisms before they enter the body
2. Used any time skin or mucous membranes is punctured, pierced, or incised

B. Basic Rules
1. Clean with clean
2. Dirty with dirty
3. Sterile with sterile
4. When in doubt, throw it out

TABLE 22-1   How to Distinguish Between Medical and Surgical Asepsis

	Medical Asepsis	Surgical Asepsis
Definition	Destruction of organisms *after* they leave the body	Destruction of organisms *before* they enter the body
Purpose	Prevent reinfection of the patient; avoid cross infection from one person to another	Care for open wounds; used in surgery
Technique	Universal blood and body-fluid precautions Isolation techniques	Sterile technique
Procedure	Clean objects are kept from contamination	Objects must be sterile
	Clean gloves and clean barriers used	Sterile gloves and articles used
	Objects disinfected as soon as possible after contact with the patient	Objects must be sterilized before contact with the patient
When used	For examinations that do not involve open wounds or breaks in the skin or mucous membranes but do involve patient blood or body fluids; isolating infected persons from others	Surgery, biopsy, wound treatment, insertion of instruments into sterile body cavities
Hand-washing technique	Hands and wrists washed for 1 to 2 minutes; soap, water, and plenty of friction used to remove oil and microorganisms from fingers	Hand and forearms scrubbed for 3 to 10 minutes; surgical soap, running water, friction, and sterile brush used; fingernails must be cleaned
	Hands held downward, running water allowed to drain off fingertips; hands dried with paper towels	Hands held up, under running water, to drain off elbows; hands dried with sterile towels

From Kinn ME, Woods MA: *The medical assistant: administrative and clinical*, ed 8, Philadelphia, 1999, Saunders.

C. Surgical Scrub
1. Hands and forearms scrubbed for 3 to 10 minutes
2. Use surgical soap with a brush
3. Clean under the fingernails
4. Hands held up; rinsed from fingertips to elbows
5. Dry with sterile towels
6. Glove immediately

D. Sterile Gloves
1. Used whenever the patient needs to be protected from microorganisms (all surgical procedures)
2. Used when handling sterile instruments or sterile supplies
3. Gloving procedure
   a. Select the proper glove size
   b. Open the package
   c. With the nondominant hand, lift the glove for the dominant hand by the folded edge of the cuff
   d. Put on the glove, keeping it above your waist
   e. Pick up the second glove by placing the gloved fingers under the cuff; insert the hand; adjust the cuffs and fingers
   f. Always keep gloved hands above your waist and away from your body

E. Sterile Field
1. Any surface on which sterile items are placed
2. Created by draping sterile towels over a Mayo stand
3. Sterile field is also a draped surgical site after the patient's skin is prepared and draped
4. Any item placed below the waist is considered contaminated
5. The 1-inch edge around the entire sterile field is considered nonsterile
6. Edges of all wrappers, packs, and towels are nonsterile
7. Sides of containers are nonsterile
8. Moisture carries bacteria from nonsterile to sterile surfaces

F. Handling Instruments and Supplies
1. Sterile forceps are used to handle sterile instruments or sterile supplies when sterile gloves are not being worn
   a. Lift forceps out of the container without touching the sides of the container
   b. Touch the tips of the forceps to sterile gauze to dry
   c. Always keep forceps tips facing down
2. Lids removed from containers are placed face up on surfaces; hold face down if not placed on surfaces
3. Pour solutions to avoid splashing; avoid touching the rim of a sterile receptacle with the bottle

4. Do not reach over the sterile field
5. Cover the setup with a sterile towel if it is not to be used immediately

G. Skin Preparation
1. Skin cannot be sterilized
2. Resident and transient bacteria must be completely removed
3. Skin preparation is performed by a gloved assistant
4. Make sure that the patient is not allergic to the surgical scrub solution used (examples: Betadine, iodine)
5. Area is cleansed in a circular motion from the inside of the circle out; repeat the cleansing with a new sponge; dry with sterile, dry sponges

VIII. WOUNDS

A. Definition
1. Interruption in continuity of internal or external body tissues

B. Types of Wounds
1. Closed wound
   a. Nonpenetrating
   b. No outward opening
   c. Underlying tissue is damaged
2. Open wound
   a. Skin is broken
   b. Underlying tissue is exposed
   c. Classified according to the appearance of the opening
      1) Laceration: jagged, irregular, breaking or tearing of tissues
      2) Puncture: skin is pierced by a pointed object (e.g., pin, nail, splinter)
      3) Abrasion: superficial wound; scraping of the skin
      4) Avulsion: tissue is torn away or separated
      5) Surgical incision: neat, clean cut
      6) Contusion: closed, nonpenetrating wound; blood from broken vessels accumulates in tissues

C. Wound Healing (see Figure 22-2)
1. All wounds go through healing (repair)
2. Three phases:
   a. Lag phase
      1) Blood vessels contract to control bleeding
      2) Platelets form a plug
      3) Fibrin is released to begin clotting (dried clot becomes the scab)
      4) White blood cells arrive at the site to clear away debris
      5) Within 1 to 4 days, fibrin threads contract and pull the edges of the wound together under the scab

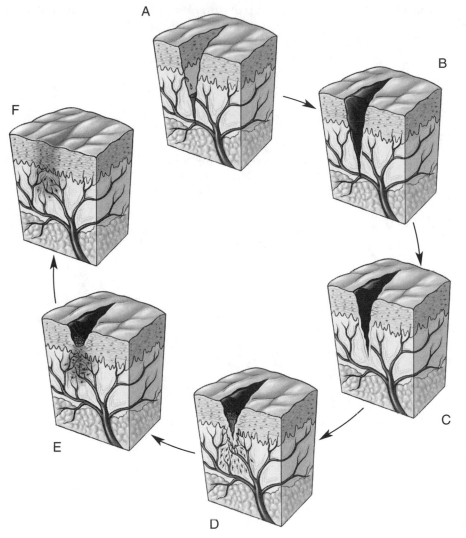

FIGURE 22-2 Steps in tissue repair. **A,** A deep wound to the skin severs blood vessels, causing blood to fill the wound. **B,** A blood clot forms, and as it dries, it forms a scab. **C** and **D,** The process of tissue repair begins. Scar tissue forms in the deep layers. **E,** At the same time, surface epithelial cells multiply and fill the area between the scar tissue and the scab. **F,** When the epithelium is complete, the scab detaches. The result is a fully regenerated layer of epithelium over an underlying area of scar tissue. (From Herlihy B: *The human body in health and illness*, ed 3, St Louis, 2007, Saunders.)

b. Proliferation phase
   1) Lasts from 5 to 20 days
   2) Tissues repair themselves
   3) Wound continues to contract and seal
c. Remodeling phase
   1) Day 21 on
   2) Scar tissue forms
   3) Scar tissue is not true skin; very strong and nonelastic
   4) Scar tissue is connective tissue without blood or nerve supply

D. Classification of Wound Repair
1. First intention
   a. Minimal tissue damage and scarring
   b. Wound may be sutured closed
2. Second intention
   a. Wound edges are not sutured or approximated
   b. Heals slowly from bottom up
   c. Large amount of scarring
3. Third intention: infected wound requires reopening

E. Wound Drainage (Exudate)
1. Serous
   a. Consists mainly of serum
   b. Clear and watery
2. Sanguineous
   a. Consists of red blood cells
   b. Bright red (fresh bleeding) or dark red (older bleeding)
3. Purulent
   a. Contains pus
   b. Thick; unpleasant odor; can be white, pink, green, or yellow
4. Serosanguineous
   a. Serum and blood mixed together
   b. Pink color; occurs postoperatively

IX. DRESSINGS AND BANDAGES

A. Dressings
1. Sterile covering placed over wound
2. Protect wound from injury and/or contamination

3. Maintain constant pressure on the wound
4. Help hold wound edges together
5. Control bleeding
6. Absorb drainage and secretions
7. Hide temporary disfigurement
8. May need to be removed periodically so that the wound can be checked for healing or suture removal
9. Always note amount and odor of any drainage in chart

B. Bandages
1. Nonsterile material used to hold dressings in place
   a. Splints and protects injured tissue
   b. Maintains pressure on the wound
   c. Aids in circulation
2. Made up of different materials and different sizes
   a. Gauze roller bandage
   b. Kling (self-adhering)
   c. Elastic cloth (Ace)
   d. Adhesive bandage (Band-Aid)
   e. Seamless tubular gauze (Tube-gauze)

X. PATIENT EDUCATION

A. General
1. Instruct the patient to contact the practitioner immediately to report:
   a. Excessive bleeding at the wound site
   b. Fever
   c. Redness, swelling, or streaking around the wound site

Clinical Lab 23

I. ORIENTATION TO THE LABORATORY

A. Laboratory Departments

1. Blood bank
   a. Analyzes blood and blood components for transfusions
   b. Examples: type and cross-match
2. Chemistry
   a. Analyzes blood and body fluids for presence and quantity of chemical substances
   b. Examples: glucose, cholesterol, and electrolytes
3. Cytology and histology
   a. Examines cells and tissues to diagnose diseases
   b. Examples: Papanicolaou (Pap) smear, biopsy
4. Hematology
   a. Performs tests on blood and blood components
   b. Examples: complete blood count (CBC), erythrocyte sedimentation rate (ESR, sed rate), and coagulation studies
5. Microbiology
   a. Identification and study of pathogenic microorganisms
   b. Includes bacteriology (bacteria), parasitology (parasites), and virology (viruses)
6. Serology
   a. Examination of blood to detect diseases through antigen-antibody reactions
   b. Examples: rubella titer and mononucleosis testing

B. Laboratory Personnel

1. Pathologist: physician in charge of the laboratory
2. Medical technologist: bachelor's degree–prepared laboratory technician
3. Medical laboratory technician: laboratory technician who has completed 1 to 2 years of training
4. Phlebotomist: obtains blood samples from patients

C. Occupational Safety and Health Administration (OSHA) Standards

1. Hazard communication standard
   a. Employer must provide information and training to employees who are exposed to hazardous agents (chemicals, noise, radiation, infectious agents)
   b. Standards must be in writing and include:
      1) Training outline
      2) List of hazards and material safety data sheet (MSDS) forms
      3) Warning and labeling system
      4) Method of informing employees
   c. MSDS
      1) Must be kept for each hazardous substance on site
      2) Prepared by the manufacturer
      3) Describes chemical and physical properties, hazards, precautions, and first aid
      4) Signs posted in laboratory
   d. All hazardous agents must be labeled showing:
      1) Name of hazardous substance
      2) Specific product warnings
      3) Name and address of manufacturer
2. Blood-borne pathogen standard
   a. Disease-causing microorganisms transmitted through blood and body fluids
   b. OSHA requires employers to ensure the safety of employees and provide training about exposure
   c. Blood-borne pathogens transmitted when contaminated blood or body fluids come into contact with nonintact skin or mucous membranes of another person
   d. Prevention includes:
      1) Engineering controls: structural and mechanical devices that minimize exposure (sharps containers, eyewash stations)

2) Work practice controls: promotion of behaviors necessary to use the engineering controls properly

3) Personal protective equipment (PPE): equipment that decreases exposure (gloves, masks, laboratory aprons)

4) Standard precautions: concept that all bodily secretions should be treated as if they are contaminated

5) Body secretions include:
   a) Blood and body fluids containing blood
   b) Semen
   c) Cerebrospinal fluid
   d) Saliva
   e) Sputum
   f) Vaginal secretions
   g) Feces
   h) Urine
   i) Sweat and tears
   j) Vomitus
   k) Unidentifiable body fluids

D. Laboratory Safety

1. Post evacuation routes
2. Post emergency telephone numbers (fire, police, poison control)
3. First-aid kit accessible and up to date
4. Safety equipment accessible and in working order, including:
   a. Eyewash station
   b. Shower
   c. Fire extinguisher
5. Laboratory coats or aprons worn at all times; remove before leaving the laboratory
6. Hair is pulled back; only minimal jewelry is allowed; fingernails are short
7. Dispose of sharps and broken glass immediately in a puncture-resistant container
8. Observe hazard identification labels
9. Work under the hood in a well-ventilated area when working with chemicals
10. Never pipette by mouth
11. Close all reagent containers when not in use
12. Label all reagent containers with name, expiration date, date of preparation, and preparer's initials
13. Pour acids into water when preparing solutions
14. Properly ground all electrical equipment
15. Wash hands after handling specimens and before leaving the laboratory
16. Do not eat, drink, smoke, apply makeup, or handle contact lenses in the laboratory
17. Do not store food in the laboratory refrigerator
18. Do not recap, break, or bend contaminated needles
19. Cap all tubes before centrifuging

20. Dispose of all contaminated nonsharps in labeled biohazard containers (red trash can or red trash bag)

E. Clinical Laboratory Improvement Act of 1988 (CLIA '88)

1. Federal legislation developed to regulate testing of specimens to diagnose, prevent, and treat diseases and disorders
2. Enforced by the Centers for Disease Control and Prevention (CDC) and Health Care Financing Administration (HCFA)
3. Laboratory must be in compliance with CLIA to receive Medicare and Medicaid reimbursement
4. Three main standards:
   a. Personnel standards
      1) Identify qualifications of persons directing or performing testing
      2) Qualifications depend on the complexity levels of the testing
   b. Testing standards: identify the tests that fall into one of three levels of complexity:
      1) Waived tests
         a) Not subject to personnel or quality assurance requirements
         b) Common in medical office (physician's office laboratory) [POL])
      2) Moderately complex tests
      3) Highly complex tests
   c. Quality assurance standards
      1) Identify quality assurance requirements for qualified laboratories
      2) Apply only to laboratories that perform moderately and highly complex testing
      3) Standards include:
         a) Written policies and standards
         b) Documented personnel training and proficiency testing
         c) Procedure manual
         d) Maintenance and documentation of the maintenance of instruments
         e) Quality control documentation

II. MICROSCOPE

A. General

1. Precision magnifying instrument used to view objects too small to be seen with the naked eye
2. Total magnification equals objective lens magnification times ocular lens magnification

B. Parts of the Microscope (see Figure 23-1)

1. Base: portion that supports the microscope
2. Arm: supports lenses and focus knobs
3. Stage: platform that holds the objects being observed; contains clips for holding the objects on the stage

FIGURE 23-1 Microscope. **A,** Base. **B,** Arm. **C,** Stage. **D,** Slide holder. **E,** Mechanical slide controls. **F,** Light source. **G,** Condenser. **H,** Condenser adjustment. **I,** Diaphragm lever. **J,** Low power objective. **K,** Nosepiece. **L,** Ocular lens. **M,** Coarse focus objective. **N,** Fine focus adjustment. (From Garrels M, Oatis CS: *Laboratory testing for ambulatory settings: a guide for health care professionals*, St. Louis, 2006, Saunders.)

4. Light source: light bulb in base that illuminates the objects; knob controls the intensity of the light
5. Condenser: lens over the light source that directs and focuses the light on the object
6. Iris diaphragm: shutter mechanism on the bottom of condenser; regulates the amount of light passing through the object
7. Ocular: one or two eyepieces; contains a lens that magnifies the image
8. Objectives: lenses mounted on a revolving nosepiece; microscope usually contains three lenses on the nosepiece
   a. Low power: usually 10×; used for initial focusing
   b. High-dry power: usually 40×; used for cellular specimens, wet preparations, and urine sediment
   c. Oil immersion: usually 100×; requires the use of immersion oil to prevent refraction; used to study cell detail and bacteria

9. Coarse adjustment: large focusing knob; moves the stage up or down for rough focus
10. Fine adjustment: small focusing knob; allows for precise focusing

C. Care
1. Transport with one hand under the base, the other on the arm
2. Wipe immersion oil off the objective immediately after use
3. Store with 10× objective over the stage; bring the stage to the lowest level and cover
4. Lenses should be cleaned only with lens paper to decrease the possibility of scratches

III. URINALYSIS

A. General
1. Physical, chemical, and microscopic examination of urine
2. Provides information about the conditions of the kidneys and urinary tract
3. Can help in the diagnosis of metabolic and systemic disorders

B. Collection of Specimens
1. Sterile liquid waste product easily obtainable
2. Volume needed is usually between 25 and 50 mL
3. Should be analyzed within 30 minutes of collection but may be refrigerated for up to 8 hours
4. Specimen types include:
   a. First-morning specimen
      1) Specimen of choice
      2) Most concentrated
   b. Random specimen: specimen collected at any time of the day
   c. Midstream specimen
      1) Used for routine urinalysis
      2) Patient is instructed to retract foreskin or labia, void the first portion of the urine stream into the toilet, collect the midportion of the stream into a sterile container, and void the remaining portion of the stream into the toilet
      3) Properly label the container
   d. Clean-catch specimen
      1) Used for culture
      2) Patient is instructed to thoroughly cleanse the glans penis or urethral meatus with an antiseptic solution, continue with the midstream specimen collection technique, and collect in a sterile container
   e. 24-hour specimen
      1) Used to measure volume
      2) Used for quantitative analysis (amount) of chemicals

3) Specimen requires a preservative and refrigeration (specimen container usually provided by laboratory)
4) Patient is instructed to void first morning urine into the toilet; collect all urine into the same container for the next 24 hours, including the first morning specimen of the next day; bring the entire specimen in the container to the laboratory

C. Physical Examination of Urine
1. Color
   a. Normal: yellow; color is due to urochrome pigment
   b. Pale (straw): dilute urine
   c. Dark yellow (amber): concentrated urine; may be seen in person with fever or dehydration
   d. Yellow-brown or green/brown: presence of bilirubin; will foam when shaken
   e. Bright orange: seen in patients taking Pyridium; will interfere with reagent strips
   f. Red: clear red may indicate hemoglobin; cloudy red indicates the presence of red blood cells (hematuria)
   g. Dark brown or black: presence of melanin
   h. Pink, green, or blue: results from foods, dyes, chemicals, or vitamins
2. Appearance/Clarity
   a. Normal: clear but becomes cloudy on standing
   b. Hazy: solid particles make urine appear hazy; print is not distorted when viewed through the sample
   c. Cloudy: solid particles make print difficult to see through the sample
   d. Turbid: solid particles make print impossible to see through the sample
   e. Normal cloudiness may be caused by:
      1) Mucus
      2) Certain crystals
      3) Epithelial cells
      4) Sperm cells
   f. Abnormal cloudiness may be caused by:
      1) Certain crystals
      2) White and red blood cells (WBCs and RBCs)
      3) Pus
      4) Epithelial cells
      5) Casts
      6) Fats
3. Specific gravity (SG)
   a. Measures the amount of dissolved solids in urine
   b. Compares weight to an equal amount of distilled water

1) Normal SG is 1.005 to 1.035: SG inverses with volume
   a) Low volume has high specific gravity (concentrated urine)
   b) High volume has low specific gravity (diluted urine)
2) Methods of measuring SG
   a) Reagent strip
   b) Urinometer
   c) Refractometer
4. Odor: may be noted if abnormal
   a. Normal: faintly aromatic; not unpleasant
   b. Ketones: sweet or fruity odor
   c. Ammonia: caused by bacterial growth that breaks down urea
   d. Food ingestion may cause strong odor

D. Chemical Examination
1. Chemical components are measured by use of a reagent strip
2. Presence of a chemical causes a color change on the reagent pad on the strip
3. Tests are qualitative
4. Specimen should be well mixed before testing
5. Completely immerse the strip into the sample
6. Remove the strip and keep it in a horizontal position (avoids cross-contamination of pads)
7. Compare the color of the reagent pad with the color on the bottle or chart at the time specified
8. Testing includes:
   a. pH: measures acidity and alkalinity of urine; normal is 5 to 7
   b. Protein: significant for renal disease; normal is *negative*
   c. Blood: significant for kidney disease or hemorrhage in the urinary tract; normal is *negative*
   d. Nitrite: significant for urinary tract infection (UTI) (some bacteria convert nitrate to nitrite); normal is *negative*
   e. Leukocytes: significant for UTI; normal is *negative*
   f. Glucose: significant for diabetes mellitus; normal is *negative*
   g. Ketones: end product of metabolism; significant for diabetes mellitus and starvation; normal is *negative*
   h. Bilirubin: by-product of RBC destruction; significant for liver disease or bile duct obstruction; normal is *negative*
   i. Urobilinogen: result of breakdown of bilirubin in the intestine; significant for anemias and malaria; normal is *small amount*
9. Automated (Clinitek) method
   a. Analyzer that automatically reads the reagent strips
   b. Based on principle of photometry
   c. Timing and color interpretation are consistent

E. Microscopic Examination
1. Consists of examining, counting, and categorizing the solid material found in urine
2. Standardized method (Kova Urine Sediment system) is used
3. Sample is centrifuged, supernatant (liquid portion) is poured off, and sediment is stained
4. Medical assistant may prepare the slide; practitioner interprets the results
   a. Examined under low power (10×)
   b. Examined under high power (40×) for cells and bacteria
   c. Examination includes:
      1) RBCs: normal is zero to two per high-powered field (HPF); cells appear small, round, and clear
      2) WBCs: normal is zero to five per HPF; cells appear two to three times the size of RBCs and round with a grainy appearance
      3) Epithelial cells
         a) Squamous epithelial cells: normal: not significant unless a large quantity per HPF; appear approximately the same size as WBCs
         b) Renal epithelial cells: normal is zero per HPF; presence indicates renal tubule destruction; appear round and grainy, approximately twice the size of WBCs
      4) Bacteria: normal is a few per HPF; more indicates UTI; appear as tiny grains
      5) Yeast: normal is a few per HPF; more indicates yeast infection (*Candida albicans*); they appear as round, clear bodies; some have buds (hyphae); may be confused with RBCs
      6) Mucous threads: wavy, threadlike structures
      7) Spermatozoa: appear as small oval bodies, with tail; normal in men after intercourse, contamination in women
      8) Casts: structures formed in nephron tubules; material solidifies in tubules and may contain cells, fat, and bacteria; normal is zero to two per LPF; appear as cylindrical bodies, longer than wide: types include:
         a) Hyaline: colorless and semitransparent
         b) Fatty cast: contains fat globules
         c) RBC cast: orange-yellow in color
         d) WBC cast: contains WBCs
         e) Granular cast: sandlike granules
         f) Waxy cast: yellowish, wide cast with irregular edges
      9) Crystals
         a) Normal crystals found in acidic urine
            (1) Uric acid: appears lemon-shaped
            (2) Calcium oxalate: square shape with an *X*
         b) Normal crystals found in alkaline urine
            (1) Triple phosphate: coffin lid–shaped
            (2) Calcium phosphate: flat plates
         c) Abnormal crystals found in acidic urine
            (1) Cystine: hexagonal plates
            (2) Tyrosine: fine needles
            (3) Leucine: yellow spheres
            (4) Sulfonamides: large needles in rosettes
            (5) Cholesterol: large, flat, hexagonal plates with notched corners

IV. HEMATOLOGY

A. General
1. Study of blood and blood components

B. Blood Components
1. Part of the circulatory system
2. Functions as transport mechanism for nutrients, waste, and defense agents to tissues and cells
3. Specimens collected by venipuncture (anticoagulated specimens) or capillary puncture
4. Plasma
   a. Liquid portion of circulating, unclotted blood
      1) If allowed to clot, the liquid portion is called serum; serum contains no clotting factors (formed clot)
      2) Appears clear and light yellow
   b. 55% of total blood volume made up of:
      1) 90% water
      2) 10% solutes (proteins, hormones, vitamins, carbohydrates, enzymes, lipids, and salts)
5. Formed elements
   a. Blood cells
   b. 45% of total blood volume made up of:
      1) Erythrocytes (RBCs)
      2) Leukocytes (WBCs)
      3) Thrombocytes (platelets)

C. Collection of Specimens
1. Sample can be separated into components by centrifuging or settling
   a. Plasma
      1) Liquid component of circulating blood
   b. Buffy coat: consists of white blood cells and platelets
   c. RBCs
2. Blood collection: Vacutainer Collection System
   a. Vacuum tubes with color-coded stoppers (Figure 23-2)
   b. Tube used depends on the test to be performed on the sample
      1) Yellow stopper
         a) Used for serum collection
         b) Contains no additive
         c) Tube is sterile and used for bacteriologic testing

FIGURE 23-2 Vacuum tube system. (Hunt SA: *Saunders fundamentals of medical assisting*, St Louis, 2002, Saunders.)

2) Red stopper
   a) Used for serum collection
   b) Contains no additives
   c) Tube must sit for 15 minutes to allow a clot to form, then centrifuge
   d) Used for samples for chemistry and serology
3) Tiger, speckled, SST (serum separator tube)
   a) Red-and-black mottled stopper
   b) Used to collect serum
   c) Tube contains a silicon gel that creates a barrier between the serum and the clotted cells when centrifuged
   d) Tube must sit for 15 minutes to allow a clot to form, then centrifuge
   e) Used for the same purpose as red stopper
4) Lavender stopper
   a) Used to collect plasma
   b) Tube contains the anticoagulant EDTA (ethylenediaminetetraacetic acid)
   c) Used for hematology
   d) Tube must be gently mixed after collection
5) Blue stopper
   a) Used to collect plasma
   b) Contains anticoagulant sodium citrate
   c) Used to perform coagulation testing
6) Green stopper
   a) Used to collect plasma
   b) Contains the anticoagulant sodium heparin
   c) Used in chemistry for immediate (stat) testing

7) Gray stopper
   a) Contains the anticoagulant sodium fluoride
   b) Used in chemistry for glucose testing and alcohol testing
3. Order of collection: when multiple tubes are to be collected, collect in the following order (see Table 23-1):
   a. Yellow stopper
   b. Blue stopper
   c. Red/SST stopper
   d. Green stopper
   e. Lavender stopper
   f. Gray stopper
4. Venipuncture (phlebotomy) (see Figures 23-3 and 23-4)
   a. Puncture of vein to withdraw blood sample
   b. Usually performed on the median cubital vein in the antecubital area
      1) Apply tourniquet approximately 3 to 4 inches above site; palpate and observe for the vein; release the tourniquet (do not leave the tourniquet on for more than 60 seconds)
      2) Assemble all equipment
      3) Reapply the tourniquet
      4) Glove; cleanse the site with an alcohol wipe, and allow it to dry
      5) Anchor the vein; insert the needle at approximately 15 degrees, bevel up
      6) Fill the syringe by slowly pulling back on the plunger or by inserting the vacuum tube onto the needle in the holder
      7) As the blood fills, release the tourniquet

TABLE 23-1   Vacuum Tube Table

Colors of the Picture and the Plastic Vacutainer Tubes Placed in Order of Draw from Top to Bottom		Additives	Laboratory Uses
Blue sky	Blue topped	Citrate	Coagulation studies
Red rays and gold rays	Red topped "clot tube"	Clot activator in plastic tubes (Note: red glass tubes do not have clot activator)	Both yield serum commonly used for testing blood chemistry
	Gold topped "SST tube"	Clot activator and gel	
Green grass	Green topped	Heparin (with lithium or sodium)	Special tests such as electrolytes
Lavender flowers	Lavender topped	EDTA	Hematology tests
Gray rocks	Gray topped	Oxalate	For glucose testing

From Garrels M, Oatis CS: *Laboratory testing for ambulatory settings: a guide for health care professionals*, St. Louis, 2006, Saunders.

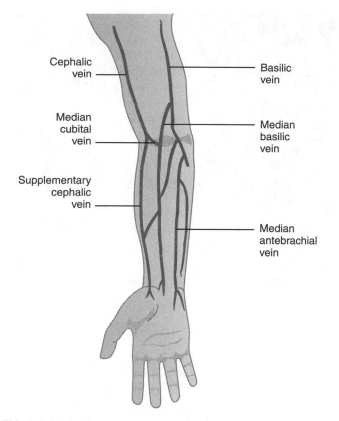

FIGURE 23-3 Antecubital veins. (From Bonewit-West K: *Clinical procedures for medical assistants*, ed 7, St Louis, 2008, Saunders.)

8) After collection is complete, place a clean cotton ball or gauze over the site, and quickly withdraw the needle; instruct the patient to apply pressure to the site; apply a pressure dressing to the site

9) Label the specimen; dispose of the needle into a sharps container

5. Butterfly-winged infusion set
   a. Used on small veins and for older adult and pediatric draws
   b. Can be attached to a Vacutainer Collection System or syringe

6. Syringe method
   a. Used on fragile veins that might collapse under the pressure of the Vacutainer
   b. Same procedure as the Vacutainer except the phlebotomist pulls back on the plunger to draw the blood into the syringe
   c. Blood can be seen entering the tip of the syringe as soon as the needle enters the vein (flash)
   d. Blood must be transferred into vacuum tubes quickly so it does not clot

7. Capillary puncture (see Figure 23-5)
   a. Used to collect small amounts of blood
   b. Sites include:
      1) Middle or ring finger of the nondominant hand
      2) Earlobe

FIGURE 23-4 Alternative venipuncture sites: the inner forearm, the wrist area above the thumb, and the back of the hand. (From Bonewit-West K: *Clinical procedures for medical assistants*, ed 7, St Louis, 2008, Saunders.)

FIGURE 23-5 Skin puncture sites for microcapillary blood collection. (Young AP, Kennedy DB: *Kinn's the medical assistant: an applied learning approach*, ed 10, St Louis, 2007, Saunders.)

    3) Heel or big toe on an infant
  c. Procedure
    1) Cleanse the site with alcohol, and allow it to dry
    2) Quickly puncture the skin with a lancet; wipe away the first drop of blood
    3) Collect a sample in the appropriate container

D. Erythrocytes
  1. Mature cells are anuclear biconcave disks
  2. Contain hemoglobin (Hgb)
    a. Heme (iron-containing portion) plus globin (protein-containing portion)
    b. Transport oxygen
  3. Color
    a. Normally appear pinkish-red (depends on Hgb concentration)
    b. Anisochromia: variations in color (depends on Hgb concentration)
  4. Size
    a. Normally 6 to 8 micrometers
    b. Anisocytosis: variation in size
  5. Shape
    a. Normally appear round
    b. Poikilocytosis: variation in shape
  6. Laboratory testing
    a. Hgb (hemoglobin) test
      1) Measures the total amount of Hgb in the blood
      2) Rapid indirect measurement of RBC count
      3) Evaluates anemic patients
      4) Routine portion of CBC
      5) Blood sample is diluted with Drabkin solution; lyses RBCs and releases Hgb into the solution; chemicals in the

reagent react with released Hgb and form the pigment cyanmethemoglobin, which can be measured by photometer
      6) Common CLIA waived methods
        a) HemoCue
        b) Hgb meter
        c) i-STAT
      7) Normal Hgb ranges:
        a) Newborn: 17 to 21 g/dL
        b) Infant: 10 to 15 g/dL
        c) Child: 11 to 16 g/dL
        d) Male adult: 15 to 18 g/dL
        e) Female adult: 12 to 16 g/dL
    b. Hematocrit (HCT, microhematocrit, crit)
      1) Direct measurement of percentage of RBCs in total blood volume
      2) Indirect measurement of RBC number and volume
      3) Rapid measurement of RBC count
      4) Routine portion of CBC
      5) Height of RBC column is measured after the blood sample is centrifuged; compared with the height of the column of whole blood (height of the column of whole blood is 100%)
      6) After centrifuging, blood separates into three layers:
        a) Plasma (top) layer
        b) Buffy coat: thin middle layer made up of WBCs and platelets
        c) RBCs (bottom) layer
      7) Hgb value multiplied by 3 gives the HCT value (±3)
      8) Procedure
        a) Two tubes needed (for comparison; to balance centrifuge; if one breaks)

b) Fill two capillary tubes three-quarters full with blood from capillary puncture or lavender-stoppered tube from venipuncture

c) Wipe the ends to remove blood from the outside of the tubes and seal with clay (Critoseal)

d) Place in a HCT centrifuge with the sealed ends facing outward; spin for 5 minutes

e) Read tubes by comparing them to the printed reading device

f) To be valid, the tubes should read within 2% of each other; report the average reading; repeat the test if not within 2%

9) Normal HCT ranges:

a) Newborn: 44% to 64%

b) Infant: 30% to 40%

c) Child: 35% to 41%

d) Female adult: 37% to 47%

e) Male adult: 42% to 52%

c. RBC count

1) Counts the number of circulating RBCs in 1 mm^3 of peripheral venous blood

2) Routine portion of CBC

3) Closely related to Hgb and HCT values

4) Normal RBC ranges (in million/mm^3):

a) Newborn: 4.8 to 7.1

b) Infant: 3.5 to 5.5

c) Child: 4.5 to 4.8

d) Female adult: 4 to 5.5

e) Male adult: 4.5 to 6

d. Indices

1) Provide information about RBC size, weight, and Hgb concentration

2) Part of automated CBC

3) Results of RBC count, HCT, and Hgb necessary to calculate indices

a) Mean corpuscular volume (MCV)

(1) Measure of average size per volume of an RBC

(2) Used to classify anemias

(3) CT (%) × 10 MCV = RBC (in million/mm^3)

(4) Normal ranges:

(a) Newborn: 96 to 108

(b) Child and adult: 82 to 98

b) Mean corpuscular hemoglobin (MCH)

(1) Measures amount per weight of Hgb within an RBC

(2) Hgb (g/dL) × 10 MCH = RBC (in million/mm^3)

(3) Normal ranges:

(a) Newborn: 32 to 34 pg

(b) Child and adult: 26 to 34 pg

c) Mean corpuscular hemoglobin concentration (MCHC)

(1) Measure of average concentration per percentage of Hgb in a single RBC

(2) Hgb (g/dL) × 100 HCT = g/dL or (%)

(3) Normal ranges:

(a) Newborn: 31 to 33 g/dL

(b) Child and adult: 31 to 37 g/dL

e. Reticulocyte count

1) Reticulocytes are immature RBCs

2) Indication of ability of bone marrow to respond to anemia and make RBCs

3) Used to classify and monitor anemia therapy

4) Count is percentage of total number of RBCs

5) Normal ranges:

a) Newborn: 0.5% to 2% of total RBCs

b) Infant: 0.5% to 3.1% of total RBCs

c) Child and adult: 0.5% to 2% of total RBCs

f. ESR (sed rate; erythrocyte sedimentation rate)

1) Nonspecific test used to detect illnesses associated with acute and chronic infection, inflammation, and neoplasms

2) Measures the rate at which RBCs settle in plasma over a specified time period (1 hour)

3) Methods include:

a) Wintrobe

b) Westergren

c) Landau-Adams

4) All methods are based on the same principle, although they vary in the amount of blood needed, the tube size, and calibration

5) Procedure

a) Fill the tube according to manufacturer's directions

b) Place the tube perfectly upright in the rack; let the tube sit for 1 hour without being disturbed

c) After 1 hour, note how many millimeters cells fall (settle)

6) Normal ranges:

a) Newborn: 0 to 2 mm/hr

b) Child: 0 to 10 mm/hr

c) Female adult: 0 to 30 mm/hr

d) Male adult: 0 to 20 mm/hr

E. Leukocytes

1. Mature cells vary in morphology depending on type

2. Neutrophil (segmented neutrophil [seg], poly, polymorphonuclear [PMN]): most numerous of granulocytes

a. Size: 10 to 15 micrometers

b. Nucleus: contains two to five lobes with constrictions (as sausage links); stains deep reddish-purple

c. Cytoplasm: abundant; stains light to medium pink, with many small granules of circulating WBCs

d. Increased number: shift to the right

3. Bands (stabs): immature form of segmented neutrophil

   a. Size: 10 to 15 micrometers

   b. Nucleus: peanut-, band-, or rod-shaped; no lobes or constrictions

   c. Cytoplasm: same as segmented neutrophil

   d. Distribution: 1% to 5% of circulating WBCs

   e. Increased number: shift to the left

4. Eosinophil (eos): granulocyte

   a. Size: 11 to 16 micrometers

   b. Nucleus: not significant; stains dark pinkish-red

   c. Cytoplasm: stains pink; contains large, reddish-orange granules

   d. Distribution: 1% to 5% of circulating WBCs; increase seen in allergic reactions, parasite infestation, and inflammation

5. Basophil (baso): granulocyte

   a. Size: 10 to 15 micrometers

   b. Nucleus: indistinct; usually occluded by granules

   c. Cytoplasm: small amount; stains purplish-blue; contains large, dark-purple-to-black granules; granules contain histamine and heparin

   d. Distribution: 0% to 1% of circulating WBCs; increase seen in allergic reactions, radiation exposure, and after splenectomy

6. Monocytes (mono): agranulocyte

   a. Size: 15 to 20 micrometers

   b. Nucleus: large, foamy, and round; stains reddish-purple to medium purple

   c. Cytoplasm: large amount; may appear foamy; stains sky-blue to blue-gray

   d. Distribution: 3% to 5% of circulating WBCs

7. Lymphocyte (lymph): agranulocyte

   a. Smallest in size of all WBCs

   b. Size: 6 to 10 micrometers

   c. Nucleus: round; fills most of the cell; stains dark purple

   d. Cytoplasm: small amount; encircles the nucleus; stains sky-blue to medium blue

   e. Distribution: 30% to 40% of circulating WBCs; infants and children normally have more than adults; increase seen in acute and chronic infections

8. Laboratory testing

   a. WBC count

      1) Measurement of total number of WBCs

      2) Routine part of CBC

      3) Helps evaluate and diagnose infection, allergy, neoplasm, or immunosuppression

      4) Normal ranges

         a) Newborn: 9000 to 30,000/mm^3

         b) Child: 5000 to 13,000/mm^3

         c) Adult: 5000 to 10,000/mm^3

   b. Differential (diff)

      1) Measurement of different WBCs in a smear

      2) Smear is stained with polychromatic stain (Wright's)

      3) Preparation of smear

         a) Small drop of blood is placed approximately ½ inch from the end of the slide

         b) Spreader slide is held at a 35- to 40-degree angle and moved back into the drop of blood slide; blood should be completely spread across the edge of the spreader's edge; push the spreader smoothly from the blood across the slide

         c) Allow to air dry; a smooth feather edge should be seen

         d) Stain the smear following the manufacturer's directions and completely air dry

      4) Normal ranges adult:

         a) Segs: 50 to 65

         b) Bands: 0 to 7

         c) Lymphs: 25 to 40

         d) Monos: 3 to 9

         e) EOS: 1 to 3

         f) BASO: 0 to 1

F. Thrombocytes

1. Platelet count test

   a. Actual count of the number of platelets in a cubic millimeter of blood

   b. Used to monitor the course of disease and therapy for thrombocytopenia and bone marrow failure

   c. Small round or oval bodies; no nucleus

   d. Stain dark blue on a different smear

   e. Normal ranges

      1) Newborn: 140,000 to 300,000/mm^3

      2) Infant: 200,000 to 473,000/mm^3

      3) Child/adult: 150,000 to 400,000/mm^3

2. Bleeding time

   a. Measures platelet function by noting the length of time required for bleeding to stop

   b. Two methods:

      1) Ivy method: small incision in the patient's arm

      2) Duke method: small incision in the patient's earlobe (not commonly performed)

      3) Normal range: 1 to 9 minutes for bleeding to stop

3. Prothrombin time (PT, pro-time)
   a. Used to evaluate clotting mechanism
   b. Used to monitor Coumadin therapy
   c. Normal range: 11 to 12.5 seconds; INR: 2 to 2.5
4. Partial thromboplastin time (PTT)
   a. Used to evaluate the pathway to clot formation
   b. Used to monitor heparin therapy
   c. Normal range: 60 to 70 seconds

G. Complete Blood Count (CBC)

1. Advanced concept
2. Consists of seven or more separate tests that reflect total count, analysis, and microscopic descriptions of the cellular elements of blood
3. Tests include:
   a. RBC count
   b. Hct
   c. RBC indices
   d. Hgb
   e. WBC count
   f. Differential smear
   g. Platelet count

V. CLINICAL CHEMISTRY

A. General

1. Testing of the chemical analytes found in various liquid body specimens (urine, whole blood, serum, plasma, synovial fluid, pleural fluid, cerebrospinal fluid)
2. Change in blood chemistry allows detection of confirmation of a diagnosis
3. Testing usually requires a serum sample
4. Tests may be ordered in groups (panels)

B. Lipids

1. Fats essential to the body
2. Before lipid testing, the patient should fast for 12 to 14 hours; the patient should consume no alcohol for 24 hours before the test; the patient should reduce fat intake for 2 weeks before the test
3. These tests can assess the risk of coronary and vascular disease
4. Lipid profile is made up of the following tests:
   a. Cholesterol
      1) Fatty compound
      2) Necessary for production of sex hormones and bile
      3) Helps in formation of cell membranes
      4) Normal reading: <200 mg/dL
   b. High-density lipoproteins (HDLs)
      1) "Good" cholesterol
      2) Removes excess cholesterol from cells and carries it back to the liver for excretions
      3) Normal reading: >50 mg/dL
   c. Low-density lipoproteins (LDLs)
      1) "Bad" cholesterol
      2) Picks up fat from liver and carries it in the blood
      3) Normal reading: <100 mg/dL
   d. Triglycerides
      1) Form fat in the bloodstream
      2) Transported in blood by LDLs
      3) Make up most of the fat in the body
      4) Normal reading: 30 to 150 mg/dL

C. Glucose

1. Simple sugar from the breakdown of carbohydrates
2. Provides energy for cells and tissues
3. Excess is stored as glycogen in the liver
4. Blood levels regulated by hormones produced by pancreas
   a. Glucagon: converts glycogen to glucose (increased blood levels)
   b. Insulin: transports glucose into cells (decreased blood levels)
5. Tests include:
   a. Fasting blood glucose (FBG)
      1) Testing done on blood sample of patient after fasting for 8 to 12 hours (water permitted)
      2) Test is commonly used in the diagnosis or evaluation of diabetes mellitus
      3) Normal range: 65 to 110 mg/dL
   b. Postprandial glucose (2-hour postprandial blood sugar [PPBS])
      1) Measures the amount of glucose in the patient's blood after a meal is ingested
      2) Blood level should return to the premeal range within 2 hours
      3) Normal range: 65 to 110 mg/dL
   c. Glucose tolerance test (GTT)
      1) Assists in the diagnosis of diabetes mellitus
      2) Patient's blood glucose levels are evaluated at fasting, then 30, 60, 120, and 180 minutes after ingestion of a standard oral glucose solution
      3) Urine samples are evaluated at the same time
      4) Patient is to fast 12 hours before the test
      5) Fasting blood sugar is drawn
      6) Patient drinks 75 g of glucose solution
      7) Collect blood samples and urine samples 30, 60, 120, and 180 minutes (or any combination of these times) after the patient takes the glucose solution

8) Patient may drink water during the test, but no coffee, tea, or tobacco
9) Normal glucose readings:
   a) Fasting: 65 to 110 mg/dL
   b) 30 min: 200 mg/dL
   c) 1 hour: 200 mg/dL
   d) 2 hours: 140 mg/dL
   e) 3 hours: 65 to 115 mg/dL

D. Electrolytes
1. Charged particles of the body
2. Includes:
   a. Cation: positively charged ions
   b. Anion: negatively charged ions
3. Found in extracellular fluids
4. Body strives for neutrality (balance of anions and cations); if balance is not achieved, can be dangerous or fatal for the patient
5. Lungs and kidneys control the electrolyte balance
6. Functions of electrolytes
   a. Maintain water balance in the body
   b. Maintain pH of the body
   c. Help with blood coagulation
   d. Control neuromuscular excitability
7. Sodium (Na^+)
   a. Major extracellular cation
   b. Helps maintain osmotic pressure
   c. Low sodium level: hyponatremia
   d. High sodium level: hypernatremia
   e. Normal range: 135 to 146 mEq/L
8. Potassium (K^+)
   a. Major intracellular cation
   b. Influences muscle activity of heart
   c. Works with sodium for acid-base balance
   d. Low K^+ level: hypokalemia
   e. High K^+ level: hyperkalemia
   f. Normal range: 3.5 to 5.3 mEq/L
9. Chloride (Cl^-)
   a. Major extracellular anion
   b. Counterbalances sodium for neutrality in body fluids
   c. Helps maintain osmotic pressure (water distribution between cells), plasma, and interstitial fluid
   d. Helps maintain acid-base balance
   e. Normal range: 98 to 108 mEq/L
10. Bicarbonate (HCO_3^-)
   a. Major anion
   b. Measured by blood carbon dioxide levels
   c. Works with Cl^-
   d. Normal range: 21 to 31 mEq/L

E. Bilirubin
1. Yellow pigment in bile
2. Comes from heme portion of hemoglobin (heme released when RBCs break down)

3. Two types:
   a. Unconjugated (indirect): transported by albumin to the liver
   b. Conjugated (direct): becomes water soluble in the liver and enters the bile; transported to the small intestine, where it is converted into urobilinogen
4. Increased levels may indicate:
   a. Destruction of RBCs
   b. Impaired liver function
   c. Obstruction of flow of bile
5. Exposure to ultraviolet light results in oxidation of bilirubin
6. Normal range: 0.1 to 1.2 mg/dL

F. Proteins
1. Make up muscles, enzymes, hormones, hemoglobin, and other important functional and structural substances in the body
2. Albumin
   a. Principal plasma protein
   b. Found in liver
   c. Functions
     1) Maintenance of osmotic pressure
     2) Transportation of drugs, hormones, and enzymes
   d. Can be a measure of nutritional status
   e. Normal range: 3.5 to 5.0 g/dL
3. Globulin
   a. Building block of antibodies, lipids, and clotting factors
   b. Transport mechanism
   c. Can be measure of nutritional status
   d. Normal range: 1.7 to 3.5 g/dL
4. Albumin to globulin (A/G) ratio
   a. Normal range: 1.1 to 2.5
5. Total protein
   a. Albumin plus globulin
   b. Component of osmotic pressure (keeps fluids within vascular system)
   c. Normal range: 6.0 to 8.5 g/dL

G. Nitrogenous Compounds
1. Forms of nitrogen in the body
2. Waste product of metabolism
3. Blood urea nitrogen (BUN)
   a. Main indicator of kidney function
   b. Urea is main nonprotein nitrogen in blood
   c. Urea is formed in the liver and is the waste product of the breakdown of protein
   d. Normal range: 8 to 26 mg/dL
4. Creatinine
   a. End product of creatine metabolism in muscles
   b. Constantly being formed; the amount has a direct relationship to muscle mass
   c. Filtered by the kidneys and excreted in urine

d. Reliable screening test for renal function
e. Normal range: 0.7 to 1.4 mg/dL
5. Uric acid
a. By-product of protein metabolism
b. Blood levels from food metabolism (high-protein diet) and muscle tissue breakdown
c. Normal range: men: 3.6 to 8.0 mg/dL; women: 2.5 to 6.8 mg/dL

H. Enzymes
1. Substances that speed up chemical reactions but remain unchanged themselves
2. Values expressed in International Units (IU)
3. Always end with the suffix -ase
4. Can originate in cells, specific organs, or tissues
5. Release may be caused by damage or disease of tissues
6. Alanine aminotransferase (ALT)
a. Formerly serum glutamic-oxaloacetic transaminase (SGOT)
b. Found in highly metabolic tissues (heart muscle, liver, skeletal muscles)
c. Levels increase post–myocardial infarction (MI) (indication of MI)
d. Normal range: men: 0 to 37 U/L; women: 0 to 31 U/L
7. Creatine phosphokinase (CPK, CK)
a. Enzyme found in mitochondria of cells
b. High concentration in the heart, skeletal muscles, and brain
c. Useful in diagnosis of MI and muscle disease
d. Normal range: 25 to 130 IU/L
8. Alkaline phosphatase (ALP)
a. High concentration in bone and liver
b. Bone growth or liver disease can cause levels to rise
c. Normal range: child: 117 to 390 U/L; adult: 39 to 117 U/L
9. Acid phosphatase
a. Largest source is the prostate gland
b. Elevated in prostate cancer
c. Normal value: 0 to 0.8I U/L

I. Minerals
1. Inorganic chemical elements needed in small amounts but essential for life
2. May be part of hormones or enzymes or work with vitamins
3. Calcium (Ca)
a. Found in bone tissue
b. Required for:
1) Bone development
2) Cardiac function
3) Blood clotting
4) Transmission of nerve impulses
5) Muscle contractions
c. Normal range: 8.5 to 11.5 mg/dL

4. Phosphorus (P)
a. Required for metabolism of protein, calcium, and glucose
b. Combines with calcium
c. Normal range: 2.5 to 4.5 mg/dL
5. Magnesium (Mg)
a. Found in bone
b. Binds with adenosine triphosphate (ATP) molecule for energy
c. Required for:
1) Muscle action
2) Nerve impulse transmission
3) Calcium regulation
4) Enzyme activity
d. Normal range: 1.2 to 2.0 mEq/L

J. Thyroid
1. Triiodothyronine (T_3)
a. Evaluates thyroid function (hyperthyroidism, hypothyroidism)
b. Monitors thyroid replacement and suppressive therapy
c. Normal range: 70 to 205 ng/dL
2. Thyroxine (tetraiodothyronine) (T_4)
a. Initial test done for assessing thyroid function
b. Used to diagnose thyroid function
c. Used to monitor replacement and suppressive therapy
d. Normal range: women: 5 to 12 µg/dL; men: 4 to 12 µg/dL

VI. SEROLOGY AND IMMUNOLOGY

A. General
1. Tests done on serum to evaluate antigen-antibody reaction
2. Helps detect disease or amount of antibodies present (titer)
3. Some tests available in kit and/or rapid forms
4. Test reactions include:
a. Precipitation: antigen-antibody complex visibly settles out of solution
b. Agglutination: type of precipitation method that creates visible clumping

B. Infectious Mononucleosis
1. Disease caused by Epstein-Barr virus
2. Body produces heterophil antibodies in response
3. Tests (Monospot, QuickVue+) are designed to detect heterophile antibody

C. Streptococcus
1. Group A beta hemolytic Streptococcus causes strep throat, rheumatic fever, and impetigo
2. Tests detect antibody antistreptolysin-O (ASO)

D. Rheumatoid Factor
1. Group of proteins (autoantibodies)
2. Causes rheumatoid arthritis
3. Test detects antibodies against factor

E. Human Chorionic Gonadotropin (HCG)

1. Hormone produced by the placenta
2. Test for hormone in blood and urine
3. Basis of pregnancy testing

F. Blood Groups

1. Blood cells are mixed with antisera; agglutination indicates the presence of antigens on RBCs
2. Can detect ABO group (A, B, AB, or O)
3. Can detect Rh (Rh+, or Rh−)

G. Syphilis

1. Antibody test for *Treponema pallidum*
2. Tests include:
   a. Rapid plasma reagin (RPR)
   b. Venereal disease research laboratory (VDRL)

H. Systemic Lupus Erythematosus

1. Testing to detect antinuclear antibodies (ANA)

I. *Helicobacter pylori*

1. Spiral-shaped bacteria believed to be the cause of the majority of peptic ulcers
2. QuickVue *Helicobacter pylori* gII Test is performed from a finger stick

J. Human Immunodeficiency Virus (HIV)

1. Virus attacks and destroys T helper (CD4) lymphocytes
2. ELISA test (enzyme-linked immunosorbent assay) detects antibodies
3. Antibodies can also be detected in oral specimens (ORA Quick)

K. Antibody Titers

1. Laboratory-based quantitative test to determine the amount of antibody in blood
2. Examples: rubella, hepatitis B, varicella

VII. MICROBIOLOGY

A. General

1. Study of microorganisms
2. Includes:
   a. Bacteria
   b. Fungi
   c. Viruses
   d. Rickettsiae
   e. Mycobacteria
   f. Parasites
3. Main objective is to identify the organism so that the practitioner can properly treat
4. Collection of most common specimens
   a. Throat culture
      1) Use a sterile swab and swab the back of throat in a *rainbow* or *figure-8* pattern
      2) Collect any material in the area
      3) Transport or send the specimen to the laboratory using a transport medium or streak immediately
   b. Urine culture
      1) Clean-catch specimen in a sterile container
      2) Use a sterile loop to streak the plate
   c. Genitourinary culture
      1) Collect a specimen using a sterile swab
      2) Roll the swab over the plate in a Z or W pattern
      3) Streak across the Z or W, using a sterile loop
   d. Blood culture
      1) Collect a specimen in a yellow-stoppered tube
      2) Cleanse the skin with Betadine before venipuncture
      3) Inject approximately 10 mL of the specimen into two separate blood culture bottles
   e. Wound culture
      1) Collect a specimen with a sterile swab
      2) Streak the plate using the Z or W method
   f. Fecal culture
      1) Collect a specimen in a clean container
      2) Streak the plate with a sterile loop

B. Classification of Organisms

1. Scientific study of classification process is taxonomy
2. Simple, orderly method
3. Places organisms into categories according to similar morphologic and biochemical properties
   a. Species: basic unit; based on reproduction (members of the same species can mate successfully)
   b. Genus: share biological likenesses
   c. Family: similar genera
   d. Order: related families
   e. Class: related orders
   f. Phylum: classes with common characteristics
4. Organisms in laboratory setting have two separate names:
   a. Genus: name is capitalized; often abbreviated, using the first initial
   b. Species: name in lowercase
5. Both names are underlined or italicized when written

C. Bacteria (Bacteriology)

1. Characteristics: help with identification of organisms in the laboratory (see Figure 23-6)
   a. Shape
      1) Cocci: round (singular: coccus)
      2) Bacilli: rod shaped (singular: bacillus)
      3) Vibrio: comma shaped
      4) Spirilla: spiral shaped (singular: spirillum)
   b. Arrangement
      1) Diplo: arranged in pairs
      2) Strepto: arranged in chains

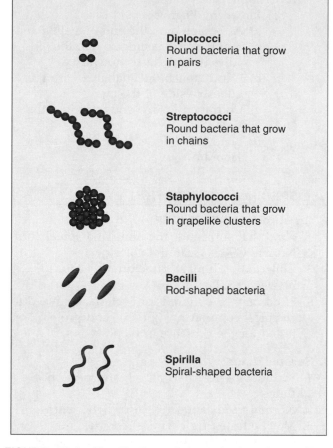

FIGURE 23-6 Classification of bacteria by shape. (From Bonewit-West K: *Clinical procedures for medical assistants*, ed 7, St Louis, 2008, Saunders.)

Near figure:
- **Diplococci** Round bacteria that grow in pairs
- **Streptococci** Round bacteria that grow in chains
- **Staphylococci** Round bacteria that grow in grapelike clusters
- **Bacilli** Rod-shaped bacteria
- **Spirilla** Spiral-shaped bacteria

      3) Staphylo: arranged in grapelike clusters
      4) Tetra: four cocci together in capsule
   c. Staining properties
      1) Gram stain
         a) Gram-positive: stain blue or dark purple
         b) Gram-negative: stain pink or red
      2) Acid-fast stain: type of stain used on bacteria that are difficult to stain with other stains
   d. Oxygen requirements
      1) Aerobic: requires oxygen to survive
      2) Anaerobic: requires no oxygen to survive
      3) Facultative: can survive in either environment
   e. Colony growth
      1) Size
      2) Color
      3) Shape
      4) Elevation
      5) Texture
      6) Margins
      7) Hemolysis (present or absent)
   f. Chemical reactions: bacteria respond differently to chemical reagents

  2. Bacterial growth requirements
   a. Nutrients: differ among species
   b. Temperature: usually thrive at normal body temperature (98.6°F, 37°C)
   c. Oxygen: differs among species (aerobic or anaerobic)
   d. pH: human pathogens thrive at 7 (neutral); blood, milk, and seawater are neutral
   e. Sterile: medium must be sterile and uncontaminated for use
   f. Moisture: most bacteria require some level of moisture
  3. Culture and sensitivity (C&S)
   a. Determines an organism's susceptibility to selected antibiotics
   b. Streak the plate with culture; cover the entire plate, rotating 45 degrees between each streak
   c. Apply antibody disks using a dispenser or sterile forceps; make sure the disk is in contact with the medium
   d. Incubate; check after 24 hours
   e. Measure the zones of inhibition around each disk; compare with the chart provided by the manufacturer
   f. Report the results

D. Mycology
  1. Study of fungus
  2. Medical mycology fungal forms
   a. Molds
      1) Multicellular organisms made up of hyphae
      2) Produce powdery, fuzzy, or fluffy colonies on media
   b. Yeasts
      1) Single-cell organisms
      2) Multiply by budding
      3) Produce moist, creamy colonies on media
  3. Identification methods
   a. Potassium hydroxide (KOH) preparation
      1) Place the specimen on a slide
      2) Mix KOH with the specimen and allow to sit for 15 to 20 minutes
      3) Observe under low power
   b. India ink
      1) Helps identify capsules
      2) Mix bodily fluid with ink on the slide
      3) Observe under low power
      4) Cells will appear to have halo around them

E. Virology
  1. Study of viruses
  2. Intracellular parasites that require a host to carry out their functions
  3. Do not have cellular structure (nucleic acid and protein layer)
  4. Reproductive by replication

F. Parasitology
1. Study of parasites
2. Organisms that live in or on a host and derive nourishment from the host
3. Can be one-celled (protozoa) or many-celled (helminths) parasites
4. Relationships
   a. Commensalism: neither organism harmed; one benefits
   b. Mutualism: both organisms benefit
   c. Parasitism: one organism benefits at the expense of the other
   d. Symbiosis: dependant relationship between two dissimilar organisms
5. Infection: invasion of microscopic parasites causing disease
6. Infestation: external or internal invasion of animal-like parasites
7. Classifications
   a. Protozoa: unicellular organisms
      1) Transmission
         a) Ingestion of cysts in fecally contaminated water or food
         b) Become adults after infection; they multiply in the intestine and are passed in feces
      2) Amoeba
         a) Move by means of pseudopods (*false foot*)
      3) Flagellates
         a) Move by flagella
      4) Ciliates
         a) Move by cilia
      5) Sporozoans
         a) Have sexual and asexual reproductive cycles
   b. Helminths: parasitic worms
      1) Nematodes: roundworms
      2) Cestodes: tapeworms
      3) Trematodes (flukes)
   c. Arthropods: organisms with exoskeletons and jointed appendages; can serve as vector or as intermediate host
      1) Insects: head and body lice
      2) Fleas
      3) Mosquitoes
      4) Arachnids: itch mite
8. Diagnostic procedures
   a. O&P: examination of feces for ova and parasites
      1) Collect a sample in a clean, dry container; do not allow the specimen to touch water or urine
      2) Scoop out an amount of specimen and place in prepared specimen containers as directed by the manufacturer
   b. Cellophane-tape test
      1) Pinworm diagnosis
         a) Affix tape onto the end of a slide and drape over the slide so that the adhesive side faces outward
         b) Gently touch the anal area with the adhesive side of the tape
         c) Undrape the tape and stick it to the slide
         d) Send the slide with tape on it to the laboratory

VIII. SPECIMEN COLLECTION

A. Cerebrospinal Fluid (CSF)
1. Fluid that surrounds the brain and spinal cord
2. Normal CSF is clear and colorless
3. Collected by lumbar puncture procedure between L3, L4, or L5
4. Fluid may be cultured for bacteria, analyzed for chemical components (glucose and protein), or tested for the presence of blood cells

B. Serous Fluids
1. Includes pericardial, plural, and peritoneal fluids
2. Normal fluids appear clear or light yellow
3. May be tested for chemical components, cultured and smeared for bacteria, or tested for cell counts

C. Synovial Fluid
1. Fluid that lines and lubricates joints
2. Normal fluid appears yellow and viscous
3. Collected through joint puncture
4. May be cultured, analyzed for cells and crystals, and tested for glucose and protein

D. Feces
1. Collected in a clean container
2. Avoid contamination from water or urine
3. Tests include:
   a. Occult blood (stool guaiac test)
      1) Detects hidden blood
      2) Helps diagnosis of cancer or bleeding
      3) Hemoccult; ColoScreen
   b. Ova and parasites (O&P): detects eggs and parasites in the intestinal tract
   c. Culture: detects microorganisms

E. Sputum
1. Secretions of trachea and bronchi
2. Avoid contamination with saliva and nasal secretions
3. Patient is instructed to cough deeply into the container for the culture

F. Other Secretions

1. Collected with sterile swabs for cultures, includes:
   a. Wound secretions
   b. Throat secretions
   c. Genital secretions

IX. REFERENCE VALUES FOR COMMON LAB TESTS

Common reference values may vary depending on the testing.

A. Normal Urine Reference Values

1. Volume (mL/24 hours)
   a. Newborn: 20 to 350 mL
   b. Child: 300 to 1500 mL
   c. Adult: 750 to 2000 mL
2. Physical and chemical components
   a. Color: straw to amber, light to dark
   b. Turbidity: clear to slightly hazy
   c. Specific gravity: 1.005 to 1.030
   d. pH: 4.6 to 8.0
   e. Protein: negative to trace
   f. Glucose: negative
   g. Ketone: negative
   h. Bilirubin: negative
   i. Blood: negative
   j. Urobilinogen: 0.1 EU/dL
   k. Bacteria (nitrates): negative
   l. Leukocytes: negative
3. Urine: sediment
   a. RBCs/HPF: rare
   b. WBCs/LPF: 0 to 4
   c. Epi/HPF: occasional
   d. Casts/LPF: occasional
   e. Bacteria: negative
   f. Mucus: negative to 2+
   g. Crystals: only cystine, leucine, and tyrosine are significant

B. Normal Blood Chemistry Reference Values

1. ALT (SGPT) (alanine transaminase): 4 to 36 U/L
2. Albumin: 3.5 to 5 g/dL
3. ALP (alkaline phosphatase): 30 to 120 U/L
4. AST (SGOT) (aspartate transaminase): 0 to 35 U/L
5. Bicarbonate: 21 to 28 mEq/L
6. Bilirubin (total): 0.3 to 1 mg/dL
7. Blood urea nitrogen (BUN): 10 to 20 mg/dL
8. Calcium: 9 to 10.5 mg/dL
9. Cholesterol: <200 mg/dL
10. Creatinine: 0.5 to 1.2 mg/dL
11. C-reactive protein: <1 mg/dL
12. GGT (gamma glutamyl transferase): 8 to 38 U/L
13. Glucose: 70 to 105 mg/dL
14. Iron: 60 to 180 µg/dL
15. Phosphorus: 3 to 4.5 mg/dL
16. Potassium: 3.5 to 5 mEq/L
17. Sodium: 136 to 145 mEq/L
18. T_3 (triiodothyronine): 75 to 220 µg/dL
19. T_4 (thyroxine): 4 to 12 µg/dL
20. Total protein (albumin/globulin): 6.4 to 8.3 mg/dL
21. Uric acid: 2.7 to 8.5 mg/dL

C. Normal Hematology Reference Values

1. Hemoglobin
   a. Adult males: 14 to 18 g/dL
   b. Adult females: 12 to 16 g/dL
2. Hematocrit
   a. Adult males: 42% to 52%
   b. Adult females: 37% to 47%
3. WBC count
   a. Adults: 5000 to 10,000/mm^3
4. RBC count
   a. Adult males: 4.7 to 6.1 million/mm^3
   b. Adult females: 4.2 to 5.4 million/mm^3
5. RBC Indices
   a. MCV (mean corpuscular volume): 80 to 90 µm^3/cell
   b. MCH (mean corpuscular hemoglobin): 27 to 31/RBC
   c. MCHC (mean corpuscular hemoglobin concentration): 32% to 36%
6. Platelet count
   a. Adults: 150,000 to 400,000/mm^3
7. Erythrocyte sedimentation rate (ESR): Wintrobe
   a. Adult males: 0 to 9 mm/hr
   b. Adult females: 0 to 20 mm/hr
8. Prothrombin time: 11 to 12.5 seconds
9. Partial thromboplastin time: 25 to 38 seconds
10. Bleeding time (Ivy): 1 to 9 minutes
11. Differential leukocyte count
    a. Neutrophil: 55% to 70%
    b. Eosinophil: 1% to 4%
    c. Basophil: 0.5% to 1%
    d. Monocyte: 2% to 8%
    e. Lymphocyte: 20% to 40%

24 First Aid and Office Emergencies

I. FIRST AID

A. General

1. Immediate, temporary care given to a person who has been injured or suddenly taken ill
2. The medical assistant, in emergencies, is covered by Good Samaritan laws at the scene of an accident
3. Keep emergency telephone numbers near telephones in the office
4. As an employee of a medical facility, keep cardiopulmonary resuscitation (CPR) and first-aid cards current
5. Do not provide care beyond your scope of training or beyond your abilities
6. Call for help or 911 when needed

II. GUIDELINES FOR PROVIDING EMERGENCY CARE

A. General

1. Know your limits and only do what is in your scope of practice
2. Stay calm; speak in normal tone of voice; explain what has happened
3. Practice Standard Precautions and follow OSHA blood-borne pathogens standards
4. Assess the situation quickly; check for possibilities of life-threatening injuries
   a. Use ABC method to assess patient
      1) Airway
      2) Breathing
      3) Circulation
5. Know how to contact emergency response (911)
6. Do not move the patient unless he or she is in harm's way
7. Keep the patient warm
8. Look for medical alert tags
9. Move bystanders away from the patient
10. Do not leave the patient until emergency medical personnel have arrived and taken over; provide information that you have observed

III. COMMON EMERGENCIES IN THE MEDICAL OFFICE

A. Fainting (Syncope)

1. Lay or sit the patient with the patient's head lower than the heart
2. Loosen the patient's tight clothing
3. Maintain an open airway
4. Apply a cool cloth to the patient's head
5. Pass aromatic spirits of ammonia under the patient's nose
6. Keep the patient supine for 10 minutes after consciousness is regained

B. Choking

1. Do not interfere if the patient can speak, cough, or breathe
2. Use the Heimlich maneuver if the victim cannot speak, cough, or breathe
3. If the patient becomes unconscious, position the patient on his or her back; call for help
4. Begin CPR after removing the foreign body

C. Chest Pain

1. Sit the patient down
2. Keep the patient quiet and warm
3. Loosen the patient's tight clothing
4. Take the apical and radial pulse
5. Administer oxygen if the practitioner orders
6. Bring the emergency (*crash*) cart into the room
7. If cardiac arrest occurs, perform CPR

D. Cerebrovascular Accident (CVA)

1. Call for help
2. Protect the patient against injury while waiting for transport
3. Keep the patient lying down
4. Maintain an open airway
5. Do not give food or water

E. Poisoning

1. Ask what was taken, how much was taken, how long ago, and whether vomiting has occurred
2. Call the Poison Control Center

3. Induce vomiting (unless a corrosive had been ingested) or dilute with 1 to 2 cups of water or milk; give 1 tablespoon of syrup of ipecac (or follow specific directions given by the Poison Control Center)

F. Animal Bites
1. Thoroughly wash the wound with soap and water
2. Report the bite to the authorities

G. Insect Bites and Stings
1. Remove the stinger by brushing it off or using tweezers
2. Apply ice to the bite area
3. Be aware of patient allergy to insect bites or stings
4. If the patient is allergic and shows signs of shock or difficulty breathing, a true emergency exists

H. Shock
1. Ensure and maintain an open airway
2. Call 911
3. While waiting for transport, place the patient on his or her back with legs elevated above the heart
4. Loosen the patient's tight clothing
5. Cover the patient with a blanket to maintain warmth

I. Asthma Attack
1. Assist the patient with an inhaler
2. Encourage and assist the patient to relax
3. Patient may breathe into a paper bag if hyperventilating

J. Seizures
1. Lay the patient on his or her back
2. Loosen the patient's tight clothing
3. Do not restrain the patient
4. Do not place anything between the patient's teeth
5. Protect the patient's head from injury
6. Give the patient nothing by mouth
7. Let the patient rest after the seizure subsides

K. Sprain
1. Begin treatment within 10 to 20 minutes of the injury (RICE)
2. Rest the injured area
3. Ice the area
4. Compress the area by wrapping with an elastic bandage
5. Elevate the injured area

L. Fractures
1. Make the patient as comfortable as possible
2. Prevent movement of the injured area
3. Apply ice
4. Control bleeding, if applicable
5. Assist the health care provider

M. Burns
1. Remove the patient's clothing from the burned area
2. Stay with the patient
3. Assist the health care provider

N. Lacerations
1. Keep the patient as calm as possible
2. Cover the area with a sterile dressing using standard precautions
3. Apply direct pressure to the wound to control bleeding using standard precautions
4. Elevate the injured area above the level of the patient's heart
5. Ask the patient about when the last tetanus injection was given
6. Cleanse the wound if it is not bleeding severely
7. Assist the health care provider

O. Nosebleeds (Epistaxis)
1. Keep the patient quiet and in a sitting position
2. Apply direct pressure to the affected nostril by pinching

P. Hemorrhage
1. Apply direct pressure over the area; do not remove the original pad when it becomes saturated; add additional pads
2. Elevate the injured part above the patient's heart
3. Apply pressure over the area's pressure point
4. As a last resort, apply a tourniquet as directed by the health care provider
5. Assist the health care provider

Q. Head Injuries
1. Lay the patient flat
2. Do not move the patient if a neck injury is suspected
3. Do not administer the patient anything by mouth
4. Keep the patient warm and quiet
5. Watch the patient's pupils for changes
6. Assist the health care provider

R. Diabetic Emergencies
1. For hypoglycemia (insulin shock): give juice, candy, or soda (a sugar source)
2. For hyperglycemia (diabetic coma): if the patient is conscious, administer fluids; if you are uncertain whether this is insulin shock or diabetic coma, give the patient a sugar source
3. Assist the health care provider

S. Foreign Body in the Eye
1. Place the patient in a darkened room
2. Apply a cool, wet compress to the affected eye; do not apply pressure
3. Assist the health care provider

IV. BASIC MEDICAL OFFICE EMERGENCY CART (CRASH CART)

A. Equipment and Supplies
1. Defibrillator
2. Oxygen tank, tubing, mask, nasal cannula
3. Airways
4. Ambu bag
5. Intravenous supplies
6. Intravenous fluids
7. Gloves (sterile, non-sterile)
8. Scissors (bandage, operative)
9. Syringes and needles
10. Biohazard containers
11. Sterile gauze squares (2 × 2, 4 × 4)
12. Penlight
13. Pen and paper
14. Pocket mask
15. Kling dressings
16. Blood pressure cuff and stethoscope

B. Medications
1. Adenosine
2. Aminophylline
3. Atropine
4. Albuterol
5. Diazepam
6. Digoxin
7. Benadryl
8. Dopamine
9. Adrenalin
10. Lasix
11. Lidocaine
12. Narcan
13. Solu-medrol
14. Dilantin
15. Sodium bicarbonate
16. Activated charcoal
17. Ammonia inhalants
18. Glucose or glucagon

V. EMERGENCY PREPAREDNESS

A. Definition
1. Act of making plans to prevent, respond to, and recover from emergencies
2. Coordinated actions to meet the needs of a community

B. Roles of Health Care Professionals
1. Each profession has special skills
2. Respond within scope of practice
3. May fill support roles
4. Training may be provided by employer

C. Natural Disasters
1. Earthquakes
2. Floods
3. Heat waves
4. Hurricanes
5. Tornadoes
6. Winter storms
7. Wildfires

D. Manmade Disasters
1. Chemicals
2. Radiation
3. Terrorism

E. Emergency Management
1. Mitigation: prevent or minimize emergencies
2. Preparedness: actions taken to enable future responses
3. Response: plans put into action
4. Recovery: activities to help a community return to normal

F. Medical Assistant's Role
1. All administrative and clinical skills can be used in an emergency
2. Communicate with patients about evacuation orders, hazards, precautions, and emergency sources of medical equipment
3. Provide medical care for chronically ill patients
4. Rearrange appointments to accommodate patients needing emergency care
5. Volunteer on response teams

GENERAL

Directions: Select the *best* response.

1. Which of the following documents applies to donation of anatomical gifts?
   A. Advanced directive
   B. Uniform Anatomical Gift Act
   C. Living will
   D. Durable power of attorney

2. In which of the following situations can a patient's medical record be released without a signed authorization?
   A. The patient's attorney requests them
   B. The patient is human immunodeficiency virus (HIV) positive
   C. An insurance company requests them
   D. Another physician requests them

3. Which of the following would be the most appropriate first step when dealing with a patient who is distraught and angry?
   A. Escort the patient to a private area
   B. Ask the patient to calm down
   C. Inform the patient that the physician will see him or her shortly
   D. Ask the patient to have a seat in the waiting room

4. A 75-year-old woman with emphysema continues to smoke and to miss appointments against the orders of her physician. What is the most appropriate next step?
   A. Notify the patient that her medical care is being terminated
   B. Instruct her family how to change her behavior
   C. Accept her behavior and adjust her treatment
   D. Refer her to a psychiatrist

5. Which of the following agencies regulates licensure for physicians?
   A. Local hospital boards
   B. Federal government
   C. Medical colleges
   D. State government

6. "Have you had this problem in the past?" is an example of which of the following types of questions?
   A. Leading
   B. Open-ended
   C. Closed-ended
   D. Nonleading

7. The best method for transmitting confidential information from one medical practice to another is by
   A. Fax
   B. E-mail
   C. Cellular telephone
   D. Answering machine

8. Ischemia is
   A. An irregular heartbeat
   B. Dilation of the aorta
   C. Lack of blood flow to tissue
   D. Infection of the myocardium

9. A patient whose husband recently passed away comes into the office because of malaise. She is unkempt and weepy. She tells the medical assistant that she wishes she were dead. Which of the following would be the most sensitive response to this patient?
   A. "Please tell me more about those feelings."
   B. "Why is that?"
   C. "You need to talk to the doctor about this."
   D. "That's natural to feel that way after the death of a spouse."

10. Tingling in the hands, numbness in the arm, and frequent episodes of blurred vision are characteristic of
    A. An aneurysm
    B. Epilepsy
    C. Tourette's syndrome

D. Lou Gehrig's disease
E. Transient ischemic attack

11. Which of the following punctuation marks is used to indicate the exact words of the patient?
    A. Semicolon
    B. Comma
    C. Quotation marks
    D. Colon

12. A mucous membrane
    A. Lines closed cavities of the body
    B. Covers the lungs
    C. Lines the abdominal cavity
    D. Lines body cavities that open to the outside of the body

13. Which of the following is the most effective way of communicating with a patient who does not speak English?
    A. Speaking slowly and loudly
    B. Encouraging nonverbal communication
    C. Maintaining eye contact with the patient
    D. Putting messages in writing

14. Spermatozoa are produced in the
    A. Epididymis
    B. Seminiferous tubules
    C. Prostate gland
    D. Vas deferens

15. The bone located in the posterior of the skull is the
    A. Frontal
    B. Ethmoid
    C. Temporal
    D. Occipital

16. According to Maslow's hierarchy of needs, which of the following is the primary motivation for human behavior?
    A. Survival
    B. Safety
    C. Love
    D. Self-actualization

17. A failure of bone marrow to produce red blood cells results in which type of anemia?
    A. Aplastic
    B. Hemolytic
    C. Pernicious
    D. Microcytic

18. Which of the following is an example of an open-ended question?
    A. "Have you been staying on your diet?"
    B. "Did you have a nice trip?"

C. "Are you single or married?"
D. "Can you tell me more about that?"

19. *Res ipsa loquitur* is best illustrated by which of the following?
    A. A physician accidentally amputates the wrong finger from a patient
    B. A physician diagnoses lung cancer but the patient continues to smoke
    C. A physician prescribes the wrong medication for a patient
    D. A physician terminates care of a patient but does notify him or her in writing

20. Release of a patient's medical records without proper authorization might result in charges of
    A. Abandonment
    B. Invasion of privacy
    C. Defamation of character
    D. Negligence

21. The alpha cells in the pancreas are responsible for the production of
    A. Insulin
    B. Glucagon
    C. Hydrochloric acid
    D. Pepsin

22. These tiny projections on the surface of the small intestines increase the surface area and allow for greater absorption of nutrients.
    A. Rugae
    B. Villi
    C. Diverticula
    D. Omenta

23. Legally, a physician
    A. May not refuse treatment in an emergency situation
    B. May refuse to provide follow-up care after initial treatment
    C. Must provide a diagnosis to a patient's employer if requested
    D. Must provide a medical history to the patient's insurance company if the insurance company requests it
    E. May refuse to accept a patient if he or she chooses

24. Professionalism may best be displayed by
    A. Keeping emotions to self
    B. Staying calm when dealing with angry patients
    C. Showing no consideration for other members of the team
    D. Referring all problems to the physician
    E. Arriving late or leaving early

25. The combining form for *uterus* is
    A. Vagin/o
    B. Hyster/o
    C. Salping/o
    D. Oophor/o

26. Personality differences are due to
    A. Age
    B. Experience
    C. Heredity
    D. Environment
    E. All of the above

27. Which of the following is a segment of the large intestine?
    A. Pylorus
    B. Cecum
    C. Duodenum
    D. Jejunum

28. Blood that is low in oxygen exits the heart through the
    A. Aorta
    B. Pulmonary artery
    C. Pulmonary vein
    D. Inferior vena cava

29. Which of the following telephone calls should be given immediately to the physician?
    A. Another physician
    B. An angry patient
    C. A patient's family member
    D. An insurance company

30. If a patient refuses to consent to treatment, the medical assistant should
    A. Schedule the patient for another appointment
    B. Force treatment on the patient
    C. Force the patient to consent
    D. Delay treatment and inform or consult with the physician

31. Which of the following is most likely to reduce patient satisfaction with a medical practice?
    A. Explaining the risks and benefits of a procedure
    B. Discussing fees
    C. Overbooking
    D. Taking notes while interviewing the patient

32. Which of the following devices has the ability to digitize and convert images into an electronic format?
    A. A keyboard
    B. A monitor
    C. A printer
    D. A scanner

33. What is the monthly net income for a medical practice whose expenses are $8500, revenue is $14,130, total assets are $263,000, and liabilities are $53,000?
    A. $5630
    B. $22,630
    C. $39,000
    D. $210,000

34. The file folder label for Jennie Holmes-Mathis should be
    A. Jennie, Holmes-Mathis
    B. Mathis, Jennie Holmes
    C. Holmes-Mathis, Jennie
    D. Mathis, Jennie (nee Holmes)

35. The date must be changed daily on which of the following?
    A. Computer
    B. Transcriber
    C. Fax machine
    D. Postage meter

36. When the word *Confidential* is to be typed on the envelope, it should be placed
    A. In the lower right corner
    B. In the lower left corner
    C. Below the return address
    D. Both B and C

37. Which of the following may be used to replace a medical record that has temporarily been removed from the filing cabinet?
    A. 3 × 5 card
    B. An OUTguide
    C. A yellow Post-it note
    D. An empty file folder

38. When is the most appropriate time to discuss payment arrangements with a new patient?
    A. When the patient calls to make an appointment
    B. When the insurance form is processed
    C. When statements are sent out
    D. At the time of the first visit

39. A *tickler file* is
    A. A guide for processing insurance claims
    B. A list of procedures for equipment maintenance
    C. A type of color-coding
    D. Future events arranged in chronological order

40. A patient has had a left thyroid lobectomy performed. In preparing the insurance claim form, coding for which of the following body systems should be selected?
    A. Sensory
    B. Integumentary

C. Endocrine
D. Nervous

41. The amount of federal tax withheld is based on the employee's exemptions, pay period, and
    A. State income tax
    B. Employee's marital status
    C. Benefits offered by the employer
    D. Disability of the employee

42. Which of the following is an example of an indirect filing system?
    A. Alphabetical
    B. Chronological
    C. Numerical
    D. Subject

43. When creating an office policy manual, it should begin with
    A. The dress code
    B. The hierarchy chart
    C. Office hours
    D. The mission statement

44. Which of the following telephone calls requires immediate transfer to the physician?
    A. A young child with a high fever
    B. A patient with a possible medical allergy
    C. Another physician
    D. An adult with a low-grade fever

45. In the double-entry accounting system, an asset would be
    A. The amount owed to a creditor
    B. Properties owned by the business
    C. Money owed to the practice by patients
    D. The amount by which liabilities exceed the equity

46. Which of the following forms indicates an employee's withholding allowance?
    A. 1099
    B. W-2
    C. W-3
    D. W-4

47. The record of the proceedings of a meeting is the
    A. Agenda
    B. "Robert's Rules"
    C. Itinerary
    D. Minutes

48. The scheduling system based on scheduling similar appointments or procedures together is called
    A. Wave
    B. Modified wave

C. Grouping
D. Double-booking
E. Open scheduling

49. Which of the following is considered to be capital equipment?
    A. Coffee maker
    B. Laboratory coats
    C. Photocopier
    D. Trash cans

50. According to CPT, E&M codes begin with which of the following two digits?
    A. 93
    B. 95
    C. 97
    D. 99

51. Which of the following circumstances would waive the need for a written release of medical records?
    A. A subpoena
    B. Attorney request
    C. Hospital request
    D. Insurance company request

52. The correct way to indicate an enclosure notation is
    A. encl:
    B. Enclosure
    C. enclosure
    D. enc
    E. encl

53. Which of the following is the purpose of records management?
    A. Storage
    B. Arranging
    C. Accessibility
    D. Classifying
    E. All of the above

54. Which is not an indexing rule?
    A. Unit 1 is the surname
    B. A hyphen is disregarded
    C. Initials come after complete names
    D. Apostrophes are disregarded
    E. Names are divided into units

55. When selecting the E&M code for CPT coding, which of the following elements is required for all levels of the history?
    A. Chief complaint
    B. Family history
    C. Social history
    D. Medical history
    E. Review of systems

56. Which of the following taxes are paid entirely by the employer?
    A. Social security
    B. Health insurance
    C. Federal income tax
    D. State income tax
    E. Unemployment tax

57. A spreadsheet would be commonly used for which of the following?
    A. Word processing
    B. Appointment scheduling
    C. Electronic mailings
    D. Accounting
    E. Desktop publishing

58. An illness that existed before an insurance policy is written is known as a(n)
    A. Special risk
    B. Exclusion
    C. Preexisting condition
    D. Waiting period
    E. Prior authorization required

59. "Radial pulses are present bilaterally."
    When entering the above information in the medical record, under which of the following headings should it be entered?
    A. Reflexes
    B. Head and neck
    C. Extremities
    D. Chest
    E. Axilla

60. Which of the following allows data that are saved on a floppy disk or compact disk to be read but not altered?
    A. Clipboard
    B. *Save As*
    C. Write-protect
    D. Read-only memory
    E. Random-access memory

61. Which of the following is the most appropriate first step in correcting a misspelled word in a patient's medical record?
    A. Apply a thin covering of correction fluid over the error
    B. Circle the misspelled word in red
    C. Draw a single line through the misspelled word
    D. Completely erase the misspelled word
    E. Mark a red X through the misspelled word

62. How often must employee payroll taxes be reported to the Internal Revenue Service?
    A. Weekly
    B. Monthly
    C. Annually
    D. Biannually
    E. Quarterly

63. An elderly patient wishes to move into a facility where she can remain autonomous. To which of the following might the medical assistant refer this patient?
    A. An assisted living community
    B. A retirement complex with individual apartments
    C. An extended care facility
    D. A nursing home
    E. A rehabilitation hospital

64. An agent that prevents the growth, development, or proliferation of malignant cells is an
    A. Antitussive
    B. Antineoplastic
    C. Anticoagulant
    D. Antidepressant

65. A type of drug that increases urinary output is a(n)
    A. Emetic
    B. Diuretic
    C. Miotic
    D. Cathartic

66. The purpose of pouring off a small amount of a sterile solution from a container with a single cap is to
    A. Rinse contaminants from the lip of the bottle
    B. Avoid staining the label of the bottle
    C. Generate an even flow so the solution does not splash
    D. Expel air bubbles from the solution

67. A postprandial blood glucose level is measured after
    A. Drinking water
    B. Exercising
    C. Fasting
    D. Eating

68. When assisting with a sigmoidoscopy, which of the following would be most appropriate to wear?
    A. Laboratory coat and goggles
    B. Nonsterile gloves and goggles
    C. Nonsterile gloves, laboratory coat, and goggles
    D. Nonsterile gloves, laboratory coat, and mouth barrier

69. A cholecystogram is used to view the
    A. Urinary bladder
    B. Liver
    C. Gallbladder
    D. Kidneys

70. 1 cc is equivalent to
  A. 1 mL
  B. 5 mL
  C. 10 mL
  D. 20 mL

71. Which of the following laboratory values might indicate cardiac muscle injury?
  A. Alanine aminotransferase (ALT)
  B. Blood urea nitrogen (BUN)
  C. Creatine kinase (CK)
  D. Bilirubin

72. To cauterize a small lesion on the oral mucosa, the physician might use an applicator with
  A. Silver nitrate
  B. Alcohol
  C. Formalin
  D. Betadine

73. This type of microorganism appears as grapelike clusters when stained and viewed microscopically.
  A. Bacilli
  B. Cocci
  C. Staphylococci
  D. Streptococci

74. A hemoglobin value of 10 g/dL is approximately equivalent to a hematocrit of
  A. 10%
  B. 20%
  C. 30%
  D. 40%

75. The physician orders an intramuscular injection of meperidine (Demerol) 50 mg for pain relief. On hand is a 30-mL, multiple-dose vial of Demerol that contains 50 mg/mL. The medical assistant would administer
  A. 0.5 mL
  B. 1.0 mL
  C. 1.5 mL
  D. 2.0 mL

76. Sanitization
  A. Destroys all pathogenic microorganisms
  B. Destroys most pathogenic organisms
  C. Reduces the number of contaminants to a safe level
  D. Replaces defective instruments with new instruments

77. During manual audiometry, the patient should be positioned
  A. Facing away from the examiner
  B. Behind the examiner
  C. Facing the examiner
  D. Next to the examiner

78. Which of the following injuries is classified as a closed wound?
  A. Puncture
  B. Laceration
  C. Ecchymosis
  D. Avulsion

79. Proventil (albuterol) is classified as a(n)
  A. Antiinflammatory
  B. Antihistamine
  C. Antihypertensive
  D. Bronchodilator

80. Controlled substances that are considered to be illegal and of no medical use are classified as
  A. Schedule I
  B. Schedule II
  C. Schedule III
  D. Schedule IV
  E. Schedule V

81. Which of the following instructions should be given to a patient who needs to collect stool specimens for occult blood screening?
  A. Eat a high-carbohydrate diet for 48 hours before collection
  B. Fast for 12 hours before the collection
  C. Do not eat red meat for 48 hours before the collection
  D. Do not eat fats for 12 hours before the collection

82. This term is used to describe a variation in the size of erythrocytes.
  A. Anisocytosis
  B. Poikilocytosis
  C. Polychromic
  D. Leukocytosis

83. Which of the following substances in urine may indicate liver dysfunction?
  A. Albumin
  B. Glucose
  C. Ketones
  D. Urobilinogen

84. On a Gram stain, gram-negative bacteria will appear
  A. Blue
  B. Pink or red
  C. Green
  D. Purple

85. The abbreviation for *both ears* is
  A. AS
  B. AD
  C. AU
  D. BE

86. The correct injection technique used to place a tuberculin (Mantoux) skin test is
    A. Intradermal
    B. Intramuscular
    C. Intravenous
    D. Transdermal

87. A patient in the medical office has a nosebleed. Which of the following would be the most appropriate action to be taken first by the medical assistant?
    A. Apply ice to the patient's nose
    B. Call 911
    C. Tell the patient to lie down
    D. Tilt the patient's head forward

88. The first group of leads to be recorded on an electrocardiogram are the
    A. Augmented leads
    B. Leads I, II, and III
    C. aVR, aVL, and aVF
    D. Leads V1 through V3
    E. Leads V1 through V6

89. Which of the following is the most effective method to clean a drop of blood from a countertop?
    A. Iodine and sterile gauze
    B. 1:10 bleach solution
    C. Alcohol and sterile cotton ball
    D. Surgical soap and water

90. The drug order *2 gtt AD q4h prn* is translated as
    A. Two drops in both ears every 4 hours as needed
    B. Two drops in both eyes every 4 hours as desired
    C. Two drops in both ears four times a day
    D. Two drops in the left eye every 4 hours if needed

91. Which of the following additives should be used when drawing a specimen for a differential smear?
    A. EDTA
    B. Heparin
    C. Potassium oxalate
    D. Sodium citrate

92. Which of the following results on a urinalysis is abnormal?
    A. Color: yellow
    B. pH: 5.2
    C. Specific gravity: 1.005
    D. Leukocytes: ++

93. A sphygmomanometer is used to perform which of the following procedures?
    A. Assess hearing

B. Examine the rectum
C. Evaluate vision
D. Measure blood pressure

94. Which of the following methods is used to listen to heart, lung, and bowel sounds?
    A. Manipulation
    B. Auscultation
    C. Mensuration
    D. Percussion

95. Which of the following terms refers to the total amount of air that is exhaled from fully inflated lungs?
    A. Forced vital capacity
    B. Forced expiratory flow
    C. Forced expiratory volume in 1 second
    D. Tidal volume

96. During a Snellen visual acuity test, the patient should stand how many feet from the chart?
    A. 5
    B. 10
    C. 15
    D. 20

97. When performing an electrocardiogram, which of the following chest leads would be placed on the fifth intercostal space at the midclavicular line?
    A. V_1
    B. V_2
    C. V_3
    D. V_4
    E. V_5

98. To set up for an examination of a patient with vaginitis, all of the following would be used *except*
    A. Vaginal speculum
    B. Microscope slide
    C. KOH (potassium hydroxide)
    D. Cytologic fixative

99. Coumadin and heparin are classified as
    A. Anticoagulants
    B. Diuretics
    C. Vasoconstrictors
    D. Vasodilators

100. Which of the following needle length and gauge would the medical assistant choose to administer an intramuscular injection?
    A. 1 inch, 25 gauge
    B. 1½ inch, 22 gauge
    C. 1 inch, 18 gauge
    D. ½ inch, 22 gauge

Pre-Test 1 Answer Key

GENERAL

1. B Atrophy

RATIONALE: The prefix *a-* means without, lack of. The suffix *-trophy* means development.

2. C Myoblast

RATIONALE: The root word *myo-* means muscle. The suffix *-blast* means immature cell, form.

3. A AD

RATIONALE: *AD* is the abbreviation for right ear (auris dextra). *AS* is the abbreviation for left ear, *AU* for both ears, *OD* for right eye, and *OS* for left eye.

4. B Inspect the exterior ear canal

RATIONALE: An otoscope is a lighted instrument used to visually examine the outer ear and tympanic membrane.

5. D Thoracentesis

RATIONALE: A thoracentesis is the surgical puncture of the chest wall and pleural space. Fluid or air can then be withdrawn.

6. B Hematocrit and hemoglobin

RATIONALE: Anemia is a disorder characterized by a decrease in hemoglobin or a decrease in the total number of red blood cells.

7. C Endocrinologist

RATIONALE: Hyperparathyroidism is an abnormal endocrine condition in which an excess of parathyroid hormone is secreted. An endocrinologist diagnoses and treats diseases and disorders of the endocrine system.

8. D Leukocytosis

RATIONALE: Leukocytosis is an increase in the total number of circulating white blood cells. *Leuko-* refers to white, *-cyt* refers to cells, and *-osis* is an abnormal condition.

9. A Hyperpnea

RATIONALE: Hyperpnea is deep or rapid breathing. The prefix *hyper-* means above. The root word *-pnea* refers to breathing.

10. D -algia

RATIONALE: The suffix *-algia* means pain or painful condition.

11. C -plasty

RATIONALE: The suffix *-plasty* means surgical repair.

12. C Breast

RATIONALE: A mammogram is an x-ray film of the soft tissue of the breast. The root word *mammo-* refers to breast. The suffix *-gram* refers to a record (x-ray).

13. D Baldness

RATIONALE: Alopecia is the partial or complete lack of hair, which can be caused by normal aging, an endocrine disorder, chemotherapy, or a skin disease.

14. A Mastication

RATIONALE: Mastication is the chewing, tearing, or grinding of food with the teeth while it becomes mixed with saliva.

15. E Mole on the inside of the elbow

RATIONALE: A nevus is a mole. The antecubital area is located on the inner aspect of the elbow.

16. D Arthritis

RATIONALE: The root word *arth-* means joint. The suffix *-itis* means inflammation.

17. B Adipose tissue

RATIONALE: Adipose tissue is made up of fat cells arranged in globules. It is found under the skin and serves as a reserve energy source and for insulation.

18. C Pathology

RATIONALE: Pathology is the study of the characteristics, causes, and effects of disease on the structure and function of the body.

19. C Smelling

RATIONALE: The olfactory nerve, cranial nerve I, is one of two pairs of nerves associated with the sense of smell.

20. **B** Ovaries
RATIONALE: An oophorectomy is the surgical removal of one or both ovaries. The root word *oophor-* means ovary. The suffix *-ectomy* means surgical removal.

21. **C** Urology
RATIONALE: Urology is the branch of medicine concerned with the urinary tract in men and women, as well as the male genital tract. The physician who specializes in urology is a urologist.

22. **D** Cystoscopy
RATIONALE: Cystoscopy is the direct visualization of the urinary tract and bladder by means of a cystoscope inserted into the urethra.

23. **A** Urticaria
RATIONALE: Urticaria is a pruritic skin eruption characterized by wheals (hives) of various shapes and sizes. This condition can be caused by allergic reactions to drugs, insect bites, and foods.

24. **C** Pericardium
RATIONALE: The pericardium is the serous membrane that surrounds the heart.

25. **D** Lines body cavities that open to the outside
RATIONALE: A mucous membrane lines body cavities or spaces of the body that open to the outside, including the mouth, digestive tract, respiratory tract, and genitourinary tract.

26. **D** Anterior
RATIONALE: The ventral area of the body is toward the front of the body (anterior).

27. **C** Abdominal
RATIONALE: The abdominal cavity is part of the ventral cavity of the body. It contains the stomach, small and large intestines, spleen, liver, gallbladder, and pancreas.

28. **C** Adduction
RATIONALE: Adduction is the movement of a limb or body part toward the body.

29. **A** Frontal
RATIONALE: The frontal plane is the vertical plane that divides the body or a structure into anterior and posterior portions.

30. **A** Can follow a viral illness in children
RATIONALE: Reye's syndrome is an acute and sometimes fatal illness characterized by fatty invasion of internal organs and swelling of the brain. The cause is unknown, but the condition has been linked to the use of aspirin and viral illnesses in children.

31. **C** Lumbar
RATIONALE: The vertebral column is divided into five sections: (1) cervical (neck), (2) thoracic (chest), (3) lumbar (lower back), (4) sacral (below the lumbar), and (5) coccygeal (tailbone).

32. **A** Impetigo
RATIONALE: Impetigo is an infection of the skin caused by staphylococci, streptococci, or a combination of the two. The lesions usually begin around the mouth and nose and spread locally. The lesions blister and crust.

33. **D** Occipital
RATIONALE: The occipital bone of the skull is located at the back of the skull. It articulates with the two parietal bones and contains the foramen magnum (opening for the spinal cord).

34. **C** Greenstick fracture
RATIONALE: A greenstick fracture is an incomplete fracture. The bone is bent but fractured only on the outer arc of the bend.

35. **E** 31
RATIONALE: The peripheral nervous system is made up of the motor and sensory nerves and ganglia located outside the brain and spinal cord. It consists of 12 pairs of cranial nerves and 31 pairs of spinal nerves.

36. **A** Brainstem
RATIONALE: The brainstem is the portion of the brain made up of the midbrain, pons, and medulla. It performs sensory, motor, and reflex functions. Vital centers that regulate internal body functions are located here.

37. **A** Aplastic
RATIONALE: Aplastic anemia results from a failure of blood cell production resulting from the failure of bone marrow to produce cells. The cause is unknown.

38. **C** Hiatal hernia
RATIONALE: A hernia is the abnormal protrusion of an organ or tissue through the structures that normally contain it. A hiatal hernia is the protrusion of the upper portion of the stomach upward through the esophageal opening in the diaphragm.

39. **D** Eardrum
RATIONALE: The tympanic membrane is the membrane between the external and middle ear. It is commonly called the eardrum.

40. **D** Aorta
RATIONALE: The aorta is the main trunk of the systemic arterial circulation. Blood is pumped out of the left ventricle through the aortic valve into the aorta. The aorta then branches and carries blood throughout the body.

41. **C** Is the pacemaker of the heart
RATIONALE: The sinoatrial node of the heart is located in the right atrium. The electrical impulse that initiates the heartbeat originates here.

42. **B** Radius and ulna
RATIONALE: The radius is the lateral lower arm bone on line with the thumb. The ulna is the medial lower arm bone.

43. E All of the above
RATIONALE: Involuntary (smooth) muscle is muscle that is not under a person's conscious or voluntary control. These muscles actions include muscles of the heart and muscles of the intestines, stomach, and other visceral organs.

44. A Liver
RATIONALE: The right upper quadrant of the abdominopelvic area contains the liver, gallbladder, part of the pancreas, and parts of the small and large intestines.

45. D Phrenic
RATIONALE: The diaphragm is stimulated by the phrenic nerve from the cervical plexus. The diaphragm aids in respiration by moving up and down.

46. C Scoliosis
RATIONALE: Scoliosis is a lateral curvature of the spine commonly seen in children. Unequal heights of hips and shoulders may be a sign of this condition.

47. B Glucagon
RATIONALE: Glucagon is a hormone produced by the alpha cells in the islets of Langerhans in the pancreas. It stimulates the conversion of glycogen to glucose in the liver.

48. C Cholecystectomy
RATIONALE: The root word *cholecyst-* means gallbladder. The suffix *-ectomy* means surgical removal.

49. E Optic
RATIONALE: The optic nerve (cranial nerve II) is a sensory nerve that is involved with the sense of vision.

50. D 32
RATIONALE: The deciduous (baby) teeth are replaced by 32 adult (permanent) teeth. These adult teeth include four central incisors, lateral incisors, cuspids, first and second premolars, first molars, second molars, and third molars (wisdom teeth).

51. E May refuse to accept a patient if he or she chooses
RATIONALE: Physicians have the right to determine whom they will accept as patients. Patient load may be as large as one person can adequately care for, and the decision may be made to limit new patients.

52. D Is a detailed outline of a trip
RATIONALE: An itinerary is detailed information about a trip. It includes the date and time of departure; flight numbers; mode of transportation to hotel; name, address, and telephone number of hotel; and the date and time of return.

53. B Staying calm when dealing with angry patients
RATIONALE: Professional qualities that a medical assistant must have include a friendly and pleasant attitude, ability to maintain confidentiality, courtesy, ability to control temper, consideration, respect and kindness, dependability, and accuracy.

54. B Empathy
RATIONALE: Empathy is the ability to recognize the emotions and state of mind of another person.

55. B The physician
RATIONALE: The physician owns the medical record, but the patient owns the information contained in the record.

56. A Denial
RATIONALE: Denial is the unconscious avoidance of the reality of an unpleasant or disturbing situation.

57. E All of the above
RATIONALE: Personality is the pattern of behavior each person develops as a means of adapting to a particular environment and its standards. Age, life experiences, heredity, and environment all play a part in this development.

58. B Impatience
RATIONALE: The professional services of a medical assistant are extremely personal, and the manner in which these services are performed can affect the health and well-being of the patient. An impatient person might negatively affect the patient.

59. E Young children react differently to stressful situations
RATIONALE: Stereotyping is a preconceived generalized belief. Young children do react differently to stressful situations than adults react.

60. C The patient must sign a release form
RATIONALE: The patient must sign a release of information form before information from the medical record can be released to anyone. This precaution preserves the patient's confidentiality.

61. E Human immunodeficiency virus
RATIONALE: The physician has a legal duty to report communicable diseases to the county health department. This requirement helps the state provide for the public's health, safety, and welfare.

62. B Vital signs
RATIONALE: Objective data are data that are determined in some way by someone other than the patient, such as the physician or medical assistant. Vital signs are considered to be objective.

63. A Another physician
RATIONALE: A call from another physician or professional colleague should be transferred to the physician immediately.

64. C Social need
RATIONALE: Maslow believed that lower-level needs must be satisfied before higher-level needs can be satisfied. These levels, from lowest to highest, include physiologic needs, safety needs, social needs, self-esteem needs, and self-actualization needs.

65. D   Delay treatment and inform or consult with the physician
RATIONALE: A physician must have consent to treat a patient even though this consent is usually implied. A physician who fails to secure some formal type of consent might be charged with assault and battery or trespass.

66. E   All of the above
RATIONALE: A contract is an agreement that creates an obligation. To be valid or enforceable, the contract must have four basic elements: (1) an offer and acceptance, (2) consideration, (3) capacity, and (4) legality.

67. D   Posterior
RATIONALE: The anterior of a structure is the front of the structure. The posterior of a structure is the back of the structure.

68. E   All of the above
RATIONALE: Informed consent must be obtained from the patient when a complex procedure is to be performed. Informed consent implies an understanding of what is to be done, why it should be done, the risks involved, the expected outcomes, and alternative treatments, including consequences of failure to treat.

69. E   Providing atypical care
RATIONALE: The license to practice medicine may be revoked or suspended under certain circumstances. Grounds for revoking or suspending a license generally falls within one of three categories: (1) conviction of a crime, (2) unprofessional conduct, and (3) personal and professional incapacity.

70. C   Nucleus
RATIONALE: The nucleus is the control center of every cell. It contains DNA, which is the genetic material.

71. E   All of the above
RATIONALE: The subcutaneous tissue is a layer of connective tissue found between the skin and the deep fascia. It contains a fatty layer. Hypodermic injections into this tissue are usually on the upper arm, thigh, or abdomen.

72. B   Humerus
RATIONALE: The humerus is the largest bone of the upper arm. The femur is the bone of the thigh; the tibia and fibula make up the lower leg; the metatarsals form the arch of the foot.

73. A   Deltoid
RATIONALE: The deltoid is a large, thick, triangular muscle that covers the shoulder.

74. B   Sinoatrial node
RATIONALE: The sinoatrial node is a cluster of specialized cells located in the right atrial wall of the heart. It generates impulses that travel throughout the muscle fibers of the atria and cause them to contract.

75. E   Alveoli
RATIONALE: The alveoli are small saclike structures at the terminal ends of the bronchioles. They are the functional units of respiration and are composed of a single layer of epithelium, which allows oxygen and carbon dioxide to be easily exchanged with the surrounding capillaries.

76. E   All of the above
RATIONALE: The liver is the largest gland of the body. Its main functions include production of bile, detoxification of toxins and wastes, metabolism of proteins and carbohydrates, storage of vitamins and glycogen, production of heparin, and recycling of worn-out red blood cells.

77. B   Endometrium
RATIONALE: The endometrium is the innermost layer of the uterus. The fertilized ovum implants into this layer where it develops until delivery.

78. B   Testes
RATIONALE: Testosterone, the male hormone, is manufactured in the interstitial cells of the testes.

79. A   Cerebrum
RATIONALE: The cerebrum is the largest portion of the brain. It is divided into two hemispheres, which are further divided into lobes. Its outer surface (cortex) is made up of gray matter.

80. E   31
RATIONALE: There are 31 pairs of spinal nerves that are connected to the spinal cord. They are numbered according to the vertebra from which they emerge.

81. A   Mouth
RATIONALE: The gustatory sense is the sense of taste. The receptors are located on the tongue within papillae (taste buds).

82. D   Decreases blood sugar levels
RATIONALE: Insulin is a hormone manufactured by the beta cells in the pancreas. Its main function is to metabolize glucose and thus reduce blood sugar levels.

83. E   Leukopenia
RATIONALE: Leukopenia is an abnormal decrease in the number of white blood cells to fewer than 5000 cells/mm^3 of blood. The root word *leuko-* means white, or white blood cell. The suffix *-penia* means a decrease.

84. B   stat
RATIONALE: The term *stat* is the abbreviation for *statim*, meaning immediately.

85. E   All of the above
RATIONALE: The physician has a legal duty to report information that may have an effect on the health, safety, or welfare of the public. This information includes births, deaths, communicable diseases, abuse, criminal acts, and professional misconduct.

86. **A** Slow

RATIONALE: The prefix *brady-* means slow.

87. **C** Deep

RATIONALE: Superficial pertains to the skin or another surface. *Deep* refers to away from the surface.

88. **C** An advance directive

RATIONALE: An advance directive is a legal document that gives persons the right to determine what medical procedures they want provided if they become unable to make those decisions.

89. **B** Denial

RATIONALE: Unconscious defense mechanisms help protect the mind from guilt or anxiety. Denial is the unconscious avoidance of the reality of an unpleasant or disturbing feeling, thought, or event.

90. **A** An open-ended statement

RATIONALE: An open-ended statement or question helps the patient decide what is relevant. It also encourages the patient to continue the discussion.

91. **C** Etiology

RATIONALE: Etiology is the study of all factors that may be involved in the development of a disease. This area can include the susceptibility of the patient, the nature of the disease-causing agent, and the way the agent invades the patient's body.

92. **E** All of the above

RATIONALE: Nonverbal communications are messages conveyed without the use of words. They are transmitted by body language. Body language involves grooming, dress, eye contact, facial expression, hand gestures, space, tone of voice, posture, and touch.

93. **B** An eating disorder

RATIONALE: Bulimia is an insatiable craving for food characterized by binge eating and self-induced vomiting.

94. **D** Stroke

RATIONALE: A cerebrovascular accident, or brain attack, is an abnormal condition of the blood vessels of the brain characterized by an occlusion that results in an ischemia of the brain tissue. Paralysis, weakness, speech defect, aphasia, or death may occur.

95. **D** Measles

RATIONALE: Measles (rubeola) is an acute, highly contagious viral infection. It involves the respiratory tract and is characterized by a spreading cutaneous rash. It is caused by the paramyxovirus and is transmitted by droplets.

96. **C** Trichomoniasis

RATIONALE: Trichomoniasis is a vaginal infection caused by the protozoan *Trichomonas vaginalis*. It is transmitted by sexual intercourse.

97. **E** Potassium

RATIONALE: Potassium is necessary to the life of all animals. It is the major intracellular cation and helps regulate neuromuscular excitability and muscle contraction.

98. **B** Emphysema

RATIONALE: Emphysema is an abnormal condition of the pulmonary system. It is characterized by overinflation and destructive changes of the alveoli, which results in a loss of lung elasticity and a decreased gas exchange.

99. **C** Mucous

RATIONALE: A mucous membrane is a major kind of body membrane that covers or lines cavities or canals that open to the outside of the body.

100. **E** Compound fracture

RATIONALE: An open or compound fracture is one in which the broken end of the bone tears open the skin.

Pre-Test 2 Answer Key

ADMINISTRATIVE

1. E Grouping

RATIONALE: Grouping is the practice of scheduling patients with the same type of examination (e.g., complete physicals), conditions (e.g., pregnancy), or procedures (e.g., Papanicolaou [Pap] smears) within a certain time frame.

2. C Envelope marked *Personal*

RATIONALE: Incoming mail should be sorted according to importance and urgency. The order of importance is the physician's personal mail, ordinary first-class mail, periodicals and newspapers, and lastly, all other pieces.

3. B Absence of punctuation after the salutation and a comma after the complimentary close

RATIONALE: Open punctuation style uses no punctuation at the end of any line outside of the body of the letter unless the line ends with an abbreviation. This type of punctuation is used with the simplified block letter style.

4. D Medicaid

RATIONALE: Medicaid is a federally funded insurance program that was set up by the federal government in 1965 to provide for the medically indigent. It is regulated by each state.

5. C Posting

RATIONALE: Posting is the transfer of information from one record to another. Transactions are posted from the day sheet to the ledger.

6. B An alphabetic cross-reference

RATIONALE: Numeric filing involves filing records, correspondence, or cards by number. It is an indirect filing system and requires the use of an alphabetical cross-reference to find a given file.

7. D Holmes-Mathis, Jennie

RATIONALE: Hyphenated elements of a name, whether first name, middle name, or surname, are considered as one unit.

8. C Physician, patient, and insurance company

RATIONALE: A third-party payor is some entity other than the patient, spouse, or parent who is responsible for paying all or part of the patient's medical costs.

9. E All of the above

RATIONALE: If a claim form is not sufficiently detailed, complete, and accurate, then the insurance company may reject the claim. Reasons for claim rejection might include missing or incomplete diagnosis; incorrectly coded diagnosis; charges not itemized; patient's group, member, or policy number missing; patient signature missing; patient's date of birth missing; dates missing or incorrect; and physician's signature missing.

10. D $0.84

RATIONALE: The first ounce would cost $0.34, and the two additional ounces would total $0.50 ($0.34 + $0.50 = $0.84).

11. D Below the return address

RATIONALE: Any notation on the envelope directed toward the addressee, such as *Personal* or *Confidential*, should be typed and underlined on the third line below the return address. It should be aligned with the return address on the left edge of the envelope.

12. A Very truly yours

RATIONALE: The complimentary close is the writer's way of saying "good-bye." The words used are determined by the formality used in the salutation.

13. D Insurance information

RATIONALE: The patient's insurance information is obtained at the time of the first visit to the office. Necessary information includes the patient's name, telephone number, reason for coming to the office, and times available for the appointment.

14. B Conference call

RATIONALE: A conference call allows more than two people to participate in a conversation at one time. Each person can hear or talk to all others who are participating.

15. C Backing up

RATIONALE: A backup is a tape or disk for storage of files to prevent their loss in the event of hard drive failure.

16. E Future events arranged in chronologic order

RATIONALE: A tickler file is a chronologic file used as a reminder that something must be done on a certain date. This type of file is frequently used as a follow-up method.

17. A Diarrhea

RATIONALE: CPT is a listing of descriptive terms and identifying codes used for reporting medical services and procedures performed by the physician. All of the choices are procedures except diarrhea.

18. E All of the above

RATIONALE: The receptionist is usually the first person in the medical office with whom the patient has contact. The appearance, professionalism, attitude, and manners of the receptionist, as well as the appearance of the reception area as a whole, can influence the patient's perception of the entire practice.

19. C See also

RATIONALE: *See also* is the coding convention that gives the direction to the coder to consider another code.

20. C Refers to factors that influence health status

RATIONALE: V-codes (V01 through V82) are codes referring to factors that influence health status. A definite diagnosis is not stated, but a valid reason for seeking medical care exists. Reasons can include annual physical examinations, well-baby checks, and preoperative physicals. These codes are part of the ICD-9-CM coding system.

21. D Resealed with tape and noted as *opened in error*

RATIONALE: All offices should have a procedure to follow regarding incoming mail. Personal mail should be left unopened. Should it be opened in error, fold and replace it inside the envelope, reseal the envelope, and write across the outside *opened in error* followed by the opener's initials.

22. E All of the above

RATIONALE: E&M descriptors include basic diagnostic and treatment services such as office visits and physical examinations. These descriptors are part of the CPT coding system.

23. B Medicare

RATIONALE: A third-party payor is any person, insurance company, or government agent other than the patient or the patient's family who pays the patient's account.

24. C A numbered list of present problems

RATIONALE: The POMR system is designed to organize the patient's medical record and the information it contains. The system uses four parts: (1) the database, (2) the problem list, (3) the treatment plan, and (4) the progress notes. The database includes the chief complaint, present illness or illnesses, and the patient profile.

25. D Ledger card totals and account-receivable balance

RATIONALE: A trial balance is a method of checking the accuracy of accounts. It should be done once a month after all posting has been completed and before preparing monthly statements. The purpose of a trial balance is to disclose any discrepancies between the ledger cards and accounts receivable. It does not prove the accuracy of the accounts.

26. C Newest to the front

RATIONALE: The medical record is a chronologic system for recording a patient's medical care. Its continuity ensures the best medical care. By filing the most current information to the front, it provides a quick current reference of the patient's care and management.

27. C Another physician

RATIONALE: The person answering the telephone is expected to screen all incoming calls. Good judgment in deciding whether to put through a call comes with experience. Calls from other physicians should be put through at once if the physician is available to take the call.

28. D In consecutive order without large gaps

RATIONALE: Appointment scheduling is the process that determines which patients will be seen by the provider, dates and times of the appointments, and how much time will be allotted to each patient based on the complaint and the availability of the provider. Most providers find that efficient scheduling and time management is one of the most important factors in the success of the practice.

29. E Diagnosis

RATIONALE: At an initial visit, the patient's diagnosis may not be made. At the first visit, the patient may complete a patient information form that will include name, address, telephone number, insurance information, business information, and referral information.

30. A 8 ½ × 11; no. 10 envelope

RATIONALE: A standard-size letter (8 ½ × 11 in) is used for general business and professional correspondence. Standard ways of folding and inserting letters are used so the letter fits properly and is easy to remove. A size no. 10 envelope is used for a standard-size letter.

31. C In a separate ledger file

RATIONALE: A ledger card is prepared for each patient (or family) at the time of the first visit. It is the record of all charges and payments for each patient and is kept in a separate file for ease of access and billing purposes.

32. A The checkbook

RATIONALE: A bank statement is periodically sent by the bank to the customer. It shows the status of the account on a given date. The bank statement balance and the checkbook balance should be the same or they will need to be reconciled (disclosure of any errors in the checkbook or bank statement).

33. D Minutes

RATIONALE: The record of the proceedings of a meeting is called the *minutes*. The minutes contain a record of what was done at a meeting, not what was said by the members. Minutes should be signed by the secretary and kept on file according to the procedure of the organization.

34. C Backing up

RATIONALE: Backing up is the process of using a tape, floppy disk, or compact disk for storage of files to prevent their loss in the event of hard drive failure.

35. C Grouping

RATIONALE: Grouping or clustering allows the provider to make good use of time by seeing patients with the same needs at the same time. An example of grouping may be that the provider only performs complete physical examinations on Wednesday mornings.

36. A Information about the scope of the practice

RATIONALE: Each office should have an attractive brochure that can be used to welcome new patients and to furnish general information about the practice. This brochure can include name and type of practice; name or names of physicians; address and location map; appointment procedures; office hours; comments on billing, charges, and insurance; and a statement concerning the confidentiality of medical records. Any more specific information should be discussed with the appropriate person.

37. B W-4 Form

RATIONALE: The W-4 Form is the Employee's Withholding Allowance Certificate. It is filled out by the employee and allows him or her to determine the number of withholding allowances.

38. D HGB

RATIONALE: The correct abbreviation for hemoglobin is Hgb.

39. C Invasion of privacy

RATIONALE: Invasion of privacy is the act of divulging patient information that has been acquired through privileged interaction (provider-patient communication) without the consent of the patient, which is an intentional tort. Information shared between the provider and the patient is confidential. A release of information form must be signed before this information can be shared.

40. A Omission of all punctuation

RATIONALE: The U.S. Postal Service attempts to read, code, sort, and cancel all mail electronically. The success of this system depends on the correct format that can be read by the automatic equipment. This format includes all addresses typed in block format in the correct area of the envelope, everything in the address capitalized, all punctuation eliminated, states abbreviated using the standard two-letter code, and ZIP code must be included in the last line.

41. B A subpoena

RATIONALE: A *subpoena duces tecum* is an order to provide records or documents to the court. Authority to release information from the medical record lies solely with the patient unless required by law.

42. B Daily log

RATIONALE: The double-entry system provides a comprehensive picture of the medical practice and its effect on the physician's net worth. It requires skill and time and is not frequently used in a small practice. The medical assistant generally maintains only the daily log.

43. B Enclosure

RATIONALE: The enclosure notation identifies any material that may be accompanying the correspondence. The notation is placed two lines below the signature line. If more than one enclosure is included, then specify the number (e.g., Enclosures 2).

44. A Insurance claim

RATIONALE: A superbill is a combination charge slip, statement, and insurance reporting form. It is completed and given to the patient at each visit.

45. E All of the above

RATIONALE: Complete and accurate records are essential to a well-managed medical practice. Health information management includes not only the assembling of the record, but also having an efficient system for saving, retrieving, protecting, transferring, storing, retaining, and destroying these records.

46. B *International Classification of Diseases,* ninth edition, Clinical Modification (ICD-9-CM)

RATIONALE: ICD-9-CM is the coding system used to code diagnosis or disease conditions. CPT, HCPCS, RVS, and RBRVS are systems used to code medical procedures.

47. C Initials come before complete names

RATIONALE: Indexing rules are standardized and are based on current business practices. The rule that applies to initials states, "that initials precede a name beginning with the same letter." For example, the chart for M. Johnson would be filed before the chart for Mary Johnson.

48. E V-codes

RATIONALE: V codes (V01 to V82) are the codes that refer to factors that influence the health status of the patient. A definite diagnosis cannot be stated, but a valid reason for seeing the provider exists (e.g., well-baby check-up, annual physical examination).

49. B Bit

RATIONALE: A bit is a binary digit. It is the smallest piece of information that can be processed by a computer.

50. D Directory

RATIONALE: The directory is the index of files on a disk. It shows the names of the documents that are saved on that disk. The operator can then choose a file and open it.

51. E B and C only

RATIONALE: The scheduling system chosen by the facility must be individualized for each specific practice. Important factors that determine the best system include patient need, physician preferences and habits, and the facilities available.

52. B Mixed punctuation

RATIONALE: Mixed (standard) punctuation is appropriate for use with block or modified block letter styles. It places a colon after the salutation and a comma after the complimentary closing. It is the most commonly used punctuation pattern.

53. C Operating manuals

RATIONALE: An inventory of all capital items (equipment) should be prepared every year. For each item, the name, serial number, date of purchase, price, and any warranty information are included. Operating manuals should be kept separate and readily accessible.

54. B Operative notes

RATIONALE: Operative notes are considered to be part of the physician's records and can only be released by the physician. Nurse's notes, laboratory reports, radiology reports, and billing are hospital-generated documents and belong to the institution.

55. C Preexisting condition

RATIONALE: A preexisting condition is a physical condition of a person that existed before the insurance policy was issued.

56. D Inactive files

RATIONALE: Inactive files generally are those of patients whom the provider has not seen for 6 months or longer. When the patient returns for care, his or her chart is moved to the active file.

57. A Patient confidentiality

RATIONALE: The patient is entitled to complete confidentiality with regard to his or her medical records and release of information. Computer technology allows for the gathering and storage of vast amounts of information. This information can then be accessible to a variety of individuals. The monitor displays information and should be positioned away from others that may be at the desk.

58. E All of the above

RATIONALE: All patients should be escorted to the examination or treatment room. All patients are generally more cooperative and less anxious if they understand what is expected of them.

59. B Name of the assisting physician

RATIONALE: Surgery is scheduled by type of procedure and availability of facilities. Important information includes the name of the procedure, expected length of the procedure in hours, type of anesthesia, and the patient's name, age, and telephone number.

60. B A copy of the letter is sent to Dr. Jones

RATIONALE: The copy notation (c:) indicates that a copy of the document was sent to a third party or parties. The notation is placed one to two lines below the enclosure notation.

61. A Results of laboratory tests

RATIONALE: The history and physical are valuable tools in diagnosis. They are a way for the physician to gather information about the physical and psychological condition of the patient. The history is the record of the information provided by the patient. The physical involves a thorough examination of the patient from head to toe. Laboratory tests may be ordered after the physical if needed for diagnosis.

62. B Accept predetermined fees

RATIONALE: Managed care is a type of prepaid health plan. It was developed to provide health care services at a low cost. Managed care includes Health Maintenance Organizations (HMOs) and Independent Practice Associations (IPAs). The traditional HMO builds a group of physicians who agree to be paid on a per-patient basis instead of a fee-for-service basis.

63. D Preferred provider organization

RATIONALE: The preferred provider organization uses a fee-for-service concept. Providers agree on a predetermined list of charges for all services. Care is not prepaid. The patient must pay deductibles.

64. A Cost of services

RATIONALE: E&M codes include basic diagnostic and treatment services such as office visits and examinations. The type of history, the type of examination, and the complexity of medical decision making must be determined to select the correct code properly.

65. E Deposit slip

RATIONALE: Deposit slips are itemized documents of cash, checks, and other funds that a depositor presents to the bank with the items to be credited to an account. All deposits must be accompanied by a deposit slip. A copy of the slip is kept on file.

66. D Patient's surname

RATIONALE: One system of color-coding files is the alphabetical color-coding system. This system uses different colored tabs to represent a different segment of the alphabet. The chart is coded by the patient's last name (surname).

67. B The patient

RATIONALE: The physician owns the medical record, but the patient owns the information contained in the record. Any information concerning the contents of the medical record requires consent from both the patient and the physician before it can be released.

68. C Times not available

RATIONALE: To develop the matrix in the appointment book, block out the times the physician or physicians will be unavailable. All else revolves around the physicians' availability.

69. D Group scheduling

RATIONALE: Grouping is scheduling similar appointments together during a day. For example, all complete physical examinations are scheduled for Friday morning. This type of scheduling is a method of time management.

70. A Extensive editing capability

RATIONALE: The computer, as a document production tool, permits efficient preparation and editing of written documents. Spell-check and column layout are simply added benefits. Storage capacity relates to the computer as a whole and is not specific to word processing.

71. A Insurance coverage is available

RATIONALE: Certified mail requires the receiver's signature as proof of delivery and receipt. Any mail in which first-class postage is paid can be accepted as certified mail.

72. D Personal letters and postcards

RATIONALE: First-class mail includes sealed or unsealed handwritten or typed material, such as letters, postcards, and business reply mail. A variety of mailing options is available for other mailable materials.

73. E   The estate is billed

RATIONALE: Estate claims are made against the estate of a deceased patient. Once the office receives notification of the patient's death, the office must submit a claim for the unpaid balance to the administrator of the estate. Each state has different rules and regulations concerning the filing of estate claims.

74. A   Immediately

RATIONALE: Endorsement is a signature or writing on the back of a check by which the endorser transfers all rights of the check to another party. All checks received as payments should be restrictively endorsed (for deposit only) immediately to safeguard against loss or theft.

75. E   Andrew Stephen

RATIONALE: In alphabetic filing, a person's name is indexed with the surname as unit 1, the given name as unit 2, and the middle name as unit 3. Names are alphabetized according to the first unit letter by letter.

76. E   David Roberts, M.D.

RATIONALE: The inside address includes the name, title, and address of the receiver. When addressing a letter to a physician, omit the courtesy title, and type the physician's name followed by his or her academic degree.

77. E   A license must be obtained from the post office

RATIONALE: A postage meter is an efficient way of stamping large amounts of mail. Postage is prepaid and applied directly to the envelope or on adhesive strips. The other choices are all true about postage meters.

78. B   NE

RATIONALE: The use of standard two-letter abbreviations aids in the reading, coding, sorting, and canceling of the mail. The U.S. Postal Service has issued a list of two-letter state abbreviations to be used with ZIP codes. None of the other choices represent a U.S. state abbreviation.

79. C   Full block style

RATIONALE: The full block style places all lines flush at the left margin. The other choices vary indentation of the margin or margins.

80. C   Complimentary close

RATIONALE: A memorandum is a written communication among persons within an office or organization. It uses guide words that indicate the date, sender, receiver or receivers, and subject.

81. C   Name, page number, and date

RATIONALE: The second and continuous pages of a letter or report are placed on plain paper that matches the letterhead in weight, color, and fiber content. The heading of the subsequent pages must contain the name of the addressee, page number, and date.

82. A   Two

RATIONALE: The complimentary close is placed on the second line below the last line of the body of the letter.

83. D   Physician charges

RATIONALE: A fee profile is established by compiling and averaging the usual charges for services of the physician over a given period. This profile is then used to determine the amount of third-party liability.

84. B   Date of birth

RATIONALE: Demographics relate to the statistical characteristics of a population. It includes the name, date of birth, marital status, children, occupation, education, and social information of the patient.

85. D   Irritable bowel syndrome

RATIONALE: ICD-9-CM assigns numeric codes to diseases, illnesses, injuries, and health-related conditions. The coding system is used to establish medical necessity to facilitate payment for health care services and to translate written terminology or descriptions into numbers to provide a universal common language.

86. B   1:00 pm

RATIONALE: The United States is divided into four time zones: (1) Pacific time (WA, OR, NV, and CA), (2) Mountain time (MT, UT, ID, WY, CO, NM, AZ, and parts of ND, SD, NE, and KS), (3) Central time (MN, WI, IA, MO, AR, OK, TX, LA, MS, IL, AL, and parts of TN, KY, ND, SD, NE, and KS), and (4) Eastern time (all others). Central, Mountain, and Pacific time zones are 1 or more hours behind Eastern time. Pacific time is 3 hours behind Eastern time; when it is 1:00 Pacific time, it is 4:00 Eastern time.

87. B   Third ring

RATIONALE: If possible, the telephone should be answered on the first ring and always by the third ring.

88. A   Refers to external causes

RATIONALE: An E-code is a classification of ICD-9-CM coding. It is used to describe environmental events, circumstances, and conditions as the external cause of injury, poisoning, and other adverse effects.

89. D   CMS-1500

RATIONALE: The CMS-1500 is a universal claim form developed by the HCFA that standardizes the data required by most insurance carriers to process insurance claims.

90. D   At the end of the day

RATIONALE: Patients who are habitually late for appointments should be scheduled at the end of the day so as not to disrupt the workflow.

91. C   Draw a single line through the error, write the word *error*, make the correction, and date and initial the entry

RATIONALE: Corrections are made in the medical record by drawing a single line through the error, writing the word *error* next to it, making the correction, and dating and initialing the correction (SLIDE rule).

92. D   Problem-oriented progress notes

RATIONALE: SOAP is an organized way of charting progress notes. SOAP stands for *subjective, objective, assessment,* and *plan.*

93. A A referral to another physician

RATIONALE: The physician must notify the patient of his or her intention to terminate the relationship to protect the physician against abandonment. The physician is not required to refer to another physician.

94. E Should be squeezed in for a brief visit so the physician can decide what the next treatment step should be

RATIONALE: If the patient requires immediate attention, then he or she should be accommodated. If the patient does not need immediate care, then a brief visit with the physician and a scheduled appointment at a later date may be the best policy. The patient should be told that the office runs on an appointment basis.

95. B Immediately offer a new appointment time

RATIONALE: Attempt to reschedule the appointment while the patient is on the telephone. Patients with advance appointments may fill canceled appointments.

96. B Low-pitched and expressive voice

RATIONALE: The telephone voice should be warm, friendly, and natural. Pronunciation and enunciation should be clear and distinct. A normal tone of voice carries best. Variance in tone brings out the meaning of words and adds vitality to what is said. The other choices present opportunities for disconcertion, confusion, or miscommunication.

97. B To deal with the collection agency

RATIONALE: After an account has been released to a collection agency, the medical office makes no further attempts at collection. No more statements are sent. The patient's ledger is marked so that the office knows it is in the hands of an agency. Refer the patient to the agency if he or she contacts the office in regard to the account. Any payments should be reported to the agency.

98. D Word processing

RATIONALE: Word processing is the system used to process written communications. It is a document production tool. Telecommunications involve verbal communication; documentation, interfacing, and formatting are not types of computer systems.

99. B Enclosed packing slip

RATIONALE: All orders received should be compared with the original purchase order and the invoice included with the shipment. The order should be checked for correct items, sizes, styles, and amounts.

100. C The patient pays in advance

RATIONALE: A credit balance is the amount of advance payment or overpayment on an account. The amount of receipts exceeds the amount charged.

CLINICAL

1. C All patients

RATIONALE: *Standard precautions* apply to the handling of all potentially infectious body fluids and tissues. Health care workers should take nondiscriminatory precautions to protect themselves.

2. E B and C

RATIONALE: Gloves are considered to be a barrier precaution and should be used when contact with blood or other body fluids is anticipated.

3. C 98.6°F

RATIONALE: Normal adult oral temperature is between 97° and 99° F.

4. B 14 to 20 breaths per minute

RATIONALE: Normal adult rate can be from 14 to 20 breaths per minute.

5. E B and C

RATIONALE: Temperature, pulse, respiration, and blood pressure are considered to be the vital signs. They are the measurements that indicate the state of general health of the patient.

6. B Usually higher in children than in adults

RATIONALE: The normal pulse rate for a child is between 80 and 120 beats per minute. Normal values for an adult are between 60 and 80 beats per minute.

7. E All of the above

RATIONALE: The pulse rate is decreased by conditions such as depression, chronic pain, central nervous system disorders, and hypothyroidism.

8. D 103° to 105° F

RATIONALE: Fever is a temperature over 100° F. A high temperature is over 103° F. Untreated high temperature can result in brain damage or death.

9. A The difference between the systolic and the diastolic blood pressure

RATIONALE: The pulse pressure is the difference between the systolic and the diastolic blood pressures. It reflects the volume of circulating blood. Less than 30 mm Hg or more than 50 mm Hg is considered normal.

10. B 99

RATIONALE: To convert kilograms to pounds, multiply the number of kilograms by 2.2 (45 kg $\times$ 2.2 = 99 lb).

11. A 6 feet

RATIONALE: Height is measured in inches. Using the conversion factor of 12 inches equals 1 foot, divide 72 inches by 12 inches (72 $\div$ 12 = 6).

12. A Chest and back

RATIONALE: Percussion is the use of tapping or striking the body to elicit sounds, usually done with the fingers or small hammer. Percussion aids in the determination of the size, position, and density of the underlying organ or cavity.

13. D Social history

RATIONALE: The social history gives information regarding the patient's lifestyle, hobbies, education, occupation, sleeping habits, methods of exercise, sex life, and coping skills.

14. D All of the above

RATIONALE: Subjective findings (symptoms) are perceptible only to the patient or known only to the patient.

15. E Clearness of vision

RATIONALE: Visual acuity using the Snellen eye chart is a common distance acuity screening test.

16. C Rectum

RATIONALE: Proctoscopy is the use of a scope to examine the rectum and the distal portion of the colon.

17. B Left side and chest, with right leg flexed

RATIONALE: The Sims' position is one in which the patient lies on the left side with the right knee and thigh drawn up toward the chest. It is sometimes called the lateral position and can be used for rectal examinations and some pelvic examinations.

18. D Prone position

RATIONALE: The prone position is one in which the patient is lying face down on the table.

19. A Ophthalmoscope

RATIONALE: The ophthalmoscope is an instrument used to inspect the inner structures of the eye. It has a handle containing batteries and an attached head equipped with a light and magnifying lenses.

20. B Sitting

RATIONALE: In the sitting position, the patient is sitting upright on the examination table. This position is useful in examining and treating the head, neck, and chest.

21. A Glucose and protein

RATIONALE: On all subsequent visits, a urine sample is obtained and tested for the presence of sugar (glucose) and albumin (protein). The presence of glucose might be a warning sign of a prediabetic state or diabetes. The presence of protein might be an early warning sign of toxemia. Both of these conditions would require careful medical supervision and treatment.

22. A 1 week after her period

RATIONALE: A monthly breast self-examination can detect early signs of breast cancer. The examination should be performed once a month and approximately 1 week after the menstrual period because the breasts are usually not tender or swollen at this time.

23. A Acute

RATIONALE: Disease is a pathologic process that in some way alters the normal function, structure, or metabolism of an organism. An acute disease process or acute infection begins abruptly with sharp intensity and then subsides after a short period.

24. C 21 to 28 days

RATIONALE: Double-wrapped sterile packs are considered sterile up to 28 days from the date of sterilization. They should be stored in a clean, dry, and dust-free place. When a pack expires, the contents must be reprocessed.

25. E Unwrap the pack, rewrap the pack, replace the indicator, and resterilize

RATIONALE: A sterilization indicator shows that the proper combination of steam, time, and temperature has been achieved. It does not prove that the contents are sterile. Failure of an indicator to change color might indicate that an error has occurred in the sterilization process. The pack should be reprocessed to correct any problem that may have caused the improper sterilization.

26. B Sanitization

RATIONALE: Instruments and other items used in the office must be carefully cleaned before proceeding with disinfection or sterilization. This cleaning process is sanitization. It is used to remove microorganisms, blood, and debris that might interfere with the sterilization process.

27. C Acquired active

RATIONALE: Immunity is the body's resistance to pathogenic microorganisms. It is classified as either natural or acquired. Natural immunity is a genetic feature specific to a person's race, sex, and ability to respond. Acquired immunity means that the body has developed an ability to defend itself. Acquired immunity can be active or passive. Active immunity results when a person has been exposed to or has had the disease. Passive immunity is gained from receiving immune substances, thus bypassing the body's immune system.

28. B Away from the body

RATIONALE: Unfolding the top flap away from the body avoids the necessity of reaching over the sterile field and causing contamination. It also helps avoid touching a person or uniform.

29. E 8-0

RATIONALE: The size or gauge of most sutures is labeled in terms of zeros; 0 is the thickest, and the number of zeros decreases up to 10-0, which is the thinnest. (The more zeros, the thinner the material.)

30. D Forceps

RATIONALE: Forceps are instruments of varied sizes and shapes used for grasping, compressing, or holding tissues and objects. They are two-pronged instruments with either a spring handle or a ring handle with a ratchet closure.

31. C Iodine

RATIONALE: Betadine is an antiseptic solution often used to disinfect the skin before a minor surgical procedure. It contains iodine, and a patient who is allergic to iodine will have a reaction to the solution.

32. E Purulent

RATIONALE: When a dressing is changed, it and the wound must be inspected for the amount and character of drainage. Drainage that is described as purulent consists of or contains pus.

33. A 10 to 15 degrees

RATIONALE: The objective of an intradermal injection is to inject a minute amount of solution between the layers of the skin. The needle is inserted at a 10 to 15 degree angle to deliver the solution to the correct area. When given correctly, the injection produces a wheal on the skin surface.

34. C Sublingual

RATIONALE: A sublingual route of administration places the drug under the patient's tongue. It is then left to dissolve and be absorbed.

35. B 1½ inch, 21 gauge

RATIONALE: The main objective when administering an intramuscular injection is to inject the medication into deep muscle tissue for gradual and optimal absorption. The longer length of the needle allows this level of administration to occur. The gauge allows for thick medications to be injected easily.

36. B Diuretic

RATIONALE: Diuretic medications promote the formation and excretion of urine. They can be prescribed to reduce the volume of extracellular fluid in the treatment of many disorders, including hypertension, edema, and congestive heart failure.

37. A 0.5 mL

RATIONALE: Use the following formula:

$$\frac{dose\ ordered}{available\ strength} \times dose\ form = dose\ given$$

$$\frac{250\ mg \times 1\ mL}{500\ mg} = 0.5\ mL$$

38. B Directly opposite from the specimen

RATIONALE: A centrifuge is a piece of laboratory equipment used to separate specimens by using centrifugal force. When a specimen tube is placed in the centrifuge, it must be counterbalanced with a tube of similar design and weight for balance. An unbalanced load can cause the centrifuge to vibrate and ruin the specimen.

39. A Within ½ hour of collection

RATIONALE: The microscopic examination of urine consists of categorizing and counting cells, casts, crystals, and miscellaneous constituents of the sediment. Chemical and cellular components change rapidly in a urine sample if they are allowed to sit at room temperature. These changes can be avoided by refrigerating the specimen if the analysis cannot be performed within 30 minutes after collection.

40. A Anuria

RATIONALE: Normal volume of urine produced every 24 hours is approximately 750 to 2000 mL, with an average of 1500 mL. Anuria is the complete suppression of urine formation by the kidney. It can be caused by renal obstruction or renal failure.

41. E 1.010 and 1.025

RATIONALE: Specific gravity is the weight of a substance compared with the weight of an equal volume of distilled water. In urinalysis, specific gravity is the rough measurement of the concentration of substances dissolved in urine. Most urine samples fall between 1.010 and 1.025. This reading indicates the ability of the kidney to concentrate the specimen, and a reading outside this range might indicate kidney disease.

42. D All of the above

RATIONALE: A complete blood count (CBC) is one of the most common laboratory tests ordered on blood. It gives a complete look at the blood components, thus giving a wealth of information about a patient's condition. Tests performed in a CBC include red blood cell count, white blood cell count, hemoglobin and hematocrit, differential, platelet number estimation, and red blood cell morphology.

43. A From a skin puncture

RATIONALE: Capillary or peripheral blood is obtained by performing a skin puncture on the fingertip, earlobe, or great toe or heel of an infant. This method allows for a minimal amount of blood to be collected but is sufficient for many laboratory tests.

44. C Gallbladder

RATIONALE: A cholecystogram is an x-ray of the gallbladder. It is made after the ingestion or injection of a radiopaque substance. The test is useful in diagnosing cholecystitis (inflammation of the gallbladder), cholelithiasis (gallstones), and tumors.

45. A Dilates blood vessels

RATIONALE: Thermotherapy (application of heat) produces local vasodilation and increases circulation. These results of heat application speed up the inflammatory process, promote local drainage, relax muscles, and relieve pain.

46. A P

RATIONALE: Electrocardiography is the procedure that records the electrical activity of the heart. The electrocardiogram records a series of waves or deflections above or below a baseline. Each wave or deflection corresponds to a particular part of the cardiac cycle. The P wave reflects contraction of the atria.

47. B Sinoatrial node

RATIONALE: The sinoatrial node is a specialized tissue found in the right atrial wall near the superior vena cava. It initiates each heartbeat and sets its pace (pacemaker).

48. D 12

RATIONALE: The standard electrocardiogram consists of 12 separate leads or recordings of the electrical activity of the heart from different angles. Each lead must be marked or coded for the physician to know which angle has been recorded. The 12 leads include leads I, II, and III (standard or bipolar leads); leads aVR, aVL, and aVF (augmented leads); and leads V_1, V_2, V_3, V_4, V_5, and V_6 (chest or precordial leads).

49. D 25 mm/sec

RATIONALE: The paper used in an electrocardiographic machine is a specialized graph paper with internationally accepted increments for measuring the cardiac cycle. As the paper advances, the heat-sensitive stylus moves along the vertical line and intersects with a vertical line. The paper advances at a speed of 25 mm/sec.

50. A Silver nitrate

RATIONALE: Silver nitrate ($AgNO_3$) is a caustic solution that is used to promote the healing process after surgery. It is available in solution form or coated on an applicator stick.

51. A Prothrombin time

RATIONALE: The drug Coumadin (warfarin sodium) is an anticoagulant and keeps the blood from clotting. The prothrombin time (pro time) is a test for detecting coagulation deficits. A prolonged pro time can indicate a deficiency in the normal blood clotting mechanism and can help monitor anticoagulation therapy.

52. C Catgut

RATIONALE: The purpose of sutures is to hold the edges of a wound together until healing can occur. Absorbable sutures, usually used on deeper tissues, do not have to be removed because they are absorbed or digested by body fluids and tissues during the healing process. An example of this type of suture material is surgical gut (catgut). Nonabsorbable sutures used on outer skin surfaces are removed after the wound is healed.

53. B 100

RATIONALE: The differential white blood cell count is a test that determines the percentage of each of the five different types of white blood cells in the blood. The procedure involves examining a specific area of a stained blood smear under the microscope. One hundred cells are counted and classified, and a tally is kept.

54. C 30%

RATIONALE: Hemoglobin and hematocrit values are related. Each 1% hematocrit contains 0.34 g of hemoglobin. The hematocrit should equal three times the hemoglobin within 3%.

55. D Erythrocyte sedimentation rate: 30 mm/hr

RATIONALE: The normal value for a sedimentation rate is 0 to 20 mm/hr. An increased erythrocyte sedimentation rate might indicate inflammation.

56. A Gram stain

RATIONALE: Because bacteria are small and possess little color, staining is necessary to observe them under the microscope. The Gram stain is used most often. The dyes in the stain are taken up differently in each type of bacterial cell, and they stain different colors. Bacteria are identified as gram negative (stain red) or gram positive (stain purple).

57. B Alkaline

RATIONALE: pH expresses the degree of acidity or alkalinity of a solution. Usually, freshly voided urine is acidic. After sitting, bacteria contaminate the sample and cause it to become alkaline.

58. D Red-stoppered (serum separator tube [SST], tiger)

RATIONALE: Blood collection tubes are color-coded, depending on the additive it contains or does not contain. Red-stoppered (SST, tiger) tubes contain no additives, therefore the blood collected in these tubes clot and serum can be removed.

59. E All of the above

RATIONALE: Surgical instruments have clearly identifiable parts and can easily be differentiated from one another. Instruments are classified according to their uses, and most belong to one of four main groups: (1) cutting and dissecting instruments, (2) grasping and clamping instruments, (3) retractors, and (4) probes and dilators.

60. A Assess the victim's airway

RATIONALE: Check the victim for responsiveness. If unconscious, assess the ABCs: airway, breathing, and circulation.

61. E All of the above

RATIONALE: A complete urinalysis is composed of three parts: (1) the physical examination that includes assessment of color, clarity, odor, amount, and specific gravity; (2) the chemical examination that can include using a reagent strip to test for the presence of glucose, ketones, leukocytes, blood, nitrates, pH, urobilinogen, protein, and bilirubin; and (3) the microscopic examination for cells, bacteria, casts, and artifacts.

62. D Liver

RATIONALE: After a drug is absorbed into the body and transported to the cells or tissues for which it is intended, it is again picked up by the bloodstream and transported to the liver, the site of metabolism and/or biotransformation. In the liver, the drug is broken down and prepared for elimination from the body.

63. C Tests for color-blindness

RATIONALE: Color-blindness is tested using Ishihara plates. The Ishihara color test uses a series of plates on which are printed round dots in a variety of colors and patterns. Patients with normal color vision are able to discern specific patterns on the plates. Patients with a deficiency in color perception cannot do so.

64. E Polyuria

RATIONALE: Signs and symptoms of a myocardial infarction (heart attack) is an occlusion of a coronary artery that results in loss of blood flow and necrosis to the myocardium. The onset is characterized by crushing chest pain. The patient becomes ashen, clammy, short of breath, and nauseated.

65. A Forceps

RATIONALE: Hemostatic forceps are a type of clamping instrument used to stop bleeding, clamp severed vessels, and hold tissue.

66. C 1 to 4

RATIONALE: A fairly constant ratio of four pulse beats to one respiration exists. As a general rule, both pulse and respiration rates normally respond to exercise or emotional upsets. Normal pulse rate for an adult is between 60 and 80 beats per minute. Normal respiratory rate for an adult is between 14 and 20 breaths per minute.

67. E All of the above

RATIONALE: Insulin shock is caused by too much insulin intake, decrease in food intake, or excessive exercise. It is characterized by sweating, trembling, chills, nervousness, irritability, hunger, hallucinations, and pallor. If uncorrected, it can progress to convulsions, coma, and death. Treatment requires an immediate dose of glucose.

68. A Kidneys

RATIONALE: The kidneys are the most important route for the excretion (elimination) of drugs from the body. Most drugs are filtered out of the circulation, broken down into harmless substances, and then excreted in the urine.

69. C Antidepressant

RATIONALE: Drugs can be classified according to their actions in the body. An antidepressant medication is used as a mood elevator and is used to treat depression. Prozac (fluoxetine) is an example of an antidepressant.

70. B Friction and running water

RATIONALE: Hands must be washed, using the correct technique, before and after each patient is examined or treated. Proper hand washing depends on two factors: (1) running water and (2) friction. Friction is the firm rubbing of skin surfaces to loosen debris. Running water washes away the debris.

71. D 12 months

RATIONALE: The vaccination for mumps, measles, and rubella is recommended that the first dose be given between 12 and 15 months of age. The second dose is recommended between ages 6 and 12 years.

72. B Migraine

RATIONALE: Migraine headaches are paroxysmal attacks of headaches that may be completely incapacitating. They are frequently characterized by nausea, vomiting, visual disturbances, throbbing pain in one side of the head, and an aura. An aura is some type of visual disturbance such as lines or spots across the visual field.

73. D To carry oxygen and carbon dioxide

RATIONALE: Hemoglobin, which is made up of iron and protein, is a main constituent of red blood cells. It carries oxygen to the cells from the lungs and carbon dioxide away from the cells to the lungs for excretion. Normal hemoglobin values vary throughout life and are affected by age, gender, diet, altitude, and disease.

74. A Ensures the accuracy of results

RATIONALE: Quality assurance is a major component of the Clinical Laboratory Improvement Acts of 1988 (CLIA '88) regulations relating to laboratory standards. It is a comprehensive set of policies and procedures developed to ensure the quality of laboratory testing and includes quality control, personnel orientation, laboratory documentation, knowledge of instrumentation, and enrollment in a proficiency-testing program.

75. B 48 to 72 hours after it is performed

RATIONALE: The Mantoux test is used for routine screening and diagnosis of tuberculosis. The test uses a purified protein derivative from a live tuberculin culture to test for antibodies. The results should be read 48 to 72 hours after the test is performed by intradermal injection. The extent of induration is measured and recorded.

76. C AU

RATIONALE: The abbreviation for both ears is AU. It comes from the Latin *auris unitas*.

77. D O

RATIONALE: Patients with type O blood are considered to be universal donors. Type O blood contains no antigens on the red blood cells, thus it will not agglutinate in the presence of anti-A and anti-B antibodies in the plasma.

78. E Colon

RATIONALE: A lower gastrointestinal series (barium enema) is an x-ray examination of the colon. Contrast medium (barium) is instilled into the colon through an enema. The colon can then be visualized by x-ray examination.

79. B Computed tomography scan

RATIONALE: A computed tomography scan is a radiographic technique that produces a film that represents a detailed cross-section of a tissue structure. The technique uses a narrow beam of x-ray that rotates in a continuous 360-degree motion around the patient. The pictures obtained from this method are highly detailed and simulate a three-dimensional appearance.

80. A Cancer

RATIONALE: Massive or excessive exposure to radiation can cause tissue damage and various side effects, which can include damage to blood cells, skin cells, eyes, and reproductive cells. Overexposure can result in decreased red and white blood cell counts, burns, and an increased incidence of cancers.

81. B Leads I, II, and III

RATIONALE: The first three leads recorded are the standard or bipolar leads (leads I, II, and III). They each use two limb electrodes to record electrical activity.

82. B Chains

RATIONALE: Bacteria may be classified by morphology (size and shape). Streptococci are bacteria that are spherical in shape and arranged in chains.

83. D Increasing age

RATIONALE: Normal pulse rates normally vary as a result of a person's gender, age, body size, posture, activity level, health status, nervous system function, emotional state, and the volume and composition of the blood. Pulse normally decreases with age.

84. D RL

RATIONALE: The leads of an electrocardiogram measure the electrical activity from the frontal and horizontal planes of the body. The right leg acts as the grounding as electrical activity is recorded from the right arm, left arm, and left leg.

85. A OSHA

RATIONALE: The Occupational Safety and Health Act was established by the federal government in 1970 to set standards and protocols for occupational health and safety. The regulations must be known and followed. They include hazard exposure plans, medical waste management, personal protective measures, general safety precautions, fire safety, staff development, and blood-borne pathogen regulations.

86. E Cost

RATIONALE: A drug reference provides information about medications. Most references include the following information about the medication: action, indication, side effects, adverse effects, precautions, contraindications, doses, and administration. These references include the *Physician's Desk Reference*, package inserts, *U.S. Pharmacopeia/National Formulary*, and other published references.

87. E All of the above

RATIONALE: An analgesic medication lessens the sensory function of the brain. They are used for pain relief. Analgesics can be classified as narcotic (morphine, codeine, Demerol) or nonnarcotic (aspirin, Tylenol, ibuprofen).

88. C Keep a written record of all daily activities

RATIONALE: A Holter monitor is a portable monitoring system used to record the cardiac activity of the patient for a

24-hour period. Keeping a written diary of all activities during the day that causes stress is important for the patient. Examples of these activities include driving in traffic, stair climbing, and bowel movements. Symptoms associated with possible heart problems should also be included.

89. D Peristalsis

RATIONALE: Peristalsis is the involuntary wavelike movement that moves food downward through the gastrointestinal tract. Peristalsis is activated when the food mass is swallowed and enters the esophagus.

90. A 2 months

RATIONALE: The schedule for childhood immunizations begins with the first doses of DTP (DtaP), IPV, *Haemophilus influenzae* type b (HiB) vaccine, and hepatitis B (HepB) vaccine being administered at age 2 months.

91. C Histology

RATIONALE: Histology involves the preparation and study of specimens of tissue from any source in the body. Changes in the tissue form and/or structure are observed microscopically.

92. C A nonsterile person entering the room

RATIONALE: Surgical asepsis, or sterile technique, is the practice used when an area and supplies in that area are to be made and kept sterile. The goal of surgical asepsis is to prevent the introduction of microorganisms into the body. Talking over the sterile field can introduce microorganisms onto it. Hair that is not pulled back or inside a cap might also introduce microorganisms. Moisture contaminates the sterile field. A 1-inch edge around the entire sterile field is considered not sterile.

93. C Benadryl

RATIONALE: An antihistamine drug counteracts the effects of histamine by blocking the action in the tissues. Antihistamines are used for relief of allergies. An example of an antihistamine is diphenhydramine (Benadryl).

94. D qod (every day)

RATIONALE: The abbreviation *qod* means every other day. The abbreviation *qd* means every day.

95. D Needle biopsy

RATIONALE: Surgical asepsis is defined as the destruction of organisms before they enter the body. The technique is used for any procedure that punctures, pierces, or incises the skin or mucous membranes. Everything that comes in contact with the patient should be sterile, including instruments, drapes, and gloved hands. A needle biopsy is a procedure that breaks the skin and thus requires surgical asepsis.

96. A Daily

RATIONALE: Quality control is the operational procedure used to implement the quality assurance program. The objective of quality control is to ensure accuracy of test results while detecting errors. It is mandated by law. Specially prepared quality control samples are tested daily. The results of these samples must be within a preestablished range before patient results can be reported.

97. B Impetigo

RATIONALE: Impetigo is a highly infectious bacterial infection of the skin. It is caused by *Staphylococcus* or *Streptococcus* and is characterized by vesicles that rupture and form a honey-colored crust. Lesions form primarily on the face, especially around the mouth and nose. Impetigo is treated with antibiotic ointment. Proper hand washing can help prevent its spread.

98. C Osteoporosis

RATIONALE: Osteoporosis is a disorder of the skeletal system characterized by porous, brittle bones. These bones then become susceptible to fractures. Osteoporosis occurs most frequently in postmenopausal women. It is treated with calcium supplements, hormone replacement therapy (estrogen), exercise, and medications.

99. D Presbyopia

RATIONALE: Presbyopia is a disorder of accommodation. It is due to the loss of elasticity of the lens of the eye as a result of aging. It can be corrected with bifocals or trifocals.

100. A Otitis media

RATIONALE: Otitis media is an inflammation (infection) of the middle ear. Fluid collects behind the tympanic membrane. Otitis media is often associated with an upper respiratory infection. The patient will experience pain and fever. The infected canal and eardrum appear red and swollen, and a purulent discharge may be present. It is treated with antibiotics and analgesics.

Post-Test Answer Key

GENERAL

1. B Uniform Anatomical Gift Act

RATIONALE: The Act states that any person of sound mind and of the age of 18 or older may give all or part of his or her body after death for research, transplantation, or placement in a tissue bank.

2. B The patient is human immunodeficiency virus (HIV) positive

RATIONALE: Even though the physician is charged with safeguarding patient confidentiality, state laws require certain disclosures. All states require sexually transmitted diseases to be reported, including confirmed cases of acquired immunodeficiency syndrome. Most states, but not all, require that patients who are HIV positive be reported.

3. B Ask the patient to calm down

RATIONALE: The medical assistant can help calm an angry patient by speaking calmly and refusing to return the emotion. Calmly ask the person to take a deep breath and stop talking for a few moments. Gradually lowering the volume of the voice will cause the angry person to lower his or her own voice so he or she can hear what the medical assistant is saying.

4. A Notify the patient that her medical care is being terminated

RATIONALE: The patient-physician relationship is an implied contract. Both parties must uphold their part of the contract. Not following physician's orders would be grounds to terminate the contract. The physician must notify the patient by sending a certified letter.

5. D State government

RATIONALE: The MD, DO, or DC degree is conferred on graduation from the medical or chiropractic school. The license to practice medicine is granted by a state board, also known as the *State Board of Medical Examiners*.

6. C Closed-ended

RATIONALE: The closed-ended question asks for specific information. It limits the answer to one or two words. A yes or no answer may be enough.

7. A Fax

RATIONALE: A fax machine is a time and labor saver in conveying patient information from physician to physician or physician to hospital. However, precautions must be taken to ensure security of the information arriving by fax. This goal can be accomplished by telephoning ahead to alert the receiver that sensitive information will be arriving.

8. C Lack of blood flow to tissue

RATIONALE: Ischemia is reduced or lack of blood flow to tissue that results in impairment of cell function.

9. A "Please tell me more about those feelings."

RATIONALE: Using an open-ended statement encourages the patient to open up and expand on his or her thoughts.

10. E Transient ischemic attack

RATIONALE: Transient ischemic attacks are temporary episodes of impaired neurologic functioning caused by inadequate flow of blood to a portion of the brain. Signs and symptoms may include sudden weakness, numbness and tingling on one side of the body, dizziness, confusion, and vision disturbances.

11. C Quotation marks

RATIONALE: The chief complaint is a concise account of the patient's symptoms explained in the patient's own words. This information is set apart from the other charting information by placing the words in quotes.

12. D Lines body cavities that open to the outside of the body

RATIONALE: Mucous membranes line all body cavities that open to the exterior of the body. They secrete mucus, a substance that keeps the membrane moist and lubricated.

13. B Encouraging nonverbal communication

RATIONALE: With non–English-speaking patients, the medical assistant may need to use gestures and more body language to convey messages. Having a bilingual staff member is always helpful.

14. B Seminiferous tubules

RATIONALE: The seminiferous tubules are tightly coiled structures located in each testis. Sperm are formed in the epithelium of these tubules.

15. D Occipital

RATIONALE: The occipital bone is located at the base of the skull. It contains a large opening (foramen magnum) where the spinal cord exits the cranium.

16. A Survival

RATIONALE: Psychologist Abraham Maslow created what he called the *hierarchy of needs*. This hierarchy categorizes these needs into five levels. The most basic of these needs are the physiologic needs: oxygen, food, water, excretion, shelter, and sexual expression.

17. A Aplastic

RATIONALE: Aplastic anemia results from the failure of the hematopoietic cells (stem cells) in the bone marrow. This condition can be caused by exposure to toxins, alkylating agents, certain drugs, and radiation.

18. D "Can you tell me more about that?"

RATIONALE: An open-ended question requires more than a "yes" or "no" answer. It forces the patient to provide additional detail and expand on his or her thoughts.

19. A A physician accidentally amputates the wrong finger from a patient

RATIONALE: *Res ipsa loquitur* means *the thing speaks for itself*. It describes a situation in which the nature of the injury can implicate negligence.

20. B Invasion of privacy

RATIONALE: Giving out patient information without the patient's consent is an invasion of the patient's privacy, which is an intentional tort.

21. B Glucagon

RATIONALE: Glucagon, which is produced in the alpha cells in the pancreas, stimulates the conversion of glycogen to glucose in the liver. Its primary function is to increase blood glucose levels.

22. B Villi

RATIONALE: The wall of the small intestine forms circular folds with finger-like projections called villi (*sing.* villus). The villi increase the amount of digested food that can be absorbed.

23. E May refuse to accept a patient if he or she chooses

RATIONALE: A physician has the right to limit the size of his or her practice or the number of patients that he or she treats.

24. B Staying calm when dealing with angry patients

RATIONALE: Professionalism is defined as exhibiting a courteous, conscientious, and business-like manner in the workplace. It is characterized by the technical and ethical standards of a certain profession.

25. B Hyster/o

RATIONALE: The combining forms for uterus include *hyster/o, metr/i, metr/o, metri/o, uter/i,* and *uter/o.*

26. E All of the above

RATIONALE: Personality is defined as the composite of the behavioral traits and characteristics by which one is recognized as an individual. A person's age, life experience, heredity, and environment all contribute to the composite.

27. B Cecum

RATIONALE: The cecum is the first division of the large intestine. It is connected to the ileum of the small intestine. The appendix (vermiform) is attached to the cecum.

28. B Pulmonary artery

RATIONALE: Blood that is low in oxygen exits the right ventricle through the pulmonary artery where it enters the lungs and picks up oxygen.

29. A Another physician

RATIONALE: A call from another physician or professional colleague should always be transferred to the physician immediately.

30. D Delay treatment and inform or consult with the physician

RATIONALE: A physician must have consent from the patient to treat the patient, even though the consent is usually implied. A patient has the right to refuse treatment at any time.

31. C Overbooking

RATIONALE: Overbooking may result in a prolonged waiting time for the patient to see the provider, and it may cause dissatisfaction with the practice.

32. D A scanner

RATIONALE: A scanner is a device that reads text or illustrations on a printed page and translates the information on the page into a form that the computer can understand.

33. A $5630

RATIONALE: Using the income statement, net income equals revenue minus expenses. An asset is anything of value that is owned, not just revenue.

34. C Holmes-Mathis, Jennie

RATIONALE: Hyphenated elements of a name, whether first name, middle name, or surname, are considered to be one unit.

35. D Postage meter

RATIONALE: The postage meter is the most efficient way of stamping the mail in a large business office. The machine can be purchases or leased; the postage is purchased from the U.S. Postal Service. The date must be changed daily.

36. C Below the return address

RATIONALE: Any notation on the envelope directed toward the addressee, such as *Personal* or *Confidential*, should be typed and underlined on the third line below the return address and aligned with the return address.

37. B An OUTguide

RATIONALE: An OUTguide is a heavy guide that is used to replace a folder that has temporarily been removed or moved from a filing space. It should be of a distinctive color for easy identification.

38. A When the patient calls to make an appointment
RATIONALE: As a business, a medical office must charge competitive and fair prices for services and must receive payment for the services in a timely fashion. Patients should be fully informed about a practice's fees and payment policies before they receive treatment.

39. D Future events arranged in chronological order
RATIONALE: A tickler file is a chronological file used as a reminder that something must be done on a certain date.

40. C Endocrine
RATIONALE: The thyroid gland is a major gland in the endocrine system.

41. B Employee's marital status
RATIONALE: The amount of money withheld from each paycheck is based on the information the employee provides on Form W-4. The Employer's Tax Guide includes tables showing how much tax must be withheld based on the pay period and the employee's marital status.

42. C Numerical
RATIONALE: In the numerical filing system, each file is assigned a number, starting with the lowest number and moving up. Files are organized in numerical order. A cross-reference with the patient's name is kept elsewhere.

43. D The mission statement
RATIONALE: A policy manual describes the office philosophy and goals. The office mission statement reflects the reasons for the existence of the practice.

44. C Another physician
RATIONALE: The person answering the telephone is expected to screen incoming calls. Calls from other physicians should be put through immediately if the provider is available to take the call.

45. B Properties owned by the business
RATIONALE: Anything not owed is an asset. Anything owed is a liability.

46. D W-4
RATIONALE: The Form W-4 is the Employee's Withholding Allowance Certificate. It is filled out by the employee and allows him or her to determine the number of withholding allowances.

47. D Minutes
RATIONALE: A record of the proceedings of a meeting is called the minutes. They contain a record of what was done at the meeting. Minutes should be signed and kept on file according to the policy of the organization.

48. C Grouping
RATIONALE: Grouping or clustering allows the provider to use time efficiently by seeing patients with the same needs at the same time.

49. C Photocopier
RATIONALE: Capital equipment is equipment used to generate revenue.

50. D 99
RATIONALE: CPT lists and codes procedures and services performed by the provider. The CPT book is divided into six sections. The E&M section codes are 99200 to 99499.

51. A. A subpoena
RATIONALE: The physician and medical assistant may never release confidential information without the consent of the patient except when it is legally required. A *subpoena duces tecum* is a legally binding request to provide records or documents to appear in court.

52. B Enclosure
RATIONALE: The enclosure notation identifies any material that may be accompanying the correspondence. The notation is placed two lines below the signature line.

53. E All of the above
RATIONALE: Complete and accurate records are essential to a well-managed medical practice. Health information management includes not only the assembling of the record, but also the saving, retrieving, protecting, transferring, storing, retaining, and destroying of these records.

54. C Initials come after complete names
RATIONALE: Indexing rules are standardized and are based on current business practices. The rule that applies to initials states, "that initials precede a name beginning with the same letter." (M. Johnson would be filed before Mary Johnson.)

55. A Chief complaint
RATIONALE: The patient's history relates to the patient's clinical picture and depends on the patient for answers to specific questions. The history is composed of the chief complaint or the reason why the patient is being seen. This information is usually in the patient's own words.

56. E Unemployment tax
RATIONALE: Federal unemployment taxes, based on the Federal Unemployment Tax Act (FUTA) are paid entirely by the employer. The FUTA tax provides unemployment payments to workers who lose their job.

57. D Accounting
RATIONALE: A spreadsheet is a software program for inputting and manipulating numerical data to facilitate a wide variety of financial activities.

58. C Preexisting condition
RATIONALE: A preexisting condition is a condition or disease that was present before an insurance policy was issued.

59. C Extremities
RATIONALE: The radial pulses are located in the wrists (extremities).

60. C Write-protect
RATIONALE: Write-protect is a process or code that prevents overwriting of data or programs on a disk.

61. C Draw a single line through the misspelled word
RATIONALE: Correct errors in charting by using the SLIDE rule: draw a single line through the entry, write *error* above the entry, correct the entry, and date and initial the entry.

62. E Quarterly
RATIONALE: Every 3 months, the employer must file an Employer's Quarterly Federal Tax Return (Form 941) with the IRS. This form lists the amounts withheld from employee paychecks.

63. B A retirement complex with individual apartments
RATIONALE: Autonomy is the quality of having the ability or tendency to function independently. A community where a senior can interact with persons of the same age and participate in activities but keep his or her own apartment would allow independence.

64. B Antineoplastic
RATIONALE: An antineoplastic agent (cancer drug) inhibits the growth of malignant cells.

65. B Diuretic
RATIONALE: A diuretic promotes or increases urination.

66. A Rinse contaminants from the lip of the bottle
RATIONALE: Pouring a small amount of the solution into a waste receptacle rinses any contaminants off the bottle lip. If the bottle has a double cap, then this step can be skipped.

67. D Eating
RATIONALE: The postprandial blood sugar (2-hr PPBS) is a screening test for diabetes mellitus. A fasting blood glucose level is obtained. If the results are within an acceptable range, then the patient eats a meal and is retested after 2 hours.

68. C Nonsterile gloves, laboratory coat, and goggles
RATIONALE: Sigmoidoscopy is used to diagnose polyps, hemorrhoids, and diverticular disorders. The sigmoidoscope is a flexible fiberoptic instrument that allows the physician to complete the examination without much discomfort to the patient. Nonsterile gloves, laboratory coat, and goggles are adequate personal protection equipment for assisting with the procedure.

69. C Gallbladder
RATIONALE: *Cholecyt/o* is the combining form for gallbladder, and -*gram* is the suffix meaning record.

70. A 1 mL
RATIONALE: The cubic centimeter (cc) and the milliliter (mL) are interchangeable units of measure in the metric system.

71. A Alanine aminotransferase
RATIONALE: Alanine aminotransferase is an enzyme found in highly metabolic tissues such as the heart muscle, liver, and skeletal muscle. Levels increase after a myocardial infarction.

72. A Silver nitrate
RATIONALE: Topical silver nitrate ($AgNO_3$) solution or an applicator coated with $AgNO_3$ can be used to stop localized bleeding. The applicators must be kept in lightproof brown containers. The applicators are convenient for use in the mouth and nose.

73. C Staphylococci
RATIONALE: Pathogenic bacteria are classified by their shape and arrangement. *Staphyl/o* means clusters or bunch (as in bunch of grapes).

74. C 30%
RATIONALE: Hemoglobin and hematocrit values are related. Each 1% hematocrit contains 0.34g of hemoglobin. The hematocrit should equal three times the hemoglobin within 3%.

75. B 1.0 mL
RATIONALE: Use the following formula:

$$\frac{\text{Dose ordered}}{\text{Available strength}} \times \text{dose form} = \text{dose given}$$

$$\frac{50 \text{ mg}}{50 \text{ mg}} \times 1 \text{ mL} = 1.0 \text{ mL}$$

76. C Reduces the number of contaminants to a safe level
RATIONALE: Sanitization is the cleansing process that decreases the number of microorganisms to a safe level as dictated by public health guidelines. This process removes debris so that later sterilization can penetrate all surfaces of the item.

77. A Facing away from the examiner
RATIONALE: Audiometry measures the lowest intensity of sound that a person can hear. The patient places headphones over both ears. A single frequency is delivered to each ear. The patient is asked to signal when he or she hears the sound. To reduce human error, the patient should be seated facing away from the examiner so the patient cannot see the examiner push the button to deliver the sound.

78. C Ecchymosis
RATIONALE: Ecchymosis is a hemorrhagic skin discoloration commonly called a *bruise*. The skin is not broken, thus the wound is closed.

79. D Bronchodilator
RATIONALE: A bronchodilator is used to manage reversible airway obstruction caused by asthma and chronic obstructive pulmonary disease. It helps relax the smooth muscle of the respiratory tract, resulting in bronchodilation.

80. A Schedule I
RATIONALE: Schedule I drugs have no accepted medical use and a high potential for abuse. Possession of these drugs is illegal. Examples of schedule I drugs include heroin, d-lysergic acid diethylamide (LSD), mescaline, and amphetamine variations.

81. C Do not eat red meat for 48 hours before the collection

RATIONALE: Eating red meat and taking iron supplements and certain medications (e.g., aspirin, vitamin C, steroids, anticoagulants) can cause a false-positive result.

82. A Anisocytosis

RATIONALE: In a diseased state, red blood cells may become altered in appearance. They can vary in size (anisocytosis), shape (poikilocytosis), and/or color (polychromia, hypochromia, hyperchromia).

83. D Urobilinogen

RATIONALE: Urobilinogen results from the breakdown of bilirubin in the intestines. It travels to the liver where it is sent back to the intestines and excreted in feces. Urine levels may be increased in conditions of the liver.

84. B Pink or red

RATIONALE: The Gram stain is the method of staining microorganisms, which serves as a primary means of classifying and identifying bacteria. Using this method, bacteria will be either gram-positive (retaining the purple color of the stain) or gram-negative (retaining the color of the counterstain).

85. C AU

RATIONALE: The abbreviation AU (aures unitas) means both ears.

86. A Intradermal

RATIONALE: An intradermal injection places the medication within the skin layers. The site is used primarily for allergy testing and tuberculin screening (Mantoux test).

87. D Tilt the patient's head forward

RATIONALE: Nosebleed (epistaxis) is a hemorrhage from the nose usually caused by the rupture of small blood vessels within the nose. Mild to moderate bleeding can be controlled by having the patient sit upright, lean forward, and applying direct pressure to the nose.

88. B Leads I, II, and III

RATIONALE: An electrocardiogram consists of 12 leads. The standard (bipolar) limb leads are recorded first. These leads each use two limb electrodes to record the heart's electrical activity.

89. B 1:10 bleach solution

RATIONALE: Disinfection is the process of killing pathogenic organisms or rendering them inactive. For equipment and countertops, the cheapest and most reliable method is the use of a 1:10 bleach solution.

90. A Two drops in both ears every 4 hours as needed

RATIONALE: The abbreviation for drops is gtt, AU is the abbreviation for both ears, q4h is the abbreviation for every 4 hours, and prn is the abbreviation for as needed.

91. A EDTA

RATIONALE: The anticoagulant ethylenediaminetetraacetic acid (EDTA) is used for hematology studies. It prevents the aggregation of platelets and allows preparation of blood smears with minimal distortion of white blood cells.

92. D Leukocytes: ++

RATIONALE: The normal range for leukocytes in a sample should be negative. The presence of white bloods cells usually indicates a urinary tract infection.

93. D Measure blood pressure

RATIONALE: The instrument used to measure blood pressure is called a *sphygmomanometer*. It consists of an inflatable cuff, an inflation bulb with a control valve, and a pressure gauge. (*Sphygm/o* means pulse; *manometer* refers to an instrument used to measure the pressure of a liquid or a gas.)

94. B Auscultation

RATIONALE: In auscultation, the examiner uses a stethoscope to listen to the sounds made by the body.

95. A Forced vital capacity

RATIONALE: The forced vital capacity (FVC) is the amount of air that can be forcefully exhaled from a maximal inhalation. FVC is measured through spirometry (pulmonary function test).

96. D 20

RATIONALE: Distance visual acuity is frequently part of a complete physical examination. It is widely used in schools and industry and is the best single test available for visual screening. The procedure uses the Snellen eye chart. The patient is positioned 20 feet from the chart (standard testing distance), either standing or sitting.

97. D V_4

RATIONALE: The chest (precordial) leads are unipolar and designated V_1, V_2, V_3, V_4, V_5, and V_6. These leads measure the electrical activity between six specific points on the chest wall and a point within the heart. Lead V_4 is placed in the fifth intercostal space at the left midclavicular line.

98. D Cytologic fixative

RATIONALE: Vaginitis is an inflammation of the vagina usually caused by a microorganism. It is characterized by an abnormal discharge. A specimen is collected and evaluated for the invading organism, usually with a wet preparation. This slide would not be fixed, therefore fixative is not needed.

99. A Anticoagulants

RATIONALE: An anticoagulant agent delays or prevents blood clotting. A diuretic promotes urine output. Vasoconstrictors cause narrowing of blood vessels. A vasodilator increases the diameter of blood vessels.

100. B 1½ inch, 22 gauge

RATIONALE: The goal of an intramuscular injection is to deliver the medication into muscle tissue. The length of the needle can be up to 2 inches, depending on the size of the patient and the consistency of the medication. The gauge of the needle can be from 22G to 25G, depending on the consistency of the medication.